Neglected Tropical Diseases and their Impact on Global Health

Neglected Tropical Diseases and their Impact on Global Health

Editor: Cyrus Hank

AMERICAN
MEDICAL PUBLISHERS
www.americanmedicalpublishers.com

AMERICAN
MEDICAL PUBLISHERS
www.americanmedicalpublishers.com

Cataloging-in-Publication Data

Neglected tropical diseases and their impact on global health / edited by Cyrus Hank.
p. cm.
Includes bibliographical references and index.
ISBN 979-8-88740-297-0
1. Tropical medicine. 2. Medical climatology. 3. Human beings--Effect of climate on.
4. World health. 5. Communicable diseases--Prevention. I. Hank, Cyrus.
RC961 .N443 2023
616.988 3--dc23

American Medical Publishers,
41 Flatbush Avenue,
1st Floor, New York,
NY 11217, USA

ISBN 979-8-88740-297-0 (Hardback)

Contents

Preface

Every book is a source of knowledge and this one is no exception. The idea that led to the conceptualization of this book was the fact that the world is advancing rapidly; which makes it crucial to document the progress in every field. I am aware that a lot of data is already available, yet, there is a lot more to learn. Hence, I accepted the responsibility of editing this book and contributing my knowledge to the community.

Neglected tropical diseases (NTDs) are a group of bacterial and parasitic diseases commonly found in various nations in Africa, Asia and Latin America. NTDs are caused by different kinds of pathogens and transmitted by vectors such as mosquitoes and black flies. Some of the common NTDs are schistosomiasis, leishmaniasis, lymphatic filariasis, mycetoma, onchocerciasis, trachoma, etc. There are several factors such as the lack of accessibility to clean water and hygienic sanitary conditions that contribute to the spread of NTDs. These diseases mainly affect the poor and are a source of tremendous suffering because of their disfiguring, debilitating, and sometimes deadly impact. NTDs also impair physical and cognitive development. This book investigates the neglected tropical diseases and their impact on global health in detail. Its aim is to present researches that have transformed the study of these diseases. The book will provide comprehensive knowledge to the readers.

While editing this book, I had multiple visions for it. Then I finally narrowed down to make every chapter a sole standing text explaining a particular topic, so that they can be used independently. However, the umbrella subject sinews them into a common theme. This makes the book a unique platform of knowledge.

I would like to give the major credit of this book to the experts from every corner of the world, who took the time to share their expertise with us. Also, I owe the completion of this book to the never-ending support of my family, who supported me throughout the project.

Editor

1

Lymphatic Filariasis Increases Tissue Compressibility and Extracellular Fluid in Lower Limbs of Asymptomatic Young People in Central Myanmar

Janet Douglass [1,*], Patricia Graves [2], Daniel Lindsay [1], Luke Becker [2], Maureen Roineau [2], Jesse Masson [2], Ni Ni Aye [3], San San Win [4], Tint Wai [3], Yi Yi Win [3] and Susan Gordon [1,5]

1 Division of Tropical Health and Medicine, James Cook University, Townsville 4811, Australia; daniel.lindsay1@jcu.edu.au (D.L.); sue.gordon@flinders.edu.au (S.G.)
2 Division of Tropical Health and Medicine, James Cook University, Cairns 4870, Australia; patricia.graves@jcu.edu.au (P.G.); luke.becker@jcu.edu.au (L.B.); maureenroineau@wanadoo.fr (M.R.); jesse.masson@my.jcu.edu.au (J.M.)
3 Department of Health, Myanmar Ministry of Health and Sports, Nay Pyi Taw 15011, Myanmar; shwewaethu@gmail.com (N.N.A.); mr.tintwaitun2013@gmail.com (T.W.); yywin2008@gmail.com (Y.Y.W.)
4 World Health Organization, Country Office, Yangon 11201, Myanmar; wins@who.int
5 College of Nursing & Health Sciences, Flinders University, Bedford Park 5042, Australia
* Correspondence: jan.douglass@my.jcu.edu.au;

Abstract: When normal lymphatic function is hampered, imperceptible subcutaneous edema can develop and progress to overt lymphedema. Low-cost reliable devices for objective assessment of lymphedema are well accepted in clinical practice and research on breast-cancer related lymphedema but are untested in populations with lymphatic filariasis (LF). This is a cross-sectional analysis of baseline data in a longitudinal study on asymptomatic, LF antigen-positive and -negative young people in Myanmar. Rapid field screening was used to identify antigen-positive cases and a group of antigen-negative controls of similar age and gender were invited to continue in the study. Tissue compressibility was assessed with three tissue tonometers, and free fluids were assessed using bio-impedance spectroscopy (BIS). Infection status was confirmed by Og4C3 antigen assay. At baseline (n = 98), antigen-positive cases had clinically relevant increases in tissue compressibility at the calf using a digital Indurometer (11.1%, p = 0.021), and in whole-leg free fluid using BIS (9.2%, p = 0.053). Regression analysis for moderating factors (age, gender, hydration) reinforced the between-infection group differences. Results demonstrate that sub-clinical changes associated with infection can be detected in asymptomatic cases. Further exploration of these low-cost devices in clinical and research settings on filariasis-related lymphedema are warranted.

Keywords: neglected tropical disease; lower extremity; lymphatic filariasis; tissue tonometry; bio-impedance spectroscopy; lymphedema

1. Introduction

Lymphatic filariasis (LF) is a parasitic disease in which thread-like worms inhabit the human lymphatic system, where they can impair normal lymphatic pumping. Classified as a neglected tropical disease and affecting many of the world's poorest populations, LF can lead to lymphedema, a progressively debilitating swelling of the skin and subcutaneous tissue in any body part, most frequently the legs [1]. Normal lymphatic pumping actively removes circulating proteins and fluid from the tissue spaces, maintaining a slightly negative interstitial pressure. When lymphatic capacity is impaired, extracellular fluid (ECF) and circulating proteins begin to accumulate in the interstitial spaces [2]. If normal lymphatic function is not restored, this initially covert edema gradually becomes overt, and the affected body part visibly enlarges. Over time, the protein-rich fluid is replaced with fat and fibrous tissue, and normal limb contours are lost. The outdated eponym 'elephantiasis' was inspired by the appearance of a grossly enlarged limb in late-stage lymphedema where the skin is thick, discolored, and formed into folds. In developed countries, lymphedema is frequently caused by surgical damage when lymph nodes are removed or irradiated during cancer treatment. Much of what is known about initiation and progression of lymphedema comes from research on breast cancer-related lymphedema (BCRL) of the arm [3].

A wide spectrum of devices and methods is used to objectively evaluate lymphedema depending on the setting. At the highly resourced end of the spectrum, nuclear imaging and other sophisticated technologies are often used to assess BCRL of the arm. Tissue tonometry to quantify tissue compressibility and portable bio-impedance spectroscopy (BIS) to track fluctuations in free fluid are also used and are relatively inexpensive. Using BIS, it has been shown that covert pathologic change due to lymphatic damage during breast cancer treatment can be detected, and that early intervention in this latent stage can prevent the onset of overt disease [4]. At the low-resourced end of the spectrum, assessment of LF related-lymphedema (LFRL) of the leg usually relies on classification of visible and palpable soft tissue changes [5], where subjectivity may lead to inconsistent classification. There is no differentiation or assessment of covert change, so subtle but important alterations in tissue composition may be missed.

In LF, mosquitoes pick up the microfilariae during a blood meal. The larvae develop to third stage within the mosquito before being transmitted by a subsequent bite. Transmission is relatively inefficient with a low risk of infection per bite, and after transmission there is a lag between being infected and the development of adult worms. This means that most children with LF will remain asymptomatic until young adulthood, which affords a long, latent period in which to implement preventive strategies [6]. Primary prevention in the Global Program to Eliminate LF (GPELF) is preventive chemotherapy, which is delivered annually via mass drug administration (MDA) in endemic regions [7]. This will eventually prevent any new cases of morbidity as infection rates fall too low to sustain transmission. However, preventive chemotherapy conveys no real benefit to advanced cases, most of whom will no longer be antigenemic, but will require life-long health care. In between the asymptomatic cases that will never progress to overt disease and the advanced cases that have irreversible lymphedema, there are many cases of latent and early stage lymphedema. There is some evidence that MDA may reverse very early tissue changes in LFRL [8], but without standardized assessment or diagnostic criteria for Stage 0, or devices sensitive enough to detect small changes in tissue composition, it is not clear at what stage or which individuals will remain at risk of disease progression. Reliable, sensitive, low-cost devices to provide objective assessment of LFRL are needed [9].

A pilot study in Papua New Guinea (PNG) found the skin over the posterior thigh was 20% more compressible in asymptomatic young people who had tested positive for LF antigen compared to antigen-negative peers, using a mechanical tonometer [10]. Subsequently, three tissue tonometers and a portable BIS device have demonstrated intra-operator reliability in assessing tissue composition in the lower limbs of young Australian and Myanmar populations without any history or risk of lymphedema [11]. It is not yet known if covert lymphedema can be detected by tissue tonometry or BIS in these populations.

There is no agreed standard for assessment of Stage 0 lymphedema, and diagnostic criteria for clinical onset are not well defined [3]. One study on BCRL used a 3% change in BIS values to trigger preventive treatment [4], and clinical lymphologists may use a percentage change in limb girth or volume to track lymphedema change, with a variation of more than 10% considered clinically relevant [12]. Variations in body composition will influence measurements with these devices as muscle holds more free fluid than fat, fat is more compressible than muscle, and the ECF in the subcutaneous compartment fluctuates slightly depending on overall body hydration. Individual characteristics that influence body composition should be considered when assessing superficial tissues of the lower limb, including expected changes associated with growth from child to young adult and gender-based differences in muscle and fat distribution. Habitual patterns of muscle use should also be considered, and significant between-leg differences in healthy young Australian and Myanmar people have been reported when using these devices [13].

This cross-sectional study on young people residing in an LF endemic region in Central Myanmar investigated whether tissue tonometry and BIS measures were altered in asymptomatic cases who tested positive for *Wuchereria bancrofti* antigen. The results will assist researchers and clinicians to objectively quantify changes occurring in early LFRL and may contribute to formal recognition and intervention for Stage 0 lymphedema of the leg.

2. Materials and Methods

2.1. Study Site Selection, Participant Recruitment, and Screening

Sentinel site records kept by the Vector Borne Disease Control (VBDC) Centre in Mandalay identified Amarapura Township as a densely populated area with a high prevalence of LF. It was also close enough to laboratory services for blood sample processing. A study site was set up in the Administration Centre in the village of Nge Toe and baseline data were collected over a two-week period in October 2014. The study was conducted in accordance with the Declaration of Helsinki and the protocol was approved by the Myanmar Ministry of Health (MoH) and James Cook University Human Research Ethics Committee (approval number H5261).

A sample size of 32 in each group was predicted to detect a 10% difference between groups with 80% power, based on a mean mid-calf value of 2.5 with SD of 0.7 using the digital Indurometer [13,14]. A convenience sample of local young people aged 10–21 years was invited to be screened for LF antigen and to participate in a longitudinal study on early detection of LFRL. Participant information sheets and informed consent forms were provided in Burmese. Staff of the VBDC and Amarapura Township Hospital, the World Health Organization (WHO) technical officer for Myanmar (SSW), and locally-trained research assistants explained all procedures to the participants, determined their eligibility to participate, and obtained informed consent. Written consent was given by young adults aged 18–21 and by a parent or guardian for minors aged 10–17. A further verbal assent for each procedure was obtained from all participants prior to performing that procedure. Participant inclusion and exclusion criteria are shown in Figure 1.

Inclusion criteria	**Exclusion criteria**
• Aged 10 – 21 years at screening • Residing in Amarapura Township • Able to give informed consent (18 – 21 year olds) • Accompanied by an adult relative able to give informed consent (10 – 17 years olds)	• Any clinical sign of lymphedema • Acute injury to the lower limb(s) • Past surgery to the trunk or lower limb(s) • Heart disease • Pacemaker or other implanted device • Pregnancy • Unable to give informed consent

Figure 1. Participant inclusion and exclusion criteria.

2.2. Screening and Baseline Data Collection

A rapid field test for the presence of LF antigen was performed using an immunochromatographic test (ICT) card (Binax Now, Alere, Waltham, MA, USA). This involved placing a 100 μL draw of blood from a fingerprick onto a test strip. The sample was allowed to flow for 10 min and the result appeared as one or two lines across the test strip. One line is a control and if this line was not visible then the test was void and if possible, repeated. Appearance of the second line indicated the presence of circulating *W. bancrofti* antigen that is produced by adult worms. The young people who tested positive by ICT (cases), and a sample of the negative participants of the same age and gender (controls), were invited to return and participate in the longitudinal study. A James Cook University (JCU) technical staff member (LB) trained the local research assistants in correct use of the ICT card and selected participants invited for follow-up.

Participants returned during the following fortnight for the blood draw and device measures. Local research assistants conducted a short interview to elicit information on current health status, prescription or traditional medications, surgical history, family history of lymphedema, time since the last drink (as a proxy for hydration), and if they had consumed preventive chemotherapy during the previous annual MDA. Leg dominance was determined by asking the question 'Which foot do you use to kick a ball?' Height was measured using a chart marked on a wooden post in centimeters and a set square, and weight in kilograms was recorded using digital scales purchased locally. Device measures were conducted in a small side office or screened off area and an adult relative was asked to be present during the measurement of minors.

2.2.1. Device Measures

Three tissue tonometers were used to assess tissue compressibility. The Indurometer (SA Biomedical Engineering, Adelaide, Australia) is a hand-held electro-mechanical device with a 1 cm diameter plunger/indenter extending through a 7 cm diameter reference plate and a built-in force sensor. The reference plate is aligned to the surface of the skin while the device is pressed evenly into the tissue. A beep is emitted once the equivalent to 200 g of force has been applied, and the degree of displacement is displayed in 0.01 increments on a light-emitting diode (LED) screen. An image of the Indurometer is shown in Figure S1. The mechanical Tonometer (SA Biomedical Engineering, Adelaide, Australia) is a similar device, in which a 1 cm diameter plunger extends beyond a 7 cm diameter reference plate. This purely mechanical device uses a 200 g mass to drive the indenter into the underlying tissue, and the degree of displacement is shown on an analogue scale. Both of these devices record the displacement of the indenter in relation to the reference plate as an indication of compliance (compressibility) of the underlying skin and tissue. The values provided by these devices are not absolute measures and can be considered as arbitrary units used to compare measures of tissue compressibility [15]. A third device, the SkinFibroMeter (Delfin Technologies, Kuopio, Finland), uses a smaller reference plate with a 1.25 mm length fixed indenter and built-in force sensors. The reference plate is pressed evenly onto the skin and the device emits a beep when the equivalent of 50 g has been applied. The device is applied five times and the average resistance in newtons is displayed on a digital screen. A tape measure and washable skin marker were used to locate and mark the midpoint of each thigh (front and back) and the back of each calf, and all tonometry measures were taken at these marks.

Extracellular and intracellular fluid loads were assessed using bio-impedance spectroscopy (BIS), which measures the resistance to multifrequency, low-level electrical currents. The difference between resistance in the intracellular (Ri) and extracellular (Re) fluid compartments was represented as a ratio Ri:Re. As the intracellular fluid (ICF) compartment is tightly regulated, any changes in the ratio usually represent changes in the extracellular fluid (ECF). Whole-leg BIS measures were recorded for each leg with the SFB7 (Impedimed, Australia) using self-adhesive electrodes applied to the skin according to manufacturer's instructions for lower limb measures.

A detailed description of data collection methods was published in a reliability study on these devices in Australia and Myanmar [11]. All devices were operated by the principal researcher (JD), who was blinded to the infection status of the participants. Tonometry scores were recorded on data collection sheets by a research assistant, and BIS data was downloaded to an Excel file (Microsoft Office 365, version 1706).

2.2.2. Blood Collection and Processing/Storage

Blood samples were collected by local research assistants, who were trained in specific blood collection and handling protocols by the JCU technician (LB). A 10 mL draw of venous blood was collected from each participant into cooled ethylenediaminetetraacetic acid (EDTA) anticoagulant vacutainers (BD Biosciences, North Ryde, Australia). The antigen test was repeated using 100 uL of the venous blood pipetted onto an ICT card, and the remaining blood was kept on ice until delivery to the Public Health Laboratory in Mandalay. Separation of plasma and red blood cells was performed using a centrifuge for 15 min at 3000 rpm; the plasma was transferred into 2-mL cryotubes by pipette in duplicate (4 mL per person) and stored at −20 °C. Once all baseline data had been collected, the plasma was transferred on dry ice to the Department of Medical Research in Yangon for long-term storage at −80 °C in a monitored freezer connected to a back-up generator and with daily monitoring. There were no thaws during plasma transportation or storage. One set of the cryotubes was aliquoted and used to conduct ELISA assay for the presence of Og4C3, an antigen marker for *W. bancrofti*, using the recommend 1:4 dilution for plasma as per the manufacturer (Cellabs, Sydney, Australia) kit instructions [16]. Samples were classified as positive if the antigen units, estimated using the standard curve of controls provided with the kit, exceeded 32 units. Detailed methods for the ELISA assays were previously published in a study on diagnostic testing for LF antigen [16].

2.3. Data Analysis

LF antigen-positive cases were defined as those who were positive by either antigen test (ICT or Og4C3). Body mass index (BMI) was calculated as kg/m^2, but adult values cannot be used for children; therefore, WHO growth charts and definitions were used to identify underweight participants, who were defined as being more than two standard deviations below the median BMI for their age [17]. Chi-squared tests, Fisher's exact tests, and independent samples *t*-tests were used to compare antigen-positive and -negative group characteristics at baseline for known moderating factors. Paired sample *t*-tests were used to compare device measures of dominant and non-dominant legs. Statistical analysis was conducted in SPSS version 23 (IBM Corp), and significance was set at 0.05 with a 95% confidence interval. Clinically-relevant difference for tonometry measures was set at >10% and for BIS measures it was set at >3%. Stepwise regression was performed for dominant and non-dominant legs separately to determine the level of variance in device measures associated with infection status (univariate) and other potential moderating factors (multivariate).

3. Results

3.1. Participants

Screening for LF found 60 antigen-positive cases among 316 volunteers, and 114 young people (57 cases and 57 controls of the same age and gender) were invited to continue in the longitudinal study (see Figure 2). Ten people either could not be found or refused to return, and 104 participants were available for baseline blood draw and physical measures. Data from six participants were excluded from the final analysis; four were found at a later measure to have been outside the target age range at baseline, one had a prosthetic leg, and another had a heart condition, neither of which had been disclosed at the screening interview. The final study population was comprised of 46 antigen-positive cases detected by ICT plus a further four cases identified as antigen positive by Og4C3 ELISA (n = 50). There were 48 antigen-negative (control) cases.

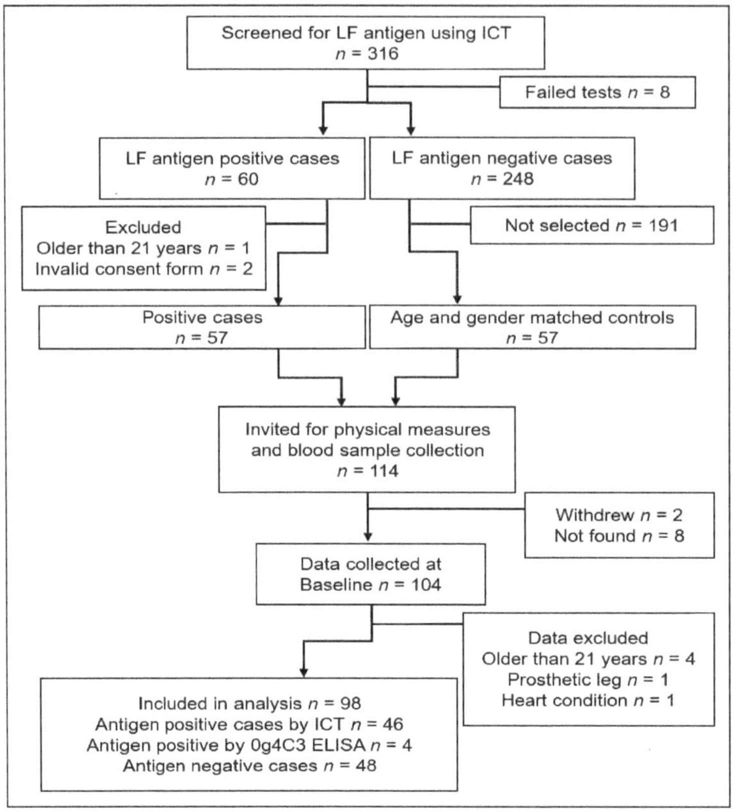

Figure 2. Flow of participants through recruitment, screening, and baseline data collection.

3.1.1. Participant Characteristics

All participants (n = 98) were aged between 10 and 21 years (mean 15.3 SD 3.4) and there were 55 females and 43 males. The mean height, weight, and BMI were 152.0 cm (SD 12.0, range 118.8–174.0), 42.3 kg (SD 11.5, range 17.5–82.7), and 18.0 kg/m^2 (SD 3.0, range 12.4–29.7), respectively. The cohort was 95.9% right leg dominant and 13.3% (n = 13) were considered underweight. Almost half (44.9%) of the participants were working in weaving workshops, 27.6% were students, 8.2% were street vendors, 2.0% were construction workers, and the remaining 17.3% worked in other occupations or did not disclose their occupation. None had a history of lymphedema in their immediate family, previous surgery or medical implants, and all were in good health. Two participants were taking prescription medications and one was using traditional medicine. One participant felt unwell on the day scheduled for taking the measures and was asked to return when feeling better. Comparing antigen-positive and antigen-negative groups, there were no significant between-group differences for any physical attribute or moderating factor. Participant characteristics at baseline are shown in Table 1.

Table 1. Group characteristics of antigen-positive and antigen-negative participants (positive by either immunochromatographic test (ICT) or Og4C3) at baseline.

	LF Antigen-Positive Cases	LF Antigen-Negative Controls	Mean Diff (95% CI)	$p=$
	$n = 50$	$n = 48$		
Age in years—mean (SD)	15.20 (3.38)	15.48 (3.46)	0.28 (−1.09, 1.07)	0.691 [a]
Gender				
Female n (%)	27 (54%)	28 (58%)		0.410 [b]
Male n (%)	23 (46%)	20 (42%)		0.410 [b]
Height in cm—mean (SD)	151.80 (12.56)	152.20 (11.52)	0.399 (−4.44, 5.24)	0.870 [a]
Weight in kg—mean (SD)	42.27 (12.81)	42.30 (10.12)	0.028 (−4.617, 4.670)	0.990 [a]
BMI in kg/m^2—mean (SD)	18.05 (3.46)	18.03 (2.65)	−0.012 (−1.239, 1.216)	0.985 [a]
Body composition n = (%)				0.976 [c]
Median weight	41 (82%)	40 (83%)		
Underweight > −2SD	7 (14%)	6 (13%)		
Overweight > +1SD	2 (4%)	2 (4%)		
Dominant leg right/left	47/3	47/1		0.324 [b]
Occupation n = (%)				0.395 [c]
Student	14 (28%)	13 (27%)		
Working/other	32/4 (72%)	34/1 (73%)		
Drank liquid n = 97				0.590 [c]
<60 min	13 (26%)	12 (26%)		
>60 min	37 (74%)	35 (74%) (1 NA)		
Consumed 2013 MDA n (%)	17 (34%)	22 (46%)		0.383 [c]

LF = lymphatic filariasis; BMI = body mass index; SD = standard deviation; [a] independent samples t-test; [b] Fishers exact test; [c] Pearson chi-square; NA = participant was not asked.

3.2. Moderating Factors Associated with Device Measures

3.2.1. Effect of Infection on Device Measures

In the antigen-positive group, tissue compressibility was higher at all measuring points, and there was more free fluid in both legs compared to that of the antigen negative group. Independent t-tests found that, at mid-calf on the non-dominant side, the increase in Indurometer measures was both clinically (11.1%) and statistically significant ($p = 0.021$). In addition, whole leg BIS measures found clinically-relevant (>3%) increases in free fluid in both legs (dominant leg, 4.9% ($p = 0.220$), non-dominant leg, 9.2% ($p = 0.053$)). Mean values and between-group differences for the Indurometer and BIS measures are shown in Table 2. Neither the mechanical Tonometer nor SkinFibroMeter found any clinically relevant or statistically significant differences between infection groups, with many differences too small to be evident at two decimal places. The only between-group difference of interest with these two devices was increased tissue compressibility with the Tonometer at the non-dominant calf (4.8% softer, $p = 0.296$). Mean values and between-group differences for all devices including the Tonometer and SkinFibroMeter are given in Table S1.

Table 2. Between-infection group differences for Indurometer and BIS measures, size, and direction of variation.

Measurement Point Indurometer	Positive $n = 50$	Negative $n = 48$	Mean Difference (%)	Direction in Positive Cases	$p=$
	Mean (SD)	Mean (SD)			
Dominant anterior thigh	4.80 (0.76)	4.72 (0.69)	0.05 (1.1%)	Softer	0.731
Non-dominant anterior thigh	5.10 (0.88)	5.00 (0.69)	0.10 (1.9%)	Softer	0.546
Dominant posterior thigh	4.13 (0.93)	4.06 (0.87)	0.07 (1.7%)	Softer	0.701
Non-dominant posterior thigh	3.88 (0.83)	3.86 (0.95)	0.02 (0.4%)	Softer	0.933
Dominant calf	2.91 (0.57)	2.70 (0.68)	0.21 (7.8%)	Softer	0.096
Non-dominant calf	2.73 (0.65)	2.46 (0.65)	0.27 (11.1%) *,#	Softer	0.021
BIS					
Dominant leg $n = 47/45$	2.44 (0.46)	2.56 (0.45)	0.12 (4.9%) #	More fluid	0.220
Non-dominant leg $n = 46/44$	2.62 (0.56)	2.86 (0.59)	0.24 (9.2%) #	More fluid	0.053

SD = standard deviation; * Significant between-group difference $p \leq 0.05$; # clinically relevant between-group difference.

3.2.2. Effect of Infection Status, Age, Gender, Body Composition, and Hydration on Device Measures

Regression was first performed with infection status (antigen positivity) alone, and then stepwise regression was used to add moderating factors. Being antigen positive was significantly associated with increased compressibility in the non-dominant calf when using the Indurometer (Table 3, step 1) which is consistent with the *t*-test results given above in Table 2. Using multivariate regression, after adjustment for other factors (gender, age, underweight, and hydration), increased compressibility remained significantly associated with being antigen positive (in the non-dominant calf) using the Indurometer, and was also significant in the dominant calf using the same device. When considering all factors, being antigen positive was significantly associated with increased fluid in the non-dominant leg using BIS (Table 3, step 2).

In the stepwise regression, being female was significantly associated with higher tissue compressibility using all three tonometers. The largest gender-related effect using the Indurometer was in calf measures where there is a relatively thin fat layer over the muscles, making small differences in fat and muscle composition more likely to be detected (dominant leg B (SE) = 0.639 (0.117), $p < 0.000$) (see Table 3). The least effect of gender was found over the anterior thighs where the relatively thicker fat layer reduces the influence of the underlying muscle tone and a small difference between the sexes is not likely to register as much change. Using BIS, being female was significantly associated with less free fluid in both legs, and this is consistent with females having relatively smaller muscle/higher fat mass (less fluid) than males of the same age. The largest coefficient was in the non-dominant leg (B (SE) = 0.485 (0.103), $p < 0.001$) (see Table 3).

Being less well hydrated, defined as not having a drink within one hour of measures, was associated with lower tissue compressibility. This was significant at the non-dominant calf (B (SE) = −0.239 (0.110), $p = 0.032$). Being older was significantly associated with a small increase in free fluid in both legs, consistent with normal growth increase in muscle mass. Being underweight was significantly associated with a small increase in free fluid in the non-dominant leg (BIS) which may be associated with reduced fat mass or an increased capillary filtrate due to proteinemia.

In summary, when accounting for known moderating factors of age, gender, BMI, and hydration, there was a highly significant association between antigen positivity and increased Indurometer measures at the non-dominant calf ($p = 0.007$). At the dominant calf, the same association was also significant ($p = 0.038$). When these factors are taken into account for BIS measures, there was a clinically relevant and significant increase in free fluid (Table 2) in the non-dominant leg ($p = 0.038$). All associations between moderating factors and device measures are given in Table S2.

Table 3. Stepwise regression for moderating factors associated with variation in Indurometer and bio-impedance spectroscopy (BIS) measures.

	Indurometer				**BIS**	
	Higher Values = Increased Tissue Compressibility				**Lower Values = Increased ECF**	
	Posterior Thigh B (SE)		Calf B (SE)		Whole Leg B (SE)	
Factor	Dominant	Non−dominant	Dominant	Non−dominant	Dominant	Non−dominant
Step 1 R^2=	*0.002*	*0.000*	*0.029*	*0.054*	*0.017*	*0.042*
Antigen Positive	0.070 (0.182)	0.015 (0.180)	0.212 (0.126)	0.272 (0.116) *	−0.117 (0.095)	−0.238 (0.122)
Step 2 R^2=	*0.189*	*0.187*	*0.283*	*0.269*	*0.283*	*0.398*
Antigen Positive	0.093 (0.168)	0.049 (0.166)	0.234 (0.111) *	0.286 (0.104) **	−0.108 (0.083)	−0.210 (0.099) *
Gender = Female	0.751 (0.178) **	0.679 (0.175) **	0.639 (0.117) **	0.492 (0.110) **	0.230 (0.087) **	0.485 (0.103) **
Older age	0.022 (0.025)	0.041 (0.025)	0.010 (0.017)	0.024 (0.016)	−0.051 (0.012) **	−0.061 (0.015) **
Underweight	0.136 (0.250)	0.277 (0.247)	−0.052 (0.165)	−0.094 (0.155)	−0.237 (0.120)	−0.302 (0.142) *
Less Recent Hydration	−0.338 (0.177)	−0.223 (0.174)	−0.139 (0.117)	−0.239 (0.110) *	0.107 (0.085)	0.124 (0.101)

ECF = extracellular fluid; SE = standard error; * $p < 0.05$; ** $p < 0.01$.

3.3. Patterns of Tissue Compressibility and Free Fluid in Dominant and Non-Dominant Legs

There was a consistent pattern of tissue compressibility at the measurement sites that held true for all devices and all subgroups by age, gender, or infection status. The most compressible tissue was located at the (relatively) fatty anterior thigh, the least compressible tissue was over the dense tendomuscular junction at mid-calf, and values for the posterior thigh fell between the two. When comparing dominant and non-dominant legs, a consistent pattern of between-leg differences was seen and can be attributed to expected muscle activity during a kick.

The skin was less compressible (more muscle tone) over the front of the 'dominant' kicking thigh and over the back of the 'non-dominant' thigh and calf muscles that propel the body forward during the kick. Using BIS, there was more free fluid (more muscle mass or less fat) in the dominant leg compared to the non-dominant leg (9.6%); this difference was both clinically relevant (>3%) and statistically significant ($p < 0.01$) using paired samples *t*-tests. Mean values and between-leg differences for the Indurometer and BIS are given in Table 4. Mean values and between-leg differences for all devices including the Tonometer and SkinFibroMeter and are given in Table S3.

Table 4. Mean values and between-leg differences using the Indurometer and BIS.

	Indurometer (n = 98)			BIS (n = 90)
	Anterior Thigh	**Posterior Thigh**	**Calf**	**Whole Leg**
Dominant leg mean (SD)	4.74 (0.72)	4.10 (0.90)	2.81 (0.63)	2.50 (0.46)
Non−dominant leg mean (SD)	5.05 (0.79)	3.87 (0.89)	2.60 (0.59)	2.74 (0.59)
Mean difference (SD)	−0.31 (0.31)	0.23 (0.23)	0.21 (0.21)	−0.24 (0.32)
95% CI of the difference	−0.41, −0.21	0.11, 0.35	0.13, 0.28	−0.31, −0.17
% difference	6.5% **	5.6% **	7.5% **	9.6% **,#
Direction (dominant leg)	Harder	Softer	Softer	More fluid

SD = standard deviation; ** Significant between-leg difference $p \leq 0.01$; # Clinically relevant between-leg difference (tonometry > 10%, BIS > 3%).

The overall pattern of between-leg differences (dominant vs. non-dominant), as demonstrated by kicking a ball, was maintained in the antigen-positive cases, but the degree of difference was altered. Figure 3 is a radar graph showing the percentage of between-leg differences in Indurometer and BIS values for the whole cohort and by infection group. In the infected group, between-thigh differences in tissue compressibility were exaggerated (closer to the outer ring in the radar chart) but only slightly, with similar percentage differences for positive (7%), negative (6.1%), and whole cohort groups (6.5%). The between-infection group differences were more pronounced at the calf where the mean between-calf difference in the positive cases (6.5%) was much smaller (closer to the middle) than that of the negative cases (9.7%) or whole cohort (7.5%). Similarly, as well as an overall increase in free fluid, BIS results indicated that positive cases had smaller between-leg differences compared to those of their negative counterparts (7.5% vs. 11.7%). Although not statistically significant, these reduced between-leg differences in the distal legs of the antigen-positive cases suggest a covert edema overlying and masking normal between-leg variations in muscle tone and mass.

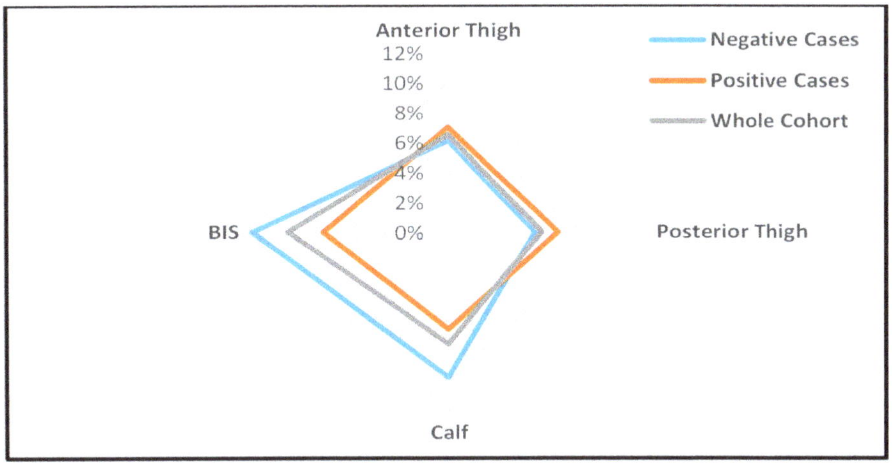

Figure 3. Percentage between-leg differences using the Indurometer and BIS in the LF antigen-negative cases, LF antigen-positive cases, and whole cohort. Data points which are closer to the outer ring indicate greater between-leg differences.

4. Discussion

In this study, tissue compressibility and free fluid loads were higher in asymptomatic young people infected with LF compared to their uninfected peers. Both groups displayed normal patterns of within-leg tissue compressibility; i.e., tissue was most compressible over the anterior thigh and least compressible at the calf, and between-leg differences were consistent with kicking a ball. However, when stratified by infection status, the size and direction of between-leg differences in the positive cases were consistent with a covert accumulation of subcutaneous fluid in the lower leg. Usually, LFRL appears distally and progresses proximally, so detectable tissue changes may occur earlier at the calf than at the thigh. The relatively thin layer of skin and tissue over the muscle of the calf may also render early tissue changes more evident than in fattier parts of the leg. Accordingly, the association with LF antigenemia and Indurometer measures was statistically significant at mid-calf, and large enough on the non-dominant side to also be clinically relevant. This early appearance of lymphatic dysfunction in the non-dominant leg is consistent with reports on BCRL, which show an increased risk of arm lymphedema if the operated side is also the non-dominant arm [18]. This tendency for fluid to accumulate more readily on the non-dominant side could be the result of differences in muscular activity that naturally promotes lymph flow and may be greater or more frequent on the dominant side.

For all devices, the significant associations between higher tissue compressibility and lower free fluid in females reflect expected variation in muscle to fat ratios between the sexes. Other moderating factors such as hydration, although not as universal as gender, did have significant associations with measures at the calf, but this could be reduced by administering a standardized drink during the assessment protocol. Increased free fluid associated with age and being underweight can be attributed to a year-by-year increase in muscle mass, or a systemic reduction in fat mass, respectively.

Results in the Myanmar study reinforce earlier findings from PNG [10], where clinically significant between-infection group differences were found in physical leg measurements. However, some differences in observations between studies were noted. In particular, in young PNG people, increased tissue compressibility was found in the posterior thighs of the infected group using the mechanical Tonometer. In the Myanmar cohort, the between-infection group differences were found using the digital Indurometer at the calf. There may be several reasons for this discrepancy. The PNG cohort had a higher proportion of females (64% vs. 54%) than the Myanmar cohort and a higher mean BMI (19.7 vs. 18.05). In addition, age, gender and hydration were not considered in that analysis. In the current study, the Tonometer did return slightly softer measures in the dominant posterior thigh and non-dominant calf in the Myanmar group, but in this cohort, the differences were not significant. (Table S1). In PNG, no MDA had been available prior to the study, after which treatment was offered to all participants; in Myanmar, MDA had been offered in 2013 and earlier, although less than half of the participants reported taking it. Taken together, these two studies provide the first empirical evidence that there are covert but measurable increases in tissue compressibility and free fluid associated with LF antigenemia, although the optimal site for assessment may differ for different populations. The advance in the current study over that done in PNG was the availability of newer, digital devices and inclusion of age, gender, BMI, and hydration in multivariate regression, which confirmed an independent effect of infection.

The proportion of all infected individuals that will progress to LFRL, while considered to be relatively small, is not well understood. It appears to depend on multiple factors including genetics, geography, exposure to infection, and worm species, and it was not possible in this cross-sectional study to determine which of the positive cases may be at risk of progression to advanced disease, if any. The fact that mean between-infection group differences can be objectively measured suggests that there is an insidious effect of LF antigenemia on skin and subcutaneous tissues in the lower limb, and this is consistent with the current understanding of the pathogenesis of lymphedema [19,20]. Follow-up on this Myanmar cohort may provide some insight into individual variation among antigen-positive persons to define who is most at risk.

The Indurometer gave the clearest indication that tonometry can be used to detect covert lymphatic change in the lower limb. While the Tonometer and SkinFibroMeter may not have detected latent changes in asymptomatic cases in this cohort, their use in assessment of established leg lymphedema from all causes warrants further study. When using these devices to track changes in the same person over time, moderating factors such as age and gender will be immaterial, hydration can be controlled for by administering a drink prior to measurement, and any change in BMI can be considered when interpreting the results, as is already the practice in BCRL. Indurometry and BIS measures may be useful in monitoring clinical progression in people at risk of lower limb lymphedema and may provide an inexpensive means to objectively measure lymphedema in LF populations.

The presence and direction of clinically-relevant changes in the antigen-positive cases in Myanmar support the hypothesis that LF can induce covert changes in the subcutaneous tissues of the lower limbs. This contributes to the case for formal recognition of a Stage 0 in the classification of LF-related lymphedema. The disparity in resources between BCRL and LFRL settings should not be a barrier to transferring reliable and effective protocols for early detection and intervention in lymphedema to LF populations.

Supplementary Materials:
Figure S1: Indurometer, SA Biomedical Engineering; Table S1: Between-infection group differences (independent samples *t*-test) for (a) Digital Indurometer, (b) Mechanical Tonometer, (c) SkinFibroMeter and (d) BIS measures, size and direction of variation; Table S2: Stepwise regression for moderating factors associated with variation in (a) Digital Indurometer, (b) Mechanical Tonometer, (c) SkinFibroMeter and (d) BIS measures; Table S3: Mean values and between-leg differences (paired samples *t*-test) for (a) Digital Indurometer, (b) Mechanical Tonometer, (c) SkinFibroMeter and (d) BIS measures.

Acknowledgments: This study formed part of the doctoral research project of Janet Douglass and received no formal institutional or grant funding and no funds were received for the cost of open access publication. All data collection activates were funded by private donors who contributed through crowdfunding. Grateful acknowledgement is given to the following individuals and organizations:

- Louise Kelly-Hope, Centre for Neglected Tropical Diseases, Liverpool School of Tropical Medicine for early advice on the study design and country selection.
- Myanmar Ministry of Health and Sports, for permission to conduct the study, translation of participant information documents and data collection support.
- Vector Borne Disease Control, Mandalay, for access to sentinel site records and providing research assistants.
- Public Health Laboratory and Staff, Mandalay, for blood separation and short-term storage of plasma.
- Department of Medical Research and Staff, Yangon, for long term storage of plasma and processing of Og4C3 ELISAQ assays.
- Impedimed Australia, for loan of an SFB7 back-up unit and donation of electrodes.
- Delfin Finland, for loan of a SkinFibroMeter.
- JCU Physiotherapy, for use of a Tonometer and Indurometer.

- Cellabs Australia, for Og4C3 reagents.
- Pentagon Freight, for provision of international freight services.
- Singapore International Airlines, for discounted airfares.
- Kyaw San Tun, Mandalay, for interpretation and transport services.

Author Contributions: J.D., S.G. and P.G. conceived and designed the experiments; J.D., L.B. and M.R. performed the experiments; N.N.A., S.S.W., Y.Y.W. and T.W. provided in-country advice and data collection; J.D., D.L. and J.M. analyzed the data; J.D. wrote the manuscript with editorial input from all co-authors.

References

1. World Health Organization. Wha50.29 elimination of lymphatic filariasis as a public health problem. In *World Health Assembly Resolutions and Decisions*, 3rd ed.; Ninth Plenary Meeting, 13 May 1997—Committee A, Third Report; Hbk, R., Ed.; World Health Organization: Geneva, Switzerland, 1997; Volume III.
2. Guyton, A.C.; Hall, J.E. *Textbook of Medical Physiology*, 11th ed.; Elselvier Inc.: Philadelphia, PA, USA, 2006.
3. International Society of Lymphology. The diagnosis and treatment of peripheral lymphedema: 2016 consensus document of the international society of lymphology. *Lymphology* **2016**, *49*, 170–184.
4. Stout Gergich, N.L.; Pfalzer, L.A.; McGarvey, C.; Springer, B.; Gerber, L.H.; Soballe, P. Preoperative assessment enables the early diagnosis and successful treatment of lymphedema. *Cancer* **2008**, *112*, 2809–2819. [CrossRef] [PubMed]
5. Dreyer, G.; Addiss, D.; Dreyer, P.; Noroes, J. *Basic Lymphoedema Management, Treatment and Prevention Problems Associated with Lymphatic Filariasis*; Hollis Publishing Company: Hollis, NH, USA, 2002.
6. Shenoy, R.K. Clinical and pathological aspects of filarial lymphedema and its management. *Korean J. Parasitol.* **2008**, *46*, 119–125. [CrossRef] [PubMed]
7. World Health Organization. *Progress Report 2000–2009 and Strategic Plan 2010–2020 of the Global Programme to Eliminate Lymphatic Filariasis: Halfway towards Eliminating Lymphatic Filariasis*; WHO: Geneva, Switzerland, 2010.
8. Addiss, D.G. Mass treatment of filariasis in New Guinea. *N. Engl. J. Med.* **2003**, *348*, 1179–1181. [PubMed]
9. Douglass, J.; Graves, P.; Gordon, S. Self-care for management of secondary lymphedema: A systematic review. *PLoS Negl. Trop. Dis.* **2016**, *10*, e0004740. [CrossRef] [PubMed]
10. Gordon, S.; Melrose, W.; Warner, J.; Buttner, P.; Ward, L. Lymphatic filariasis: A method to identify subclinical lower limb change in PNG adolescents. *PLoS Negl. Trop. Dis.* **2011**, *5*, e1242. [CrossRef] [PubMed]
11. Douglass, J.; Graves, P.; Gordon, S. Intrarater reliability of tonometry and bioimpedance spectroscopy to measure tissue compressibility and extracellular fluid in the legs of healthy young people in Australia and Myanmar. *Lymphat. Res. Biol.* **2017**, *15*, 57–63. [CrossRef] [PubMed]
12. Lawenda, B.D.; Mondry, T.E.; Johnstone, P.A.S. Lymphedema: A primer on the identification and management of a chronic condition in oncologic treatment. *CA Cancer J. Clin.* **2009**, *59*, 8–24. [CrossRef] [PubMed]
13. Douglass, J.; Graves, P.; Gordon, S. Moderating factors in tissue tonometry and bio-impedance spectroscopy measures in the lower extremity of healthy young people in Australia and Myanmar. *Lym. Res. Biol.* **2017**. in submit.
14. Biomath. Available online: http://biomath.info/power/ttestnoninf.htm (accessed on 14 August 2017).
15. Pallotta, O.; McEwen, M.; Tilley, S.; Wonders, T.; Waters, M.; Piller, N. A new way to assess superficial changes to lymphoedema. *J. Lymphoedema* **2011**, *6*, 34–40.
16. Masson, J.; Douglass, J.; Roineau, M.; Aye, K.; Htwe, K.; Warner, J.; Graves, P. Relative performance and predictive values of plasma and dried blood spots with filter paper sampling techniques and dilutions of the lymphatic filariasis Og4c3 antigen ELISA for samples from Myanmar. *Trop. Med. Infect. Dis.* **2017**, *2*, 7. [CrossRef]
17. Onis, M.D.; Onyango, A.W.; Borghi, E.; Siyam, A.; Nishida, C.; Siekmann, J. Development of a WHO growth reference for school-aged children and adolescents. *Bull. World Health Organ.* **2007**, *85*, 660–667. [CrossRef] [PubMed]
18. Hayes, S.C.; Janda, M.; Cornish, B.; Battistutta, D.; Newman, B. Lymphedema after breast cancer: Incidence, risk factors, and effect on upper body function. *J. Clin. Oncol.* **2008**, *26*, 3536–3542. [CrossRef] [PubMed]

19. Nutman, T.B. Insights into the pathogenesis of disease in human lymphatic filariasis. *Lymphat. Res. Biol.* **2013**, *11*, 144–148. [CrossRef] [PubMed]
20. Carlson, J.A. Lymphedema and subclinical lymphostasis (microlymphedema) facilitate cutaneous infection, inflammatory dermatoses, and neoplasia: A locus minoris resistentiae. *Clin. Dermatol.* **2014**, *32*, 599–615. [CrossRef] [PubMed]

2

Assessing Climate Change Impact on Ecosystems and Infectious Disease: Important Roles for Genomic Sequencing and a One Health Perspective

Kenneth B. Yeh [1,*], Jeanne M. Fair [2], Woutrina Smith [3], Teresa Martinez Torres [1], Julie Lucas [1], Corina Monagin [3], Richard Winegar [1] and Jacqueline Fletcher [4]

1 Global Health Surveillance and Diagnostics, MRIGlobal, Gaithersburg, MD 20878, USA; tmartineztorres@mriglobal.org (T.M.T.); jlucas@mriglobal.org (J.L.); rwinegar@mriglobal.org (R.W.)
2 Biosecurity and Public Health, Los Alamos National Laboratory, Los Alamos, NM 87545, USA; jmfair@lanl.gov
3 One Health Institute, University of California, Davis, CA 95616, USA; wasmith@ucdavis.edu (W.S.); cmonagin@gmail.com (C.M.)
4 National Institute for Microbial Forensics & Food and Agricultural Biosecurity, Oklahoma State University, Stillwater, OK 74078, USA; jacqueline.fletcher@okstate.edu
* Correspondence: kyeh@mriglobal.org;

Abstract: Changes in the Earth's climate and weather continue to impact the planet's ecosystems, including the interface of infectious disease agents with their hosts and vectors. Environmental disasters, natural and human-made activities raise risk factors that indirectly facilitate infectious disease outbreaks. Subsequently, changes in habitat, displaced populations, and environmental stresses that affect the survival of species are amplified over time. The recurrence and spread of vector-borne (e.g., mosquito, tick, aphid) human, animal, and plant pathogens to new geographic locations are also influenced by climate change. The distribution and range of humans, agricultural animals and plants, wildlife and native plants, as well as vectors, parasites, and microbes that cause neglected diseases of the tropics as well as other global regions are also impacted. In addition, genomic sequencing can now be applied to detect signatures of infectious pathogens as they move into new regions. Molecular detection assays complement metagenomic sequencing to help us understand the microbial community found within the microbiomes of hosts and vectors, and help us uncover mechanistic relationships between climate variability and pathogen transmission. Our understanding of, and responses to, such complex dynamics and their impacts can be enhanced through effective, multi-sectoral One Health engagement coupled with applications of both traditional and novel technologies. Concerted efforts are needed to further harness and leverage technology that can identify and track these impacts of climate changes in order to mitigate and adapt to their effects.

Keywords: biosecurity; climate change impact; One Health; genome; sequencing; infectious disease

---

Climate change impacts transcend international borders and geographic areas of responsibility.

CNA Military Advisory Board, National Security and the Accelerating Risks of Climate Change.

1. Introduction

As part of a panel discussion at the 2019 Sequencing, Finishing, and Analysis for the Future (SFAF) conference (21–23 May, 2019, Santa Fe, New Mexico, USA), we explored the importance of using genomic sequencing in a One Health context to study climate change impacts on natural and managed ecosystems and their infectious diseases (Figure 1). We summarize key discussion topics in which the application of genomic sequencing technologies can enhance our understanding of climate change and infectious diseases using a One Health approach. The topics included an array of scientific applications including current sequencing tools, genomics and environment, science of signatures and conservation genomics, plant ecosystems, a research case study, and outcomes of human behavior such as data and material sharing. The importance of integrating these applications across One Health, a multi-disciplinary, and multi-sectoral approach helps demonstrate how the entire work can be related and interact. Recent effects of relevant infectious diseases linking our discussion to the importance of neglected tropical diseases are also addressed.

Unprecedented opportunities for studying microbial populations have been created by current sequencing technologies [1]. For pathogens with comparatively low per-site mutation rates, such as DNA viruses and bacteria, Biek et al. [1] point out at that whole-genome sequencing can reveal the accumulation of novel genetic variation between population samples taken at different times. The concept of "measurably evolving populations" and related analytical approaches have provided powerful insights for fast-evolving RNA viruses, and sequencing technologies are now economical enough to apply to other DNA microbial pathogens [1]. These methodologies provide unprecedented windows to understanding how pathogens are adapting or evolving in real time in the face of climate change.

Climate change due to higher global temperatures and changing precipitation patterns affects the environment, altering coastlines and exacerbating flooding, and contributes to extreme weather patterns, all of which are influenced by the type, magnitude, and rate of change [2]. Here, climate change impact is defined as those effects resulting from climate change drivers such as deviations from average temperature and precipitation over several decades of time. For example, human, animal and plant systems are affected by rising atmospheric (greenhouse) gases coupled with globalization and other influences including cultural, economic, political, and technological factors [3,4]. Climate change is already affecting populations and infectious disease dynamics among wildlife, plants, insects and other living things, altering host and disease vector life cycles, shifting vector, pathogen and host ranges as well as migratory patterns, along with disease spread and its attributable impacts. The fact that neither transboundary infectious disease agents nor climate impacts respect international borders [5,6] reinforces the need for regional and global approaches that encourage open communication and transparency.

There are multiple scales of impact of changing climatic conditions—the habitats and plants that are responding to a changing climate, the vertebrate organisms that are adapting to the changing habitats and climate, and the microbes that are evolving to the new conditions at each level. The core thread between each of these biological scales is the genome. Genomes in all organisms evolve and adapt to new conditions over time. The genome may change by gene expressions in response to the environment or there may be modifications in the genetic code itself. Following the changes in the genomes of organisms at the multiple scales in response to changing conditions requires the measurement of the genome, which is primarily accomplished through next generation sequencing. In the One Health construct of considering the health of humans, animals, and the environment together, the genome is a foundational element for measuring the adaptation these systems over time.

Environmental changes caused by natural disasters and human-made accidents raise risk factors that indirectly increase infectious human disease outbreaks as a result of displaced human populations, constrained resources, and damaged infrastructure [7]. When variables including health, socio-economic, and political factors are considered together, climate change and its impacts can be thought of as "threat multipliers" [8,9]. Addressing these challenges through a holistic One Health approach recognizes and integrates perspectives related to animals, humans, and environment [8]. Key to the environmental aspect of the One Health concept is the importance of plant systems, which provide food and fiber and support the economy, contributing to socio-economic and political stability [3,10]. Both agricultural and environmental change are inextricably linked to climate change and, like higher vertebrate species, microbial pathogens will either adapt or not.

The design of effective programs for scientific inquiry, modeling, response to and mitigation of climate change impacts on biological systems will require a multi-sectoral, cross-disciplinary approach. For example, plant systems are often omitted from One Health considerations despite their direct nutritional and ecological relationships to animals and humans. Here, we note that plants and their phytobiomes have critical roles in both food security and climate change. One consequence is that the loss of agricultural productivity resulting from climate change can impact food security directly (reduced food production) or indirectly (the impact of rising global temperatures on food access, utilization, and safety) [11]. Furthermore, there is a link between food security, social stability and national security [3], as inadequate food supplies may trigger social unrest and/or human movement and migration. The impacts of these changes may be most severe among populations that are less affluent and those in the tropics [3,11,12]. Addressing these issues must involve key players from the climate, environmental, and genomics sciences and members of the security sector. In addition, public-private partnerships will help to galvanize national government level activity with those of industry and civil society.

2. Current State of Sequencing Tools

Tools and associated methods available for One Health-based responses to climate change impacts include both gold standard quantitative real-time PCR (qPCR) and current metagenomics sequencing approaches, which are less biased [13]. Their application can provide increased ability to detect and identify emerging and new pathogens and biological invasion by invasive species that are expected to increase due to climate impact [14,15]. Recently, the newly emerged coronavirus, which was first called the 2019-novel coronavirus (2019-nCoV) and now designated as the severe acute respiratory syndrome coronavirus-2 (SARS-CoV-2), was first reported in four cases associated with a wholesale market in Wuhan, China on 29 December 2019; [16]. The speed and transparency of the early work to understand this newly emerged coronavirus is remarkable; the full genome was released to the world on 10 January 2020. The release of the SARS-CoV-2 genome led to an almost real-time understanding of the viral phylogenetics, and the deduction that it came from a wildlife wet market, jumping from animal species [17] commonly bought at the market for consumption. With human populations, wildlife reservoirs, vectors, and microbes adapting in response to rapidly changing environmental conditions, outbreaks of pandemic potential such as that caused by SARS-CoV-2, will occur more regularly.

Genomic sequencing can be applied across many disciplines which are also relevant to climate change impacts, One Health, and biosecurity. A chart detailing a framework of how a variety of genomic tools can be applied to better understand various aspects of biological invasions [15,17] can help to facilitate outbreak response, enhance understanding of the role of changing environment and facilitate management of priorities through each stage of the invasion process. This framework of tools is also relevant to tracking certain neglected tropical diseases such as schistosomiasis, which is caused by parasitic flatworms and transmitted by exposure to contaminated water sources. Freshwater snails serve as the intermediate host of the flatworms. Climate change is expected to continue drier and hotter conditions across many parts of Africa, which should decrease the incidence of schistosomiasis by reducing the extent and availability of snail habitats [18]. Genomic sequencing can be applied here to track and multiple organisms and detect the presence of various species within a given habitat.

Developing high-quality pathogen detection methods used in clinical diagnostics, infectious disease surveillance, and forensics requires an understanding of the true genetic diversity of the pathogens, their ecology, geographic distribution, reservoirs, hosts, vectors, and genetically related organisms. Using a priori approaches to design molecular detection assays can lead to signature erosion. In the H1N1 influenza pandemic of 2009, for example, a genetic shift in the pathogen resulted in the inability of existing PCR assays to detect that strain [19]. The more we look at the genetic diversity of a particular pathogen, the more we discover, including unique sequences that reduce the sensitivity or specificity of existing diagnostics or detection methods.

Pathogen genetic diversity can be a hindrance to assay development as in the case of Lassa fever, which has symptoms similar to malaria and viral hemorrhagic fevers such as Ebola, and related co-infections among patients. Due to the complex diversity of the Old World arenavirus causing Lassa fever, PCR assays specifc for detection of this virus are difficult to design despite their single transmission mode via contact with rodent reservoirs [20]. This is due to the large genetic diversity of viral sequences in the reservoir population. Each cluster of human disease outbreak appears to derive from a single rodent-to-human transmission event that randomly samples a small portion of the true viral genetic diversity. Therefore qPCR assays are often designed using a snapshot of the viral genetic diversity known available at the time. Subsequent disease outbreaks may reveal new genetic diversity, eroding the performance of existing assays. A comprehensive surveillance of the rodent reservoir would be needed to understand the true level of genetic diversity that assays should be designed to detect. The need for proper biosafety controls from secure sample transport to laboratory biocontainment especially in low resource areas reinforce the need for effective, timely, and low-cost diagnostics [21].

3. Genomics and a Changing Environment

Although both climate change impacts and the research needed to understand and mitigate them are long term, time is no longer on our side and our approaches to solving such complex problems will require creativity and expediency. In epidemiological or climatological modeling, for example, data collection is traditionally completed first, followed by model development. However, a recent trend is for the two to be implemented concurrently so that data gaps are recognized immediately and data collection can target those gaps in real time. Estimating population spread and impacts of scenarios for changing environments or newly emerging viruses is now possible given advances in ecologic and epidemiologic models [22,23]. Genetic research and sequencing analyses have shown correlations suggesting that invasive species (weeds) moving into agricultural landscapes require less flexibility and less genetic diversity than those moving within the natural environment [15]. Tracking plant movements can help to inform the development of tools for predicting future plant invasions and migrations, which are expected to increase as climate change-induced habitat disturbances become more widespread [15]. Such approaches increase our ability to predict shifts and trends, whether in climate changes or pathogen spillover.

With regard to sequencing technology and meeting the challenge of climate change, there are two primary ways that genomics can be applied immediately. The first, as mentioned above, is understanding host, vector and pathogen range shifts due to environmental change. The second is incorporating sequencing of archived sample sets to investigate how pathogens are both evolving and shifting into new hosts and ranges. Recent evidence finds climate change is already affecting wildlife populations and disease dynamics [24–27], altering host and disease vector life cycles as in case of certain NTDs, shifting vector and host ranges and migratory patterns [26,28], and changing disease spread and its impacts. The consequences of these climatically induced changes are poorly understood, generating the need for comprehensive research involving both genomics [27] and predictive modeling of infectious disease and species distributions [29]. A multitude of factors may influence how both hosts and vectors of infectious diseases respond to changing climates. Finding signatures of environmental change in biological communities, as well as fusing and analyzing multi-scale data across species, time, and latitude, will be key.

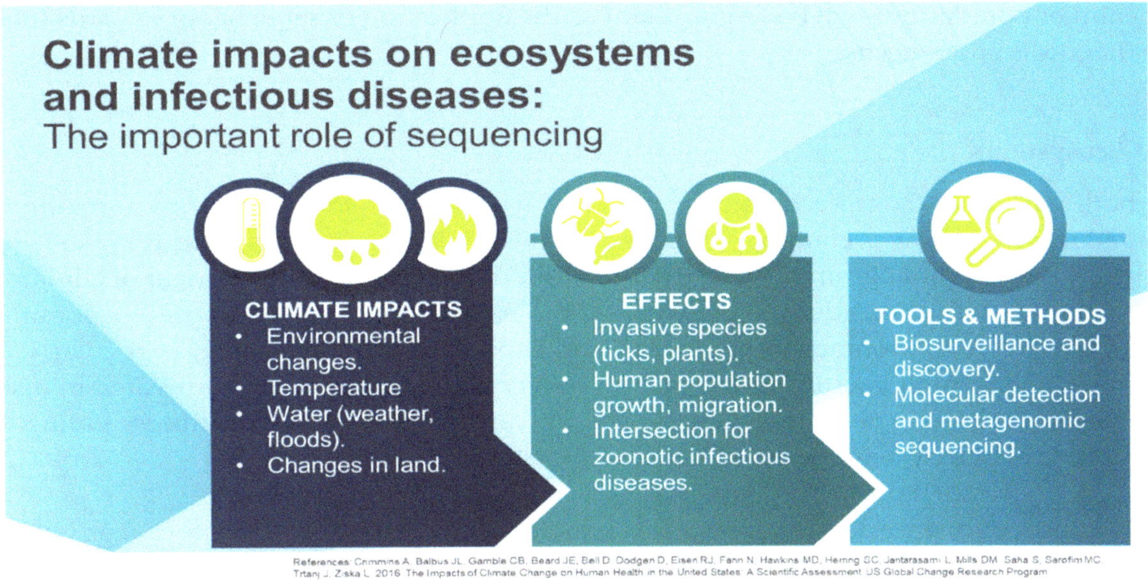

Figure 1. Climate impacts [30] whose effects on ecosystems and infectious diseases can be investigated using a variety of tools.

Combining sequencing and modeling will allow us to better understand how climate may be affecting geographic ranges of hosts, human migration, vectors, and parasites. The following questions can be asked using newly collected or archived samples from freezers around the world: How have pathogens in vectors and hosts changed over the last several decades? How do pathogens differ, at the genomic scale as well as in prevalence, geographically in both the hosts and vectors? Answering these sorts of questions is possible by simultaneously using sequencing with epidemiological models to make predictions that incorporate characteristics of pathogens, populations, and environmental variables.

4. Science of Signatures and Conservation Genomics

In order to understand the natural world, we must first find patterns that are otherwise invisible or indistinguishable from the chaos of natural systems. Finding such patterns can reveal signatures of long-term or short-term impacts of environmental events, evolutionary processes, or other idicators of environmental health. Using genomic sequences and bioinformatics to find and measure signatures in organisms can contribute to enhanced understanding of these complex systems and to better prediction of future impacts. In understanding the impacts of climate change on species, scientists are working to understand and predict which species will be able to adapt locally and which species will not be able to adapt [31,32]. Many of these adaptations will be through genetic adaptation to a changing environment [33].

Both marine and terrestrial ecosystems are under pressure, not only from climate change, but from over-exploitation, habitat loss and degradation, growing human populations, and ultimately species imperilment. Global climate change is altering our ecosystems at an unprecedented rate, threatening plants, animals, and the habitats in which they live. According to five coordinated reports in 2019 from the Intergovernmental Science-Policy Platform on Biodiversity and Ecosystem Services (IPBES), sponsored by the United Nations, over 1 million species are threatened with extinction [34]. Conservation genomics, which is closely linked to understanding the health of individuals and populations, can inform our efforts to manage infectious diseases and animal and plant health under these new environmental challenges. Understanding how ecosystems, and the populations within them, are likely to respond under different climate scenarios is essential for planning future conservation strategies and mitigations for infectious diseases. Modernizing our approach to natural resource management will ensure that we are utilizing the best available science to help make complex and difficult management decisions, and embracing sequencing where appropriate to find those signatures of the health of populations will be as important as the application of sequencing towards infectious disease diagnosis and detection.

5. Plant Ecosystems

In both natural and agro-ecosystems, plants play critical ecological roles by utilizing carbon dioxide and releasing oxygen, emitting substrates into the soil and atmosphere, modifying soil moisture, and reducing the amount of rainfall reaching the ground [35]. Effective assessment of climate issues related to plants should consider the plant as a complex "phytobiome" composed of communities of species within an environmental niche [36], and aspects of climate change, particularly altered temperatures and rainfall, modify community diversity [3]. Crop plants are cultivated in disturbed ecosystems and, at least in developed nations, are typically planted in monocultures, adding to their vulnerability to attack by new species of invasive pests or pathogens.

Since infectious disease develops only in a conducive environment [37], climate change will be a key driver of changes in plant disease epidemiology. For example, even a small increase in the length of a growing season can significantly increase the amount of pathogen inoculum produced [38]. Some genes encoding host plant disease resistance factors are less effective at higher temperatures, and higher cool-season temperatures may favor the survival of insect vectors of some plant pathogens [38]. Changes in climate (e.g., higher temperatures, lack of water, increased carbon dioxide, and other environmental changes) impact each of these elements in different ways including environmental hardiness, changes in developmental rates and flowering times, productivity, shifts in geographic ranges, and virulence (for pathogens and other microbes) or disease susceptibility (for plants) [15,35].

6. Research Example and Case Study of One Health Approaches to Using Sequencing to Understand and Mitigate Climate Change Impacts

Sequencing can provide a unique opportunity to derive new information from archived sample sets, especially when historical and recent samples are compared directly. Investigation can focus on genomic changes in individual microbes or microbiomes, or from host organisms. Targeted approaches can select specific pathogens and identify how they are associated with environmental change.

Vibrio cholerae is a well-known model for studying water-borne diseases and as part of an ecosystem, combined with environmental dynamics has been termed as biocomplexity [39]. When combined with genomic sequencing, epidemiology, and remote sensing, non-cholera vibrios such as *Vibrio parahaemolyticus* and *Vibrio vulnificus* represent a microbial barometer for climate change [40]. In 2016–2017, genomic sequencing showed that isolates in Yemen were *V. cholerae* serotype Ogawa isolates from a single sublineage of O1 El Tor [41]. This outbreak in Yemen which resulted in over one million cases and over 2000 deaths exemplifies the intersection of climate change, human disease, and related social factors of conflict and migration.

Zoonotic dieases such as plague and hantavirus caused by *Yersinia pestis* bacterium and Sin Nombre virus, respectively, are endemic in the US Four Corners region (Utah, Colorado, Arizona, and New Mexico). While the transmission of plague and hantavirus are different, the incidence of these viruses depends on rodent reservoirs and vectors (e.g., fleas). The occurrence of heavy precipitation in a given year often results in a larger rodent population, which increases risk of hantavirus transmission through interaction with humans. Models for predicting zoonotic diseases include diverse reservoirs of rodents in Central Asia, the Middle East, and the US Midwest which is adjacent to the Four Corners region [42]. Overall, the ability to collect and reconcile historical data with predictive modeling will be very powerful to understand transmission dynamics.

Case-Study: Expanding New Sequencing Technology Across the Globe to Detect Animal to Human Disease Spillover

Climate and health are intertwined with the effects of climate shifts that are currently manifesting globally. New technology, specifically in sequencing and metagenomics, must be implemented in geographically diverse regions around the globe in order to maximize impact. These newly developed or newly implemented technologies have the capacity to benefit even remote populations, who are often the most impacted by these health shifts. In addition to the identification of new pathogens, training on use of these technologies will have long-term impact by building local capacity to detect and respond to emerging health threats on a routine basis.

The USAID-funded PREDICT program [43,44] was implemented in over 30 countries around the globe from 2009–2020, aimed to strengthen capacity for surveillance and detection of viral threats transmitted from animals to humans. In order to address challenges of building and sustaining laboratory viral detection capacity in low-resource partner countries, the PREDICT approach built laboratory platforms based on conventional PCR methods to identify potential pathogens in wildlife and humans. Building upon this approach, the project also integrated more complex sequencing technology to empower local partner universities and governments to increase their viral detection capacity at the local level. Partner countries who successfully adopted this approach identified over 1000 new viruses at the human-animal interface. Recognition of the significant scientific and economic benefits of discovering high-consequence pathogens before evidence of spill-over into human populations, participating countries are now starting to realize the power and importance of sequencing and prioritize this technology as a key component to future capacity building [45]. This new focus in low-resource, viral hot-spot regions of the world promotes the potential for additional high-level metagenomic skills to be added to the cadre of possibilities. A critical piece of continuing the work of PREDICT is to encourage countries to store sample repositories for the long-term so that further work can be done utilizing mores powerful metagenomic approaches as they become available. As these countries are particularly impacted by drivers such as climate shifts, human and animal movement, and population growth, we anticipate continuing viral spillover at the human-animal interface, making the need for a continued increase and investment in pathogen detection capacity [46].

The sequencing technologies discussed in this paper, which expand our ability to detect pathogens of pandemic potential, should be deployed locally and globally in areas where spillover and disease spread continue to occur. The challenge is to continue a global dialogue to encourage development of affordable platforms and training that can lead to discovery of known and novel viruses with pandemic potential [47]. The One Health Institute at the University of California, Davis, led the PREDICT Project and is also home of the University of California Global Health Institute's Planetary Health Center of Expertise that works to raise awareness about climate and health issues as well as sustainable solutions and platforms (https://ohi.vetmed.ucdavis.edu). With the help of such centers, the global population at large is beginning to appreciate the importance of understanding local predictions for environmental change and disease spillover to utilize adaptation and mitigation measures. It has become well known that understanding drivers of pathogen spillover and risk, and utilizing state-of-the art technology for management of these threats, are critical. The authors are optimistic that there is a true space for development of easily accessible technologies that are farm, clinic or animal/human-specific, resulting in rapid, real-time on-site diagnostic care utilizing the new sequencing technologies discussed herein.

7. Importance of Trust and Sharing of Data and Material

There is a continued need to earn and build trust between partners at the working level of research groups in universities, companies and institutes, and the top level of government partners especially in host countries where work is being implemented. It is critical to invest time to build a collaborative network that respectfully supports trust through transparency and partnership. The ability to collaborate professionally with various partners is critical to generate and provide the various forms of data and technology (from field to lab), including the models and sequencing methods discussed herein. More frequently, funding and donor agencies are requiring data be made available in a public and open source manner. Occasionally frameworks for data sharing are provided, but other times the research team needs to develop an approach that works best to meet the requirements and needs. The ability to work in a global society beyond any individual research lab, or any individual organization to generate a solution by working together should be recognized. One key to success is to have strong partnerships on the ground with protocols for data sharing in place from the beginning.

8. Conclusions

Through our discussion, we draw attention to the power of genomic sequencing that complements expertise and tools across disciplines and sectors to address climate change impacts on ecosystems and infectious diseases. Using a One Health approach is important to view the problem on a larger scale, and beyond the scientific and technical work the government policies developed in some countries are now starting to take a coordinated One Health multi-sectoral approach to implement change. We described some examples of climate change impacts on animal and human infectious disease that exist in vector-borne, zoonotic, and neglected tropical diseases. Climate change is also a key driver of multiple changes in plant epidemiology, affecting disease susceptibility and resistance as well as environmental hardiness, developmental and flowering rates, productivity, and geographical range. Genetic tools facilitate the prediction of such changes and help in the development of management options. Shaping human behavior is key to positive and practical outcomes. Besides the importance of shared goals and trust-building as related to setting research agendas and sharing intellectual resources, another critical theme that arose is the need to increase partnering, especially for engaging public and private partners that can help incorporate a multi-sectoral approach with a diverse audience of stakeholders who will form policy. This audience goes beyond public and animal health specialists and targets traditional biotechnology as well as social and life scientists that have expertise in behavior change, food safety and security, the environment, hydrology, climate, and meterology. The practice and policies developed will shape funding which, in turn, will leverage the commercial partnerships that are challenged with pursuing markets with varying returns on investments and are also critical in sustaining programs through the economy and enterprise. This combination of resources and expertise contributes to a more open and collaborative approach to understanding the links between infectious disease and climate.

Author Contributions: Conceptualization, K.B.Y., J.M.F., W.S., C.M., and J.F.; resources, K.B.Y., J.M.F., W.S., R.W. and J.F.; data curation, T.M.T. and J.L.; original draft preparation, K.B.Y. and J.M.F.; writing—review and editing, W.S., T.M.T., J.L., R.W., C.M., and J.F. All authors have read and agreed to the published version of the manuscript.

Acknowledgments: We are grateful to organizers of the 14th annual Sequencing, Finishing, and Analysis in the Future conference held 21–23 May 2019 in Santa Fe, New Mexico, USA. Special thanks to Tina May for her figures and graphics.

References

1. Biek, R.; Pybus, O.G.; Lloyd-Smith, J.O.; Didelot, X. Measurably Evolving Pathogens in the Genomic Era. *Trends Ecol. Evol.* **2015**, *30*, 306–313. [CrossRef] [PubMed]
2. Marjoram, T. Silk Roads for the 21st Century: Engineering Mega-Infrastructure for Development and Sustainability. *Front. Eng. Manag.* **2016**, *3*, 187–196. [CrossRef]
3. Stack, J.P.; Fletcher, J.; Gullino, M.L. Climate Change and Plant Biosecurity: A New World Disorder? In *Global Environmental Changes: New Drivers for Resistance, Crime and Terrorism*; Mass, A., Bodó, B., Burnley, C., Comardicea, I., Roffey, R., Eds.; Nomos: Baden-Baden, Germany, 2013; pp. 161–181, ISBN 978-383-296-894-6.
4. Mirski, T.; Bartoszcze, M.; Bielawska-Drózd, A. Impact of Climate Change on Infectious Diseases. *Pol. J. Environ. Stud.* **2012**, *21*, 525–532.
5. CNA Military Advisory Board. National Security and the Accelerating Risks of Climate Change. Available online: https://www.cna.org/cna_files/pdf/MAB_5-8-14.pdf (accessed on 20 November 2019).
6. Siembieda, J.L.; Kock, R.A.; McCracken, T.A.; Newman, S.H. The Role of Wildlife in Transboundary Animal Diseases. *Anim. Health Res. Rev.* **2011**, *12*, 95–111. [CrossRef]

7. Kouadio, I.K.; Aljunid, S.; Kamigaki, T.; Hammad, K.; Oshitani, H. Infectious Diseases Following Natural Disasters: Prevention and Control Measures. *Expert Rev. Anti. Infect. Ther.* **2012**, *10*, 95–104. [CrossRef]
8. Essack, S.Y. Environment: The Neglected Component of the One Health Triad. *Lancet Planet. Health* **2018**, *2*, e238–e239. [CrossRef]
9. Black, P.F.; Butler, C.D. One Health in a World with Climate Change. *Rev. Sci. Tech.* **2014**, *33*, 465–473. [CrossRef]
10. Fletcher, J.; Franz, D.; Leclerc, J.E. Healthy Plants: Necessary for a Balanced "One Health" Concept. *Vet. Ital.* **2009**, *45*, 79–95.
11. Brown, M.E.; Antle, J.M.; Backlund, P.; Carr, E.R.; Easterling, W.E.; Walsh, M.K.; Ammann, C.; Attavanich, W.; Barrett, C.B.; Bellemare, M.F.; et al. *Climate Change, Global Food Security and the U.S. Food System*; U.S. Global Change Research Program: Washington, DC, USA, 2015. [CrossRef]
12. Ghini, R.; Bettiol, W.; Hamada, E. Diseases in Tropical and Plantation Crops as Affected by Climate Changes: Current Knowledge and Perspectives. *Plant Pathol.* **2011**, *60*, 122–132. [CrossRef]
13. Yeh, K.B.; Wood, H.; Scullion, M.; Russell, J.A.; Parker, K.; Gnade, B.T.; Jones, A.R.; Whittier, C.; Mereish, K. Molecular Detection of Biological Agents in the Field: Then and Now. *mSphere* **2019**, *4*, 1–11. [CrossRef]
14. Mansfield, K.L.; Jizhou, L.; Phipps, L.P.; Johnson, N. Emerging Tick-Borne Viruses in the Twenty-First Century. *Front. Cell. Infect. Microbiol.* **2017**, *7*, 1–11. [CrossRef] [PubMed]
15. Chown, S.L.; Hodgins, K.A.; Griffin, P.C.; Oakeshott, J.G.; Byrne, M.; Hoffmann, A. Biological invasions, climate change and genomics. *Evol. Appl.* **2015**, *8*, 23–46. [CrossRef] [PubMed]
16. Qun, L. An outbreak o f NCIP (2019-nCoV) infection in China—Wuhan, Hubei province, 2019–2020. *China CDC Wkly.* **2020**, *2*, 79–80.
17. Ji, W.; Wang, W.; Zhao, X.; Zai, J.; Li, X. Cross-species Transmission of the Newly Identified Coronavirus 2019-nCoV. *J. Med. Virol.* **2020**, *92*, 433–440. [CrossRef] [PubMed]
18. Blum, J.A.; Hotez, P.J. Global 'worming': Climate change and its projected general impact on human helminth infections. *PLoS Negl. Trop. Dis.* **2018**, *12*, 1–6. [CrossRef] [PubMed]
19. Klungthong, C.; Chinnawirotpisan, P.; Hussem, K.; Phonpakobsin, T.; Manasatienkij, W.; Ajariyakhajorn, C.; Rungrojcharoenkit, K.; Gibbons, R.V.; Jarman, R.G. The impact of primer and probe-template mismatches on the sensitivity of pandemic influenza A/H1N1/2009 virus detection by real-time RT-PCR. *J. Clin. Virol.* **2010**, *48*, 91–95. [CrossRef]
20. Mazzola, L.T.; Kelly-Cirino, C. Diagnostics for Lassa fever virus: A genetically diverse pathogen found in low-resource settings. *BMJ Glob. Heal.* **2019**, *4*, 1–10. [CrossRef]
21. Taboy, C.H.; Chapman, W.; Albetkova, A.; Kennedy, S.; Rayfield, M.A. Integrated Disease Investigations and Surveillance Planning: A Systems Approach to Strengthening National Surveillance and Detection of Events of Public Health Importance in Support of the International Health Regulations. *BMC Public Health* **2010**, *10*, 1–6. [CrossRef]
22. Plowright, R.K.; Eby, P.; Hudson, P.J.; Smith, I.L.; Westcott, D.; Bryden, W.L.; Middleton, D.; Reid, P.A.; McFarlane, R.A.; Martin, G.; et al. Ecological dynamics of emerging bat virus spillover. *Proc. R. Soc. B.* **2014**, *282*, 1–9. [CrossRef]
23. Riou, J.; Althaus, C.L. Pattern of early human-to-human transmission of Wuhan 2019 novel coronavirus (2019-nCoV), December 2019 to January 2020. *Eurosurveillance* **2020**, *25*, 1–5. [CrossRef]
24. Matthysen, E.; Adriaensen, F.; Dhondt, A.A. Multiple Responses to Increasing Spring Temperatures in the Breeding Cycle of Blue and Great Tits (Cyanistes Caeruleus, Parus Major). *Glob. Chang. Biol.* **2011**, *17*, 1–16. [CrossRef]
25. Melles, S.J.; Fortin, M.J.; Lindsay, K.; Badzinski, D. Expanding Northward: Influence of Climate Change, Forest Connectivity, and Population Processes on a Threatened Species' Range Shift. *Glob. Chang. Biol.* **2011**, *17*, 17–31. [CrossRef]
26. Carey, C. The Impacts of Climate Change on the Annual Cycles of Birds. *Philos. Trans. R. Soc. B Biol. Sci.* **2009**, *27*, 3321–3330. [CrossRef]

27. Ruegg, K.; Bay, R.A.; Anderson, E.C.; Saracco, J.F.; Harrigan, R.J.; Whitfield, M.; Paxton, E.H.; Smith, T.B. Ecological Genomics Predicts Climate Vulnerability in an Endangered Southwestern Songbird. *Ecol. Lett.* **2018**, *21*, 1085–1096. [CrossRef]
28. Bridge, E.S.; Kelly, J.F.; Bjornen, P.E.; Curry, C.M.; Crawford, P.H.C.; Paritte, J.M. Effects of Nutritional Condition on Spring Migration: Do Migrants Use Resource Availability to Keep Pace with a Changing World? *J. Exp. Biol.* **2010**, *213*, 2424–2429. [CrossRef] [PubMed]
29. Bartlow, A.W.; Manore, C.; Xu, C.; Kaufeld, K.A.; del Valle, S.; Ziemann, A.; Fairchild, G.; Fair, J.M. Forecasting Zoonotic Infectious Disease Response to Climate Change: Mosquito Vectors and a Changing Environment. *Vet. Sci.* **2019**, *6*, 40. [CrossRef] [PubMed]
30. USGCRP. *The Impacts of Climate Change on Human Health in the United States: A Scientific Assessment*; Crimmins, A., Balbus, J.L., Gamble, C.B., Beard, J.E., Bell, D., Dodgen, D., Eisen, R.J., Fann, N., Hawkins, M.D., Herring, S.C., et al., Eds.; U.S. Global Change Research Program: Washington, DC, USA, 2016. Available online: https://health2016.globalchange.gov (accessed on 19 November 2019).
31. Atkins, K.E.; Travis, J.M.J. Local Adaptation and the Evolution of Species' Ranges under Climate Change. *J. Theor. Biol.* **2010**, *266*, 449–457. [CrossRef]
32. Macfadyen, S.; McDonald, G.; Hill, M.P. From Species Distributions to Climate Change Adaptation: Knowledge Gaps in Managing Invertebrate Pests in Broad-Acre Grain Crops. *Agric. Ecosyst. Environ.* **2018**, *253*, 208–219. [CrossRef]
33. Somero, G.N. The Physiology of Climate Change: How Potentials for Acclimatization and Genetic Adaptation Will Determine "Winners" and "Losers". *J. Exp. Biol.* **2010**, *213*, 912–920. [CrossRef]
34. Intergovermental Science-Policy Platform on Biodiversity and Ecosystem Services. IPBES Global Assessment. Available online: https://ipbes.net/news/ipbes-global-assessment-preview (accessed on 24 November 2019).
35. Dutta, H.; Dutta, A. The Microbial Aspect of Climate Change. *Energ. Ecol. Environ.* **2016**, *1*, 209–232. [CrossRef]
36. Phytobiomes Writing Team. Phytobiomes: A Roadmap for Research and Translation. Available online: http://www.phytobiomes.org/roadmap/Pages/default.aspx (accessed on 19 November 2019).
37. Agrios, G. *Plant Pathology*, 5th ed.; Academic Press: Cambridge, MA, USA, 2005; ISBN 978-012-044-565-3.
38. Garrett, K.A.; Forbes, G.A.; Savary, S.; Skelsey, P.; Sparks, A.H.; Valdivia, C.; van Bruggen, A.H.C.; Willocquet, L.; Djurle, A.; Duveiller, E.; et al. Complexity in Climate-Change Impacts: An Analytical Framework for Effects Mediated by Plant Disease. *Plant Pathol.* **2011**, *60*, 15–30. [CrossRef]
39. Constantin de Magny, G.; Colwell, R.R. Cholera and climate: A demonstrated relationship. *Trans. Am. Clin. Climatol. Assoc.* **2009**, *120*, 119–128. [PubMed]
40. Baker-Austin, C.; Trinanes, J.; Gonzalez-Escalona, N.; Martinez-Urtaza, J. Non-Cholera Vibrios: The Microbial Barometer of Climate Change. *Trends Microbiol.* **2017**, *25*, 76–84. [CrossRef] [PubMed]
41. Weill, F.X.; Domman, D.; Njamkepo, E.; Almesbahi, A.A.; Naji, M.; Nasher, S.S.; Rakesh, A.; Assiri, A.M.; Sharma, N.C.; Kariuki, S.; et al. Genomic insights into the 2016–2017 cholera epidemic in Yemen. *Nature* **2019**, *565*, 230–233. [CrossRef] [PubMed]
42. Han, B.A.; Schmidt, J.P.; Bowden, S.E.; Drake, J.M. Rodent reservoirs of future zoonotic diseases. *Proc. Natl. Acad. Sci. USA* **2015**, *112*, 7039–7044. [CrossRef]
43. Kelly, T.R.; Karesh, W.B.; Johnson, C.K.; Gilardi, K.V.K.; Anthony, S.J.; Goldstein, T.; Olson, S.H.; Machalaba, C.; Mazet, J.A.; Predict Consortium. One Health proof of concept: Bringing a transdisciplinary approach to surveillance for zoonotic viruses at the human-wild animal interface. *Prev. Vet. Med.* **2017**, *137*, 112–118. [CrossRef]
44. Bird, B.H.; Mazet, J.A.K. Detection of Emerging Zoonotic Pathogens: An Integrated One Health Approach. *Annu. Rev. Anim. Biosci.* **2018**, *6*, 121–139. [CrossRef]
45. Montecino-Latorre, D.; Goldstein, T.; Gilardi, K.; Wolking, D.; Van Wormer, E.; Kazwala, R.; Ssebide, B.; Nziza, J.; Sijali, Z.; Cranfield, M.; et al. Reproduction of East-African bats may guide risk mitigation for coronavirus spillover. *One Health Outlook* **2020**, *2*, 1–13. [CrossRef]

46. Carroll, D.; Daszak, P.; Wolfe, N.D.; Gao, G.F.; Morel, C.M.; Morzaria, S.; Pablos-Méndez, A.; Tomori, O.; Mazet, J.A.K. The Global Virome Project. *Science* **2018**, *359*, 872–874. [CrossRef]
47. Goldstein, T.; Anthony, S.J.; Gbakima, A.; Bird, B.H.; Bangura, J.; Tremeau-Bravard, A.; Belaganahalli, M.N.; Wells, H.L.; Dhanota, J.K.; Liang, E.; et al. The discovery of Bombali virus adds further support for bats as hosts of ebolaviruses. *Nat. Microbiol.* **2018**, *3*, 1084–1089. [CrossRef]

3

Control Strategies for Scabies

Daniel Engelman [1,2,3,4,*] and **Andrew C. Steer** [1,2,3,4]

1 Tropical Diseases, Murdoch Children's Research Institute, Parkville VIC 3052, Australia; Andrew.Steer@rch.org.au
2 Department of Paediatrics, University of Melbourne, Parkville VIC 3052, Australia
3 Department of General Medicine, Royal Children's Hospital, Parkville VIC 3052, Australia
4 International Alliance for the Control of Scabies, Parkville VIC 3052, Australia
* Correspondence: Daniel.Engelman@rch.org.au;

Abstract: Scabies is a neglected tropical disease of the skin, causing severe itching and stigmatizing skin lesions. Further, scabies leads to impetigo, severe bacterial infections, and post-infectious complications. Around 200 million people are affected, particularly among disadvantaged populations living in crowded conditions in tropical areas. After almost 50 years, research into scabies control has shown great promise, particularly in highly-endemic island settings, but these findings have not been widely adopted. Newer approaches, utilizing ivermectin-based mass drug administration, appear feasible and highly effective. Inclusion of scabies in the WHO portfolio of neglected tropical diseases in 2017 may facilitate renewed opportunities and momentum toward global control. However, further operational research is needed to develop evidence-based strategies for control in a range of settings, and monitor their impact. Several enabling factors are required for successful implementation, including availability of affordable drug supply. Integration with existing health programs may provide a cost-effective approach to control.

Keywords: scabies; neglected tropical diseases; impetigo; mass drug administration; ivermectin

---

1. Introduction

Scabies is a skin disease caused by infestation with the mite, *Sarcoptes scabiei* var. *hominis*. The female mite, measuring less than 0.5 mm, burrows into the skin, where antigens on the exoskeleton of the mite, along with its saliva, excreta, and eggs, elicit a hypersensitivity reaction [1]. The resulting skin lesions most commonly affect the hands, wrists, ankles, and feet (Figure 1). In the vast majority of cases of common scabies (also known variably as ordinary, classical, or typical scabies) there is a low number of mites on the patient's body (5 to 15). Crusted scabies (formerly known as Norwegian scabies) is a rare form of the disease characterized by hyperinfestation with thousands to millions of mites and hyperkeratotic 'crusted' skin [2].

Transmission of scabies is predominantly via skin-to-skin contact. Transmission from bedding or clothes is rare in ordinary scabies, but can occur in crusted scabies because of its tremendous mite burden. The risk of transmission of scabies increases with higher levels of population density, reflected by the high endemicity observed in communities living in poverty with associated crowded housing conditions, and by outbreaks in in residential care facilities, prisons, schools, and refugee camps. Patients with underlying immunodeficiency from any cause, such as human immunodeficiency virus, human T-lymphotropic virus type 1 or corticosteroid treatment, or those with neurological conditions, are at an increased risk of crusted scabies [2–4].

Scabies causes considerable suffering due to the intense itch and associated scratching, leading to sleep disturbances which, in turn, impact on school and work attendance and performance, and ultimately the economic productivity of whole communities [5]. Like many infections that affect the skin, scabies is associated with social stigma and leads to social exclusion because of the appearance of the affected individual and attendant feelings of shame, as well as fears within the community of spread of infection [5,6]. Scabies can have a marked impact on quality of life measures, similar to the recognized psychological impact caused by other skin conditions such as psoriasis and vitiligo [7].

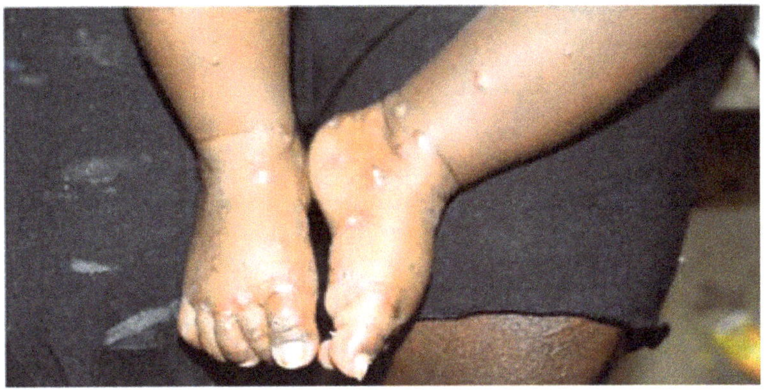

Figure 1. Infant with typical rash of scabies.

In endemic settings, scabies lesions are often super-infected with the bacteria *Streptococcus pyogenes* and *Staphylococcus aureus.* Bacterial infection occurs due to breaches in the skin barrier as a result of mite burrows and associated scratching [8], as well as direct effects of the scabies mite in downregulating host immunity and optimising conditions for bacterial growth [9,10]. These bacteria can cause local soft tissue infections such as impetigo, cellulitis, and abscesses, and can lead to life-threatening diseases including sepsis, and in the case of *S. pyogenes*, post-streptococcal glomerulonephritis [11], and possibly acute rheumatic fever (this link is epidemiologically associated but, as yet, unproven) [12,13].

This review aims to re-examine the rationale for public health control of scabies, evaluate the available evidence for scabies control interventions, and identify the barriers and future research priorities needed to develop and scale-up implementation of scabies control activities.

2. Burden of Disease

Scabies occurs worldwide, and is estimated to affect over 200 million people at any single time [14]. The highest prevalence of scabies occurs in tropical areas, especially in disadvantaged populations, and especially among children and the elderly. The Global Burden of Disease (GBD) study reported that scabies directly accounts for 0.21% of global disability-adjusted life years [15]. However, there are substantial gaps in our knowledge of the epidemiology of scabies and its complications.

First, many countries have no available data on scabies prevalence, including countries where disease burden is likely to be high, based upon known risk factors (poverty and overcrowding). For example, in a systematic review of prevalence studies of scabies published 1985 to 2015, only five sub-Saharan African countries were represented among the 48 studies included [16]. Where data do exist, they may be outdated and not representative of the current burden.

Second, routinely-collected data, and therefore GBD data, do not reflect actual disease burden. In countries where community-based prevalence survey data are available, the prevalence of scabies observed in these surveys is frequently substantially higher than the burden reported at the clinic level, and by the GBD study. For example, in the Solomon Islands, routine Ministry of Health clinic data identified 4759 cases of scabies in 2016 (total population of 584,000, corresponding to an incidence of 0.79% per year), in contrast to a detailed community-based survey in one province in the same year in which the prevalence was 19.2% [17]. This discrepancy may be because individuals within communities may not present with scabies (perhaps because it is 'normalized' or because effective treatments are often unavailable), or because there is under-diagnosis at clinics when patients do present [18].

Third, even when prevalence surveys are conducted, there is substantial heterogeneity in design and methods across studies. A key issue is the method used to diagnose scabies, which ranges from recovery of live mites by scraping of the skin, to a clinical diagnosis based on varying combinations of diagnostic features. This variability, noted even among scabies treatment trials [19], limits comparison of disease burden estimates across studies.

Fourth, there is limited evidence to determine the magnitude of the association between scabies and its complications. Available epidemiologic data suggest that, in highly endemic settings, at least 40% of impetigo lesions can be attributed to scabies, and an even higher proportion among younger children (71% in one study) [17,20–22]. The high attributable risk observed in epidemiologic studies is supported by trials of community control of scabies, as outlined below, where impetigo prevalence has been shown to fall consistently and substantially with reductions in scabies prevalence.

3. The Need for Surveillance and Control

The World Health Organization Department of Neglected Tropical Disease (NTD) Control designated scabies as an NTD for large-scale disease control action in 2017. This designation was in recognition of: (1) the large known burden and impact of scabies, justifying a global response; (2) the geographic distribution of scabies among disadvantaged populations living in tropical and subtropical regions; (3) the amenability of scabies to public health control efforts, especially noting the success of mass drug administration (MDA) for scabies (detailed below); and (4) the broad neglect of scabies across multiple research domains [23]. In 2018, the ninth meeting of the WHO NTD Strategic Technical Advisory Group Global Working Group on Monitoring and Evaluation of NTDs recognized that there is a priority need to develop resources to aid defining the global burden of scabies, and to provide guidance for countries and regions for public health approaches for scabies control, including in outbreak situations [24].

Guidance is required for assessment of disease burden at local, national and regional levels, and should include guidelines for standardised diagnosis and surveillance methodology. Consensus criteria for the diagnosis of scabies were recently developed using a four-round Delphi process among 34 international experts, under the auspices of the International Alliance for the Control of Scabies (IACS) [25]. The IACS Criteria include three levels and eight subcategories such that the criteria can be applied across a range of situations, from a dermatologist's office to a field survey in a resource-limited setting (Table 1) [26].

Table 1. Summary of 2018 IACS [1] criteria for the diagnosis of scabies [26].

Level	Criteria
A. Confirmed scabies	At least one of the following: A1: Mites, eggs or faeces on light microscopy of skin samples A2: Mites, eggs or faeces visualized on individual using high-powered imaging device A3: Mite visualized on individual using dermoscopy
B. Clinical scabies	At least one of the following: B1: Scabies burrows B2: Typical lesions affecting male genitalia B3 Typical lesions in a typical distribution and two history features
C. Suspected scabies	One of the following: C1: Typical lesions in a typical distribution and one history feature C2: Atypical lesions or atypical distribution and two history features
History features	H1: Itching H2: Close contact with an individual who has itching or typical lesions in a typical distribution
Notes:	*Diagnosis can be made at one of the three levels (A, B, or C)* *A diagnosis of clinical or suspected scabies should only be made if differential diagnoses are considered less likely than scabies.*

[1] IACS: International Alliance for the Control of Scabies.

The approach to community control for scabies is best aligned with the core strategies utilized by WHO Department of NTD Control: preventive chemotherapy using MDA, and/or innovative and intensified case management. Guidance around which approach to use will depend upon a number of factors, particularly disease burden at the community level. Therefore, feasible and accurate assessment of scabies prevalence will be crucial to inform an appropriate public health response, and also to monitor the effectiveness of this response. Below we outline the evidence to inform community control strategies for scabies, particularly MDA.

4. Community Control

The first reported public health initiatives to control scabies came from the San Blas islands (now known as the Guna Yala region) of Panama in the 1970s and 1980s. Scabies was introduced to the Guna populations and rapidly became endemic, with reported prevalences of 40–70% [27]. In a landmark series of studies, Taplin and colleagues compared approaches to scabies control in the islands. They found that treatment of all community members with 1% lindane resulted in a 98% cure rate at 10 weeks, whereas treatment of only those with clinically evident scabies had a lower effectiveness of 50% [28]. In areas where the entire community could not be treated, scabies was noted to return rapidly, leading the authors to conclude that, in those highly-endemic settings, 'treatment of individual patients without regard to community epidemiology is time consuming, and unlikely to have a significant impact in epidemic situations' [27]. Suspicion of developing mite resistance and the adverse effects profile of lindane then prompted the investigation of topical permethrin 5% for 756 residents on the island of Ticantiki. Following a MDA campaign with very high coverage, new arrivals to the island were treated and ongoing surveillance identified and treated new cases [27]. Scabies prevalence was reduced from 32% to below 2% and maintained for 3 years. Bacterial skin infection (impetigo) also declined from 32% to 1% in children without use of antibiotics. The permethrin-based MDA was well tolerated with few adverse events, but required a large project team for implementation. The team used directly observed applications, including to genital and breast areas, which may not be acceptable by some communities.

Drawing on the work in Panama, a control program commenced in five small, densely-populated islands in the Solomon Islands from 1997 to 2000 [29]. Use of topical treatments in this setting was considered 'so difficult as to be unacceptable and impractical'. Reports of the effectiveness of ivermectin for the individual and mass treatment of scabies [30], and knowledge of safety as a MDA strategy for lymphatic filariasis and onchocerciasis [31,32], led to selection of oral ivermectin as the main treatment, offered to the whole population as MDA. Permethrin 5% cream was given to children weighing less than 15 kg and pregnant women. Henceforth, we refer to this strategy of using topical treatments for ivermectin-contraindicated groups as 'ivermectin-based MDA'. Children (but not adults) were then re-examined at 6-monthly intervals and those with scabies and their household contacts were re-treated. Returned travelers and visitors were also treated, even if asymptomatic. No additional antibiotics were used. Over the three years of observation, the prevalence of scabies in children reduced from 25% to less than 1%. The proportion of children with open sores, the median number of sores, and the proportion of children with microscopic hematuria also reduced significantly. In contrast to the Panama experience, where scabies resurgence was observed after disruption of permethrin supply, when 338 residents of the same communities in the Solomon Islands were examined for scabies more than 15 years later, only a single case of scabies was found [33].

An ecological study from northern Australia aimed to reduce scabies and secondary bacterial skin infection in five remote communities from 2004 to 2007 [34]. Permethrin 5% was offered annually to all community members, but application was not directly observed. Children aged less than 15 years were screened regularly and referred for treatment if scabies or impetigo were identified. Whereas the prevalence of bacterial skin infection reduced during the project, there was little effect on scabies. A nested study found that actual use of permethrin was low, with only 44% of contacts applying the cream. Those households that did apply the cream had a much lower rate of scabies transmission [35].

The first controlled study of MDA for scabies control was conducted in Fiji in 2012. Three small island groups were randomized to one of ivermectin-based MDA (with permethrin for contraindicated groups), permethrin-based MDA, or 'standard-care' (where all community members were screened and referred for treatment if diagnosed with scabies). The trial found that at 12 months after MDA, the prevalence of scabies reduced in the ivermectin group by 94% (from 32% to 2%), in the permethrin group by 62% (42% to 16%) and in the standard-care group by 49% (37% to 19%). Once again, a considerable reduction was observed in the prevalence of impetigo without additional use of antibiotic therapy, most notably in the ivermectin group, where impetigo prevalence fell by 67% (25% to 8%).

Similar results were seen in two recent studies in the Solomon Islands. A before-and-after study evaluated a single round of ivermectin-based MDA, offered to a population of 26,000, in combination with azithromycin MDA for trachoma control. The co-administration was well tolerated with no serious adverse events [36]. A smaller study, from a different region of the Solomon Islands, reported a reduction in scabies prevalence of greater than 90%, 12 months after ivermectin-based MDA [37].

However, in a single cohort study in a remote island community of Australia, ivermectin-based MDA was less effective. Two MDA campaigns were implemented, 12 months apart, for a population of approximately 1000. Scabies prevalence fell from a baseline of 4% to less than 1%, 6 months after MDA, then increased to 9% after 12 months. A second MDA was conducted at this time, and scabies prevalence fell to 2% when measured 6 months later. Factors identified that may have contributed to the results included a lower than anticipated baseline prevalence, a highly mobile population with many new arrivals to the community after the first MDA, and a cluster of new cases associated with a case of crusted scabies.

Ivermectin-MDA programs for other NTDs also provide opportunities to study the effect on scabies [38]. In Zanzibar, Tanzania, annual MDA with ivermectin and albendazole for lymphatic filariasis from 2001–2005 resulted in a 68–98% reduction in clinic presentations for scabies [39]. However, in a recent, prospective study from the Kongwa District of Tanzania, where the baseline prevalence of scabies was 4.4%, annual ivermectin MDA for lymphatic filariasis was associated with a smaller reduction in scabies prevalence, to 2.9% after 4 years [40]. The authors concluded that a greater effect on scabies prevalence may not have been observed because of the relatively low prevalence and because only a single dose was given.

In addition to these community control strategies, there is increasing evidence of the use of MDA for management of scabies outbreaks within closed institutions such as schools, prisons, hospitals, aged care facilities and refugee and displaced person camps [30,41–43]. Scabies outbreaks in these settings are often difficult to diagnose and manage [44–46]. Ivermectin-based MDA has also been employed in the control of large-scale, open outbreaks, such as the current, drought-associated epidemic in Ethiopia, where more than one million people have been affected, although evaluation of this public health intervention is not currently available [47].

5. Outstanding Issues

The combined evidence of these control strategies reveals several common themes. First, in contrast to treating individuals and contacts, MDA strategies appear highly effective in reducing the burden of both scabies and impetigo. This strategy has been particularly successful in island communities with a very high baseline prevalence. With adequate community consultation, ivermectin-based MDA has been widely accepted by communities, well tolerated by individuals, and appeared more effective than permethrin-based MDA. Second, the benefit of MDA in communities with a lower baseline prevalence is less clear, and suggests that a different strategy may be appropriate for communities with lower prevalence (for example, less than 5%). Third, the most effective strategies have been those where active surveillance and treatment of new cases and new arrivals to the community have been incorporated, but it remains unclear to what extent these additional measures are required to ensure sustainable program success. Finally, environmental control measures (such as the washing of linen and clothing, or insecticide spraying) have not formed a component of the most successful strategies, suggesting this labor-intensive and costly strategy may not be required for community control. For control of institutional outbreaks, particularly where individuals have crusted scabies, environmental measures, if feasible, may be warranted.

Despite the promise of studies on community control for scabies, there remain several important operational questions about how their findings should be implemented, and the expected impact of such interventions. As noted, MDA appears less successful in lower-prevalence settings, and it is not clear what prevalence of scabies, or other measure, should trigger consideration of MDA. Further investigation is required to determine the optimal strategy for MDA. It is unclear whether one dose of ivermectin per MDA round is sufficient, or whether a second dose is required after 7–14 days, as is clinically recommended when using ivermectin for individual case treatment, due to its inability to kill the mite eggs [48]. The number and frequency of MDA rounds, when to stop, and duration of surveillance after stopping are all unknown. Modelling research could play an important role in this area, as for other NTDs [49–51]. The treatment of young children and pregnant women is critical for reducing transmission because these groups harbor a disproportionate burden of disease. However, because of current limitations on ivermectin use, they can only receive topical treatments, which are less practical. There is some evidence that ivermectin may be safe in these groups [52,53], but definitive research and development of pediatric-friendly formulations are needed. Further work on the feasibility and acceptability of MDA programs by communities in various settings is also required.

Standardized methods for diagnosis and mapping are required, possibly building on the 2018 IACS criteria, which need validation and testing in a variety of settings [26]. Investment into basic scientific research is required, including the development of diagnostic tests, ideally point of care tests for low-resource settings [54,55]. In lower-prevalence settings, or where MDA may be unrequired or infeasible, different strategies need to be developed and evaluated, including mass treatment of high-risk groups, or enhanced surveillance and intensified case management. Simplified, integrated clinical care pathways [56,57], and strategies such as teledermatology [58–60] may have an important role in providing high quality care to remote areas. Distinct strategies are also required for closed outbreaks in both developed and resource-limited settings. Although MDA programs do not place huge selective pressures on the microorganisms they target, ongoing monitoring for potential mite resistance to ivermectin and topical agents is important [61–64].

The impacts of scabies control programs need further evaluation, as this will inform policy makers and stakeholders of the likely health and economic benefits of the program. In particular, understanding the impact of reducing scabies and impetigo on improving quality of life and reducing downstream health complications such as skin and soft tissue infections, sepsis, and rheumatic heart disease [25]. Understanding these outcomes will facilitate cost-effectiveness evaluations in a range of settings. Research into the understanding and conception of scabies and impetigo within communities, followed by community awareness and engagement strategies, will be crucial for programmatic success.

While MDA with ivermectin appears highly effective, there are disadvantages to its use, including the apparent need for two doses, as outlined above. Moxidectin is an oral compound related to ivermectin, and was recently approved by the United States Food and Drug Administration for treatment of onchocerciasis [65]. Moxidectin has a much longer half-life than ivermectin, spanning the entire life cycle of the scabies mite [66,67]. In a preclinical treatment study using a porcine model for scabies, a single dose of moxidectin was more effective than two doses of ivermectin [68]. Clinical studies in humans are now planned, with a view to developing moxidectin as a single-dose treatment for scabies [67,69]. If clinical development is successful, moxidectin would be a very attractive option for community control of scabies because it would obviate the need for a second dose and reduce the risk of early re-infestation. Alternative topical treatments may also be required if resistance to permethrin becomes problematic [64,70].

Finally, scabies control should not occur in a vacuum. There are a number of opportunities for integration of scabies control with other NTDs, especially around the use of ivermectin [71,72]. Examples include successful co-mapping of scabies prevalence with other NTDs [17,73], and co-administration of ivermectin and azithromycin MDA with evaluation of multiple endpoints [36,37]. The roll-out of triple therapy (ivermectin, diethylcarbamazine, and albendazole) for the control of lymphatic filariasis [74,75] presents further opportunities to integrate evaluation of impact of this strategy on scabies.

6. Conclusions

In 2018, WHO recognized the need for 'a global strategy for scabies control' [24]. Such a strategy would align with the United Nations Sustainable Development Goals, including Target 3.3 to end the epidemic of NTDs (among other diseases) by 2030 [76]. Community control will be a central component of such a strategy, but broader progress will require consideration of several interrelated issues, including: engagement with key stakeholders at national, regional, and global levels to develop a coordinated, international framework; integration with existing NTD programs to leverage efficiency and cost-effectiveness of scabies control; provision of guidelines for monitoring and evaluation of programs; securement of drug supply at large scale; development of funding partnerships; and advancement of a research agenda, including operational research as outlined above, and research into improved diagnostics, new treatments (including moxidectin), and mite resistance monitoring.

Author Contributions: Conceptualization, D.E.; Writing—Original Draft Preparation, D.E. and A.C.S.; Writing—Review and Editing, D.E. and A.C.S.

Acknowledgments: We acknowledge the contribution of Myra Hardy. The clinical photograph is provided courtesy of Daniel Mason. Informed consent was obtained and confidentiality maintained in accordance with the ethical review committee requirements.

References

1. Hay, R.J.; Steer, A.C.; Engelman, D.; Walton, S. Scabies in the developing world—Its prevalence, complications, and management. *Clin. Microbiol. Infect.* **2012**, *18*, 313–323. [CrossRef] [PubMed]
2. Chosidow, O. Clinical practices. Scabies. *New Engl. J. Med.* **2006**, *354*, 1718–1727. [CrossRef] [PubMed]
3. Davis, J.S.; McGloughlin, S.; Tong, S.Y.; Walton, S.F.; Currie, B.J. A novel clinical grading scale to guide the management of crusted scabies. *PLoS Negl. Trop. Dis.* **2013**, *7*, e2387. [CrossRef] [PubMed]
4. Walton, S.F.; Beroukas, D.; Roberts-Thomson, P.; Currie, B.J. New insights into disease pathogenesis in crusted (Norwegian) scabies: The skin immune response in crusted scabies. *Br. J. Dermatol.* **2008**, *158*, 1247–1255. [CrossRef] [PubMed]
5. Worth, C.; Heukelbach, J.; Fengler, G.; Walter, B.; Lisenfeld, O.; Feldmeier, H. Impaired quality of life in adults and children with scabies from an impoverished community in Brazil. *Int. J. Dermatol.* **2012**, *51*, 275–282. [CrossRef] [PubMed]
6. Hofstraat, K.; van Brakel, W.H. Social stigma towards neglected tropical diseases: A systematic review. *Int. Health* **2016**, *8* (Suppl. 1), i53–i70. [CrossRef]
7. Olsen, J.R.; Gallacher, J.; Finlay, A.Y.; Piguet, V.; Francis, N.A. Quality of life impact of childhood skin conditions measured using the Children's Dermatology Life Quality Index (CDLQI): A meta-analysis. *Br. J. Dermatol.* **2016**, *174*, 853–861. [CrossRef] [PubMed]
8. Steer, A.C.; Jenney, A.W.; Kado, J.; Batzloff, M.R.; La Vincente, S.; Waqatakirewa, L.; Mulholland, E.K.; Carapetis, J.R. High burden of impetigo and scabies in a tropical country. *PLoS Negl. Trop. Dis.* **2009**, *3*, e467. [CrossRef] [PubMed]

9. Swe, P.M.; Zakrzewski, M.; Kelly, A.; Krause, L.; Fischer, K. Scabies mites alter the skin microbiome and promote growth of opportunistic pathogens in a porcine model. *PLoS Negl. Trop. Dis.* **2014**, *8*, e2897. [CrossRef] [PubMed]
10. Swe, P.M.; Fischer, K. A scabies mite serpin interferes with complement-mediated neutrophil functions and promotes staphylococcal growth. *PLoS Negl. Trop. Dis.* **2014**, *8*, e2928. [CrossRef] [PubMed]
11. Hay, R.J.; Steer, A.C.; Chosidow, O.; Currie, B.J. Scabies: A suitable case for a global control initiative. *Curr. Opin. Infect. Dis.* **2013**, *26*, 107–109. [CrossRef] [PubMed]
12. Parks, T.; Smeesters, P.R.; Steer, A.C. Streptococcal skin infection and rheumatic heart disease. *Curr. Opin. Infect. Dis.* **2012**, *25*, 145–153. [CrossRef] [PubMed]
13. Thornley, S.; Marshall, R.; Jarrett, P.; Sundborn, G.; Reynolds, E.; Schofield, G. Scabies is strongly associated with acute rheumatic fever in a cohort study of Auckland children. *J. Paediatr. Child Health* **2018**, *54*, 625–632. [CrossRef] [PubMed]
14. GBD 2015 Disease and Injury Incidence and Prevalence Collaborators. Global, regional, and national incidence, prevalence, and years lived with disability for 310 diseases and injuries, 1990–2015: A systematic analysis for the Global Burden of Disease Study 2015. *Lancet* **2016**, *388*, 1545–1602. [CrossRef]
15. Karimkhani, C.; Colombara, D.V.; Drucker, A.M.; Norton, S.A.; Hay, R.; Engelman, D.; Steer, A.; Whitfeld, M.; Naghavi, M.; Dellavalle, R.P. The global burden of scabies: A cross-sectional analysis from the Global Burden of Disease Study 2015. *Lancet Infect. Dis.* **2017**, *17*, 1247–1254. [CrossRef]
16. Romani, L.; Steer, A.C.; Whitfeld, M.J.; Kaldor, J.M. Prevalence of scabies and impetigo worldwide: A systematic review. *Lancet Infect. Dis.* **2015**, *15*, 960–967. [CrossRef]
17. Mason, D.S.; Marks, M.; Sokana, O.; Solomon, A.W.; Mabey, D.C.; Romani, L.; Kaldor, J.; Steer, A.C.; Engelman, D. The prevalence of scabies and impetigo in the solomon islands: A population-based survey. *PLoS Negl. Trop. Dis.* **2016**, *10*, e0004803. [CrossRef] [PubMed]
18. Yeoh, D.K.; Anderson, A.; Cleland, G.; Bowen, A.C. Are scabies and impetigo 'normalised'? A cross-sectional comparative study of hospitalised children in northern Australia assessing clinical recognition and treatment of skin infections. *PLoS Negl. Trop. Dis.* **2017**, *11*, e0005726. [CrossRef] [PubMed]
19. Thompson, M.J.; Engelman, D.; Gholam, K.; Fuller, L.C.; Steer, A.C. Systematic review of the diagnosis of scabies in therapeutic trials. *Clin. Exp. Dermatol.* **2017**, *42*, 481–487. [CrossRef] [PubMed]
20. Romani, L.; Whitfeld, M.J.; Koroivueta, J.; Kama, M.; Wand, H.; Tikoduadua, L.; Tuicakau, M.; Koroi, A.; Ritova, R.; Andrews, R.; et al. The epidemiology of scabies and impetigo in relation to demographic and residential characteristics: Baseline findings from the Skin Health Intervention Fiji Trial. *Am. J. Trop. Med. Hyg.* **2017**, *97*, 845–850. [CrossRef] [PubMed]
21. Romani, L.; Koroivueta, J.; Steer, A.C.; Kama, M.; Kaldor, J.M.; Wand, H.; Hamid, M.; Whitfeld, M.J. Scabies and impetigo prevalence and risk factors in Fiji: A national survey. *PLoS Negl. Trop. Dis.* **2015**, *9*, e0003452. [CrossRef] [PubMed]
22. Aung, P.T.Z.; Cuningham, W.; Hwang, K.; Andrews, R.M.; Carapetis, J.R.; Kearns, T.; Clucas, D.; McVernon, J.; Simpson, J.A.; Tong, S.Y.C.; et al. Scabies and risk of skin sores in remote Australian Aboriginal communities: A self-controlled case series study. *PLoS Negl. Trop. Dis.* **2018**, *12*, e0006668. [CrossRef] [PubMed]
23. World Health Organization. Report of the Tenth Meeting of the WHO Strategic and Technical Advisory Group for Neglected Tropical Diseases. 2018. Available online: http://www.who.int/neglected_diseases/NTD_STAG_report_2017.pdf?ua=1 (accessed on 17 March 2018).
24. World Health Organization. 9th NTD-STAG Global Working Group Meeting on Monitoring and Evaluation of Neglected Tropical Diseases. 2018. Available online: http://www.who.int/neglected_diseases/events/STAG_Working_Group_on_Monitoring_Evaluation/en/ (accessed on 12 August 2018).
25. Engelman, D.; Kiang, K.; Chosidow, O.; McCarthy, J.; Fuller, C.; Lammie, P.; Hay, R.; Steer, A. Members of the International Alliance for The Control of Scabies. Toward the global control of human scabies: Introducing the International Alliance for the Control of Scabies. *PLoS Negl. Trop. Dis.* **2013**, *7*, e2167. [CrossRef] [PubMed]
26. Engelman, D.; Fuller, L.C.; Steer, A.C. Consensus criteria for the diagnosis of scabies: A Delphi study of international experts. *PLoS Negl. Trop. Dis.* **2018**, *12*, e0006549. [CrossRef] [PubMed]
27. Taplin, D.; Porcelain, S.L.; Meinking, T.L.; Athey, R.L.; Chen, J.A.; Castillero, P.M.; Sanchez, R. Community control of scabies: A model based on use of permethrin cream. *Lancet* **1991**, *337*, 1016–1018. [CrossRef]

28. Taplin, D.; Arrue, C.; Walker, J.; Roth, W.; Rivera, A. Eradication of scabies with a single treatment schedule. *J. Am. Acad. Dermatol.* **1983**, *9*, 546–550. [CrossRef]
29. Lawrence, G.; Leafasia, J.; Sheridan, J.; Hills, S.; Wate, J.; Wate, C.; Montgomery, J.; Pandeya, N.; Purdie, D. Control of scabies, skin sores and haematuria in children in the Solomon Islands: Another role for ivermectin. *Bull. World Health Organ.* **2005**, *83*, 34–42. [PubMed]
30. Leppard, B.; Naburi, A.E. The use of ivermectin in controlling an outbreak of scabies in a prison. *Br. J. Dermatol.* **2000**, *143*, 520–523. [CrossRef] [PubMed]
31. Pacque, M.; Munoz, B.; Greene, B.M.; White, A.T.; Dukuly, Z.; Taylor, H.R. Safety of and compliance with community-based ivermectin therapy. *Lancet* **1990**, *335*, 1377–1380. [CrossRef]
32. Pacque, M.C.; Dukuly, Z.; Greene, B.M.; Munoz, B.; Keyvan-Larijani, E.; Williams, P.N.; Taylor, H.R. Community-based treatment of onchocerciasis with ivermectin: Acceptability and early adverse reactions. *Bull. World Health Organ.* **1989**, *67*, 721–730. [PubMed]
33. Marks, M.; Taotao-Wini, B.; Satorara, L.; Engelman, D.; Nasi, T.; Mabey, D.C.; Steer, A.C. Long term control of scabies fifteen years after an intensive treatment programme. *PLoS Negl. Trop. Dis.* **2015**, *9*, e0004246. [CrossRef] [PubMed]
34. Andrews, R.M.; Kearns, T.; Connors, C.; Parker, C.; Carville, K.; Currie, B.J.; Carapetis, J.R. A regional initiative to reduce skin infections amongst aboriginal children living in remote communities of the Northern Territory, Australia. *PLoS Negl. Trop. Dis.* **2009**, *3*, e554. [CrossRef] [PubMed]
35. La Vincente, S.; Kearns, T.; Connors, C.; Cameron, S.; Carapetis, J.; Andrews, R. Community management of endemic scabies in remote aboriginal communities of northern Australia: Low treatment uptake and high ongoing acquisition. *PLoS Negl. Trop. Dis.* **2009**, *3*, e444. [CrossRef] [PubMed]
36. Romani, L.; Marks, M.; Sokana, O.; Nasi, T.; Kamoriki, B.; Wand, H.; Whitfeld, M.; Engelman, D.; Solomon, A.W.; Steer, A.C.; et al. Feasibility and safety of mass drug co-administration with azithromycin and ivermectin for the control of neglected tropical diseases: A single-arm intervention trial. *Lancet Glob. Health* **2018**, in press.
37. Marks, M.; Toloka, H.; Baker, C.; Kositz, C.; Asugeni, J.; Puiahi, E.; Asugeni, R.; Azzopardi, K.; Diau, J.; Kaldor, J.M.; et al. Randomised trial of community treatment with azithromycin and ivermectin mass drug administration for control of scabies and impetigo. *Clin. Infect. Dis.* **2018**, in press. [CrossRef] [PubMed]
38. Engelman, D.; Martin, D.L.; Hay, R.J.; Chosidow, O.; McCarthy, J.S.; Fuller, L.C.; Steer, A.C. Opportunities to investigate the effects of ivermectin mass drug administration on scabies. *Parasit Vectors* **2013**, *6*, 106. [CrossRef] [PubMed]
39. Mohammed, K.A.; Deb, R.M.; Stanton, M.C.; Molyneux, D.H. Soil transmitted helminths and scabies in Zanzibar, Tanzania following mass drug administration for lymphatic filariasis—A rapid assessment methodology to assess impact. *Parasit Vectors* **2012**, *5*, 299. [CrossRef] [PubMed]
40. Martin, D.; Wiegand, R.; Goodhew, B.; Lammie, P.; Mkocha, H.; Kasubi, M. Impact of ivermectin mass drug administration for lymphatic filariasis on scabies in eight villages in Kongwa District, Tanzania. *Am. J. Trop. Med. Hyg.* **2018**, in press. [CrossRef] [PubMed]
41. Cassell, J.A.; Middleton, J.; Nalabanda, A.; Lanza, S.; Head, M.G.; Bostock, J.; Hewitt, K.; Jones, C.I.; Darley, C.; Karir, S.; et al. Scabies outbreaks in ten care homes for elderly people: A prospective study of clinical features, epidemiology, and treatment outcomes. *Lancet Infect. Dis.* **2018**, *18*, 894–902. [CrossRef]
42. Agrawal, S.; Puthia, A.; Kotwal, A.; Tilak, R.; Kunte, R.; Kushwaha, A.S. Mass scabies management in an orphanage of rural community: An experience. *Med. J. Armed Forces India* **2012**, *68*, 403–406. [CrossRef] [PubMed]
43. Beeres, D.T.; Ravensbergen, S.J.; Heidema, A.; Cornish, D.; Vonk, M.; Wijnholds, L.D.; Hendriks, J.J.H.; Kleinnijenhuis, J.; Omansen, T.F.; Stienstra, Y. Efficacy of ivermectin mass-drug administration to control scabies in asylum seekers in the Netherlands: A retrospective cohort study between January 2014–March 2016. *PLoS Negl. Trop. Dis.* **2018**, *12*, e0006401. [CrossRef] [PubMed]
44. White, L.C.; Lanza, S.; Middleton, J.; Hewitt, K.; Freire-Moran, L.; Edge, C.; Nicholls, M.; Rajan-Iyer, J.; Cassell, J.A. The management of scabies outbreaks in residential care facilities for the elderly in England: A review of current health protection guidelines. *Epidemiol. Infect.* **2016**, *144*, 3121–3130. [CrossRef] [PubMed]
45. Hewitt, K.A.; Nalabanda, A.; Cassell, J.A. Scabies outbreaks in residential care homes: Factors associated with late recognition, burden and impact. A mixed methods study in England. *Epidemiol. Infect.* **2015**, *143*, 1542–1551. [CrossRef] [PubMed]

46. Mounsey, K.E.; Murray, H.C.; King, M.; Oprescu, F. Retrospective analysis of institutional scabies outbreaks from 1984 to 2013: Lessons learned and moving forward. *Epidemiol. Infect.* **2016**, *144*, 2462–2471. [CrossRef] [PubMed]
47. WHO Africa. Ethiopia-Scabies Outbreak Response in Amhara Regional State. Available online: https://www.afro.who.int/news/ethiopia-scabies-outbreak-response-amhara-regional-state (accessed on 6 July 2018).
48. Currie, B.J.; McCarthy, J.S. Permethrin and ivermectin for scabies. *New Engl. J. Med.* **2010**, *362*, 717–725. [CrossRef] [PubMed]
49. Stolk, W.A.; Walker, M.; Coffeng, L.E.; Basanez, M.G.; de Vlas, S.J. Required duration of mass ivermectin treatment for onchocerciasis elimination in Africa: A comparative modelling analysis. *Parasit Vectors* **2015**, *8*, 552. [CrossRef] [PubMed]
50. Irvine, M.A.; Stolk, W.A.; Smith, M.E.; Subramanian, S.; Singh, B.K.; Weil, G.J.; Michael, E.; Hollingsworth, T.D. Effectiveness of a triple-drug regimen for global elimination of lymphatic filariasis: A modelling study. *Lancet Infect. Dis.* **2017**, *17*, 451–458. [CrossRef]
51. Lydeamore, M.J.; Campbell, P.T.; Regan, D.G.; Tong, S.Y.C.; Andrews, R.M.; Steer, A.C.; Romani, L.; Kaldor, J.M.; McVernon, J.; McCaw, J.M. A biological model of scabies infection dynamics and treatment informs mass drug administration strategies to increase the likelihood of elimination. *Math. Biosci.* **2018**, in press. [CrossRef] [PubMed]
52. Wilkins, A.L.; Steer, A.C.; Cranswick, N.; Gwee, A. Is it safe to use ivermectin in children less than five years of age and weighing less than 15 kg? *Arch. Dis. Child* **2018**, *103*, 514–519. [CrossRef] [PubMed]
53. Gyapong, J.O.; Chinbuah, M.A.; Gyapong, M. Inadvertent exposure of pregnant women to ivermectin and albendazole during mass drug administration for lymphatic filariasis. *Trop. Med. Int. Health* **2003**, *8*, 1093–1101. [CrossRef] [PubMed]
54. Walton, S.F.; Currie, B.J. Problems in diagnosing scabies, a global disease in human and animal populations. *Am. Soc. Rev.* **2007**, *20*, 268–279. [CrossRef] [PubMed]
55. Peeling, R.W.; Boeras, D.I.; Nkengasong, J. Re-imagining the future of diagnosis of neglected tropical diseases. *Comput. Struct. Biotechnol. J.* **2017**, *15*, 271–274. [CrossRef] [PubMed]
56. Mitjà, O.; Marks, M.; Bertran, L.; Kollie, K.; Argaw, D.; Fahal, A.; Fitzpatrick, C.; Fuller, C.; Garcia-Izquierdo, B.; Hay, R.; et al. Integrated control and management of neglected tropical diseases. *PLoS Negl. Trop. Dis.* **2017**, *11*, e0005136. [CrossRef] [PubMed]
57. World Health Organization. Recognizing Neglected Tropical Diseases through Changes on the Skin: A Training Guide for Front-Line Health Workers. 2018. Available online: http://apps.who.int/iris/bitstream/handle/10665/272723/9789241513531-eng.pdf (accessed on 12 August 2018).
58. Estrada, R.; Chavez-Lopez, G.; Estrada-Chavez, G.; Paredes-Solis, S. Specialized dermatological care for marginalized populations and education at the primary care level: Is community dermatology a feasible proposal? *Int. J. Dermatol.* **2012**, *51*, 1345–1350. [CrossRef] [PubMed]
59. Hay, R.; Estrada, R.; Grossmann, H. Managing skin disease in resource-poor environments-the role of community-oriented training and control programs. *Int. J. Dermatol.* **2011**, *50*, 558–563. [CrossRef] [PubMed]
60. Faye, O.; Bagayoko, C.; Dicko, A.; Cissé, L.; Berthé, S.; Traoré, B.; Fofana, Y.; Niang, M.; Traoré, S.; Karabinta, Y.; et al. A teledermatology pilot programme for the management of skin diseases in primary health care centres: Experiences from a resource-limited country (Mali, West Africa). *Trop. Med. Infect. Dis.* **2018**, *3*, 88. [CrossRef]
61. Currie, B.J.; Harumal, P.; McKinnon, M.; Walton, S.F. First documentation of in vivo and in vitro ivermectin resistance in *Sarcoptes scabiei*. *Clin. Infect. Dis.* **2004**, *39*, e8–e12. [CrossRef] [PubMed]
62. Mounsey, K.E.; Holt, D.C.; McCarthy, J.; Currie, B.J.; Walton, S.F. Scabies: Molecular perspectives and therapeutic implications in the face of emerging drug resistance. *Future Microbiol.* **2008**, *3*, 57–66. [CrossRef] [PubMed]
63. McNair, C.M. Ectoparasites of medical and veterinary importance: Drug resistance and the need for alternative control methods. *J. Pharm Pharmacol.* **2015**, *67*, 351–363. [CrossRef] [PubMed]
64. Khalil, S.; Abbas, O.; Kibbi, A.G.; Kurban, M. Scabies in the age of increasing drug resistance. *PLoS Negl. Trop. Dis.* **2017**, *11*, e0005920. [CrossRef] [PubMed]

65. Opoku, N.O.; Bakajika, D.K.; Kanza, E.M.; Howard, H.; Mambandu, G.L.; Nyathirombo, A.; Nigo, M.M.; Kasonia, K.; Masembe, S.L.; Mumbere, M.; et al. Single dose moxidectin versus ivermectin for *Onchocerca volvulus* infection in Ghana, Liberia, and the Democratic Republic of the Congo: A randomised, controlled, double-blind phase 3 trial. *Lancet* **2018**, in press. [CrossRef]
66. Cotreau, M.M.; Warren, S.; Ryan, J.L.; Fleckenstein, L.; Vanapalli, S.R.; Brown, K.R.; Rock, D.; Chen, C.Y.; Schwertschlag, U.S. The antiparasitic moxidectin: Safety, tolerability, and pharmacokinetics in humans. *J. Clin. Pharmacol.* **2003**, *43*, 1108–1115. [CrossRef] [PubMed]
67. Mounsey, K.E.; Bernigaud, C.; Chosidow, O.; McCarthy, J.S. Prospects for moxidectin as a new oral treatment for human scabies. *PLoS Negl. Trop. Dis.* **2016**, *10*, e0004389. [CrossRef] [PubMed]
68. Bernigaud, C.; Fang, F.; Fischer, K.; Lespine, A.; Aho, L.; Dreau, D.; Kelly, A.; Sutra, J.F.; Moreau, F.; Lilin, T.; et al. Preclinical study of single-dose moxidectin, a new oral treatment for scabies: Efficacy, safety, and pharmacokinetics compared to two-dose ivermectin in a porcine model. *PLoS Negl. Trop. Dis.* **2016**, *10*, e0005030. [CrossRef] [PubMed]
69. Medicines Development for Global Health. Moxidectin Program. 2018. Available online: https://www.medicinesdevelopment.com/development-programs.htm (accessed on 3 August 2018).
70. Thomas, J.; Christenson, J.K.; Walker, E.; Baby, K.E.; Peterson, G.M. Scabies - An ancient itch that is still rampant today. *J. Clin. Pharm. Ther.* **2017**, *42*, 793–799. [CrossRef] [PubMed]
71. Engelman, D.; Fuller, L.C.; Solomon, A.W.; McCarthy, J.S.; Hay, R.J.; Lammie, P.J.; Steer, A.C. Opportunities for integrated control of neglected tropical diseases that affect the skin. *Trends Parasitol.* **2016**, *32*, 843–854. [CrossRef] [PubMed]
72. Hay, R. Skin NTDs: An opportunity for integrated care. *Trans. Royal Soc. Trop. Med. Hyg.* **2016**, *110*, 679–680. [CrossRef] [PubMed]
73. Yotsu, R.R.; Kouadio, K.; Vagamon, B.; N'Guessan, K.; Akpa, A.J.; Yao, A.; Ake, J.; Abbet, R.; Tchamba Agbor Agbor, B.; Bedimo, R.; et al. Skin disease prevalence study in schoolchildren in rural Cote d'Ivoire: Implications for integration of neglected skin diseases (skin NTDs). *PLoS Negl. Trop. Dis.* **2018**, *12*, e0006489. [CrossRef] [PubMed]
74. Thomsen, E.K.; Sanuku, N.; Baea, M.; Satofan, S.; Maki, E.; Lombore, B.; Schmidt, M.S.; Siba, P.M.; Weil, G.J.; Kazura, J.W.; et al. Efficacy, safety, and pharmacokinetics of coadministered diethylcarbamazine, albendazole, and ivermectin for treatment of bancroftian filariasis. *Clin. Infect. Dis.* **2016**, *62*, 334–341. [CrossRef] [PubMed]
75. Fischer, P.U.; King, C.L.; Jacobson, J.A.; Weil, G.J. Potential value of triple drug therapy with ivermectin, diethylcarbamazine, and albendazole (IDA) to accelerate elimination of lymphatic filariasis and onchocerciasis in Africa. *PLoS Negl. Trop. Dis.* **2017**, *11*, e0005163. [CrossRef] [PubMed]
76. Fitzpatrick, C.; Engels, D. Leaving no one behind: A neglected tropical disease indicator and tracers for the Sustainable Development Goals. *Int. Health* **2016**, *8*, i15–i18. [CrossRef] [PubMed]

4

An Integrated Study of *Toxocara* Infection in Honduran Children: Human Seroepidemiology and Environmental Contamination in a Coastal Community

Sergio A. Hernández [1], José A. Gabrie [1], Carol Anahelka Rodríguez [2], Gabriela Matamoros [1,2], María Mercedes Rueda [2], Maritza Canales [2], Ronald Mergl [3] and Ana Sanchez [1,2,*]

1 Department of Health Sciences, Brock University, St. Catharines, ON L3S 2A1, Canada; hernandez@brocku.ca (S.A.H.); jgabrie@brocku.ca (J.A.G.); gm18@brocku.ca (G.M.)
2 Department of Parasitology, School of Microbiology and Institute of Microbiology Research, National Autonomous University of Honduras, Tegucigalpa, Honduras; carol.rodriguez@unah.edu.hn (C.A.R.); maria.rueda@unah.edu.hn (M.M.R.); maritza.canales@unah.edu.hn (M.C.)
3 Niagara Falls Animal Medical Centre, Niagara Falls, ON L2E 6Z8, Canada; mergl.ron@gmail.com
* Correspondence: ana.sanchez@brocku.ca

Abstract: (1) Background: Infections caused by *Toxocara canis* and *T. cati* are considered zoonoses of global importance. Reports from North and South America indicate that human infections are widespread in both continents, but epidemiological information from Central America is still lacking. (2) Methodology: In the present cross-sectional multi-year study, we aimed to undertake the first seroepidemiological and environmental study on toxocariasis in Honduras. This included the determination of seroprevalence of anti-*Toxocara* spp. antibodies in children using a *Toxocara* spp. purified excretory-secretory antigens enzyme-linked immunosorbent assay (TES-ELISA) and a confirmatory Western blot. As well, through statistical analysis including logistic regression we aimed at identifying relevant biological and epidemiological factors associated with seropositivity. The study also entailed detection of parasites' eggs in the soil samples both through Sheather's concentration method and a nested polymerase chain reaction-restriction fragment length polymorphism (PCR-RFLP) method. (3) Results: The study was undertaken in a coastal community of Honduras in 2 different years, 2015 and 2017. A total of 88 healthy schoolchildren completed the study, with participation of 79% (73/92) and 65% (46/71) of the student body in 2015 and 2017, respectively. Thirty-one children participated in both years (i.e., dual participants). Through both serological tests, seropositivity was confirmed in 88.6% (78/88) of children. Due to the high number of seropositives, logistic regression analysis was not possible for most socio-economic and epidemiological variables. Eosinophilia, on the other hand, was associated with seropositivity, independently of other intestinal helminthic infections. Continued seropositivity was observed in most of the dual participants, while seroconversion was determined in 8 of these children. Microscopic examination of soil samples did not yield any positive results. Through nested PCR-RFLP, 3 of the 50 samples (6%) were positive for *Toxocara* spp.; two were identified as *T. canis* and one as *T. cati*. (4) Conclusions: This work documents for the first time, high levels of human exposure to *Toxocara* spp. in Honduras. These findings, along with the country's favorable epidemiological conditions for this zoonosis, emphasize the need for more research to determine whether this infection is underreported in the country.

Keywords: *Toxocara*; toxocariasis; zoonosis; seroepidemiology; neglected tropical diseases; Honduras

1. Introduction

Toxocara spp. are cosmopolitan zoonotic parasites that utilize dogs, cats, foxes and other canids and felids as definitive hosts. When harboring adult worms in their intestine, these animals extensively contaminate their surroundings with their stools containing parasite ova [1]. *Toxocara* species are distributed worldwide, with higher prevalence where infected domestic dogs and cats are allowed to defecate in public spaces [2]. Once fully developed in the environment, *Toxocara* eggs are infectious to definitive hosts as well as to humans. In the latter, however, the parasites do not reach adult stages but rather lodge in tissues as larval stages causing a wide spectrum of pathologies grouped under the clinical term toxocariasis (also called 'toxocarosis') [3].

The significance of human toxocariasis as a disease remains enigmatic, partly due to the multifaceted, nonspecific and cryptic nature of symptoms, making this an insidious disease more closely related to disability and infirmity than mortality. Further, toxocariasis can lead to significant and irreversible damage such as blindness and fibrotic lesions in visceral organs. Recent research suggests that this infection may partially account for cognitive deficits and other neurological complications seen among socioeconomically disadvantaged children [1,4]. There is a strong body of research from Europe and South America and a recent interest resurgence in the United States [5,6].

Conversely, the epidemiological situation of toxocariasis in Central America is largely unknown [7,8]. Even in Latin America and the Caribbean (LAC) nations, where other neglected tropical diseases (NTDs) are well-characterized, toxocariasis has not been consistently studied and no estimates of regional prevalence have been calculated [8]. Despite that data show that *Toxocara* is an important infection in dogs and probably in cats in Central America [9], a recent review by Ma et al. brings to light the paucity of research on human *Toxocara* infection in this particular geographic region [10].

Among Central American countries, Honduras is a country that, due to its climatic and socio-economic characteristics, is endemic for several NTDs and other infections [8]. With over 60% of the population living in poverty (i.e., earning < $2 USD/day) [11–13], and with a large uncontrolled population of domestic cats and dogs, the country offers optimal conditions for *Toxocara* spp. transmission; yet data on toxocariasis is almost non-existent [4,7,8].

In the present study, we aimed to undertake the first seroepidemiological and environmental study on toxocariasis in Honduras. Firstly, we set out to determine the seroprevalence of anti-*Toxocara* spp. antibodies in children as an indicator of exposure to the parasite. Secondly, we sought out to investigate potential associations between seroprevalence and relevant biological and epidemiological factors. Finally, we conducted an environmental sampling to confirm that soil in public spaces could be one source of infection for the study population.

2. Materials and Methods

2.1. Study Design and Population

The present investigation was designed as an exploratory, cross-sectional study. A non-probability, purposive sampling method (based on expert knowledge of the population) was used to obtain the study sample. A minimum sample size was not calculated. Rather, research participants were recruited from a primary school population with high prevalence of soil-transmitted helminth (STH) infections. Two data collection visits took place: in August 2015 and October 2017.

The study was conducted in the village of Santa Cruz del Junco, within the municipality of Tela, department of Atlántida, on the northern Caribbean coast of Honduras.

The municipality has an area of 1196 km^2 and an elevation of 3 m above sea level. The most recent census (2013) by the Honduran National Institute of Statistics recorded a population of 96,758 inhabitants, of which 48.8% were rural residents and 32.8% were $\leq$14 years old. The same census also documented a poverty index of 51%, with 42% of Tela's inhabitants listing agriculture, animal husbandry or fishing as their main source of income [14]. According to the Köppen Climate Classification, Tela exhibits a tropical rainforest climate, characterized by a lack of dry or wet seasons, as all months present at least 60 mm of precipitation; a condition that contributes to high levels of humidity. There is also no defined summer or winter in Tela, and it is typically hot and wet year-round [15].

The city of Tela, named after the municipality, is located between 15°47′00″ North latitude and 87°28 00″ West longitude, placing it approximately 67 km north-east of the city of San Pedro Sula, the primary industrial center in Honduras and the nation's second largest city after the capital [14]. The study village is located approximately 11 km from the city's center.

A national survey investigating prevalence and intensities of soil-transmitted helminths (STH) in Honduran schoolchildren had identified Tela as an area with an STH prevalence close to 50% [12]. These conditions are ideal for the transmission of a variety of parasites, including *Toxocara* spp. [16,17].

2.2. Study Sample

Schoolchildren from the village's only public primary school (consisting of grades one through six), were invited to participate in the study, with no exclusion criteria. We focused on school-age children to determine exposure to *Toxocara* spp. based on their known contact with soil and propensity to harbor STH more than adults [8]. It is widely known that *Toxocara* infection is markedly more associated with children, a finding related to certain determinants such as geophagia, playing habits and hygienic practices [18–20].

2.3. Data Collection

Each participant's parent/guardian partook in a face-to-face interview that used a pre-developed questionnaire as a guideline for data collection. The questionnaire was structured into different categories aiming to gather information including demographic and epidemiological data, domestic animal presence in the household, relevant patterns of child behavior and knowledge of parasites.

2.4. Blood Sample Collection and Analysis

Sera collected from each participating child was tested for the detection of anti-*Toxocara* IgG antibodies by way of a commercially available ELISA kit (Diagnostic Automation, Inc./Cortez Diagnostics, Calabasas, CA, USA). According to manufacturer instructions, any sample that yielded an absorbance ≥ 0.3 optical density (OD) units was considered seropositive. All positive ELISA results were confirmed by a Western blot (WB) assay, as well as 3 out of the 8 ELISA-negative samples. As per manufacturer instructions, the presence of two or more bands of low molecular weight were regarded as a positive result (LDBIO Diagnostics, Lyon, France). All assays were conducted according to manufacturer instructions. During the 2015 phase of the study, an eosinophil count was performed by an independent laboratory (Hospital CEMESA clinical laboratory), located in San Pedro Sula city, 1 h-drive from the study site. Eosinophilia was defined as ≥500 eosinophils/µL [21].

2.5. Stool Sample Collection and Analysis

In order to rule out potential serum cross-reactivity due to *Ascaris lumbricoides* infection as well as other parasitic infections characterized by eosinophilia, we analyzed children's stool samples for STH. A single stool sample was collected from each child and analyzed the same day at the local hospital laboratory using the Kato-Katz technique (Vestergaard Frandsen, Lausanne, Switzerland). With a Kato-Katz template delivering 41.7 mg of sample, we used a factor of 24 to obtain the number of eggs per gram (epg) of stool. Kato-Katz smears were microscopically examined after 30 min of clarifying time. Any insufficient or unsuitable (not formed) stool sample was analyzed by direct wet mount examination.

2.6. Soil Sample Collection and Analysis

A total of 50 soil samples, each approximately weighing 30 g, were collected from 5 different sites in the community of Santa Cruz del Junco in 2017 (10 samples per site). Samples were collected from the superficial layer of soil, up to a depth of 5 cm, avoiding any pebbles or grass. Soil samples were exported according to international regulations to Brock University in Canada for further microscopic and molecular analysis (permit number P-2018-00845).

Each sample was dried overnight at 37 °C, sieved with a 150 μm pore size sifter and the resulting refined soil was kept at room temperature in 50 mL conical tubes. Volumes obtained through this process varied from 3 to 13 mL.

The detection of *Toxocara* spp. in the refined samples, was done through a centrifugation/passive flotation technique (i.e., Sheather's) and a nested PCR-RFLP. For the Sheather's technique, samples were analyzed in duplicates as follows: 1 g of soil was transferred to a 15 mL centrifuge tube, mixed with 9 mL of distilled water, vortexed for one minute and then centrifuged at 1500× *g* for 5 min. The resulting supernatant was discarded, and a flotation sucrose solution (Specific Gravity, SG~1.27) was added to the pellet to complete a volume of 10 mL. Tubes were vortexed and filled with the same sucrose solution until a positive meniscus formed. Cover slips were placed on top of the tubes and, after a 60-min period of passive flotation, were examined microscopically at 10× and 40× magnifications for the presence of *Toxocara* spp. eggs.

For the molecular detection of *Toxocara* spp., DNA was extracted from a 250 mg aliquot of the refined soil using a commercial kit (Norgen Soil DNA Isolation Plus Kit cat# 64040, Norgen Biotek Corp., Thorold, ON, Canada). Extraction was performed according to the manufacturer's protocol, with two modifications: (i) a preparatory step consisting of thermal stress, and (ii) a substitution of the beads provided with the kit. The thermal stress procedure entailed three rounds of a freeze-heat cycle, whereby samples were placed at −80 °C for 10 min followed by dry incubation at 90 °C for 10 additional minutes. This thermal stress step was followed by overnight incubation with proteinase K at 56 °C. For the second modification, the plastic beads in each bead tube were replaced with a medley of sterile stainless-steel beads measuring 3 mm, 2 mm and 1.5 mm.

A nested PCR approach, targeting segments of the 18S rRNA gene, was performed using the following primers: PCR 1: NC5f 5′–GTAGGTGAACCTGCGGAAGGATCATT–3′ and NC2r 5′–TTAGTTTCTTTTCCTCCGCT–3′ and PCR 2: FM1f 5′-TTGAGGGGAAATGGGTGAC-3′ and FM2r 5′–TGCTGGAGGCCATATCGT–3′. Each PCR mix contained 10 μM for both forward and reverse primers and 2 μL of template DNA, with a final volume of 25 μL. The cycling conditions for PCR 1 were as follows: 94 °C for 3 min; followed by 35 cycles of 94 °C for 45 s, 60 °C for 1 min, 72 °C for 1 min and a final extension of 72 °C for 6 min. For PCR 2, the cycle involved 94 °C for 3 min; 35 cycles of 94 °C for 30 s, 60 °C for 30 s and 72 °C for 1 min and a final extension of 72 °C for 5 min. The PCR was optimized for the detection of DNA originating from a single egg using spiked soil samples as well as soil negative controls.

Two restriction enzymes, SalI and Mval, were used to differentiate between *T. canis* and T. *cati* [13]. For this, amplicons were digested at 37 °C for 3 h. Digestion of the product by SalI 1500 U (ThermoScientific ER0641, ThermoFisher Scientific, Waltham, MA, USA) produced 2 fragments of ~320 bp and ~394 bp in *T. canis* and an undigested band of 736 bp for *T. cati*. While digestion by Mval (BstNI) 2000 U (ThermoScientific ER0551, ThermoFisher Scientific) yielded 2 fragments of ~600 bp and ~100 bp in *T. cati* and an undigested band of ~700 bp for *T. canis*. Both PCR products and digested fragments were separated in 1.5% agarose gels with ethidium bromide.

2.7. Statistical Analyses

Data were inputted into a Microsoft Excel 2016 spreadsheet (Microsoft Corp., Redmond, WA, USA), cleaned for errors or missing values and exported for analysis to the STATA 13 software package (StataCorp LP., College Station, TX, USA).

For characterization of the study population, we used descriptive statistics for both continuous and categorical variables. Seroprevalence of anti-*Toxocara* antibodies was calculated with the confirmatory test. Assessment of the significance of univariate associations with positive serology (as confirmed by WB) was done by Fisher's exact test. A logistic regression model was applied to investigate the relationship between the various epidemiological risk factors with anti-*Toxocara* antibody presence. Odds ratios (OR) were determined with 95% confidence intervals (CI).

Sensitivity, specificity, positive predictive, and negative predictive values were calculated for the ELISA, compared to the Western blot. The kappa statistic for level of agreement between both diagnostic tools was also evaluated. The level of agreement was interpreted as moderate, strong or almost perfect if the value of kappa was 0.60–0.79, 0.80–0.90 or >0.90, respectively [22]. For the eosinophilia measured in the first phase of the study, a Mann–Whitney *U* test was employed to determine if there was a significant difference in circulating eosinophil counts in seropositive vs. seronegative individuals. Level of significance was established at $\alpha = 0.05$.

2.8. Ethics Statement

Both phases of the present study received ethics clearance from both participating institutions, in Canada (Brock University; file number: 17-032-Sanchez, clearance received 12 September 2017; file number: 14-224-Sanchez, clearance received: 8 May 2015) and Honduras (National Autonomous University of Honduras, Tegucigalpa M.D.C, Honduras. Committee of Ethics, Master's program in Zoonotic and Infectious Diseases School of Microbiology; file number: 04-2017, clearance received: 21 September 2017; file number: 01-2015, clearance received: 1 August 2015). In addition, approval for the implementation of this study was requested from the participating school's principal and grade teachers. Both parental consent and children's assent were also required prior to an individual's participation.

3. Results

3.1. Study Participation and Characterization of the Study Population

A total of 88 different children completed the study. Enrolments were 73 and 46 for 2015 and 2017, respectively, but there were 31 children coincidentally enrolled in both years. These participants were deemed "dual participants". Study participation varied between years: in 2015, participation was 79% of the school enrolment (73/92) whereas for 2017 it was only 65% (46/71). The reason for the latter was a widespread outbreak of hemorrhagic conjunctivitis in Honduras (and throughout Latin America and the Caribbean) due to coxsackievirus A24, which prevented children's attendance to school and their potential enrolment in the study.

The final study sample was comprised of students between the ages of 6–15 years (mean 9.83 years ± 2.25) and 45 (51.1%) girls. A summary of the epidemiological and serological data and children's behavior is displayed in Table 1. An important proportion (71.6%) of interviewed participants reported dog ownership by their family (Table 1). Additionally, most participants with household pets, either dogs or cats, specified that these animals strayed from the household freely (72.6% and 66.7%, respectively). Among the behaviors listed, it is important to mention that 80.4% of children said they had some sort of contact with soil, mostly with soil from the playground adjacent to the school.

3.2. Seroprevalence of Anti-Toxocara Antibodies

Of the 88 serum samples, 80 were ELISA-positive. Western blot results (WB) confirmed that 78 out of the 80 sera were indeed positive for anti-*Toxocara* antibodies and hence, an overall seroprevalence of 88.6% was documented (Table 1). As a manner of internal quality control, we tested with WB 3 out of the 8 (37.5%) ELISA-negative samples. The WB confirmed the absence of specific antibodies in these 3 samples. This was in addition to including the kit's negative controls.

Table 1. Study sample characteristics and laboratory results by year of study. Since there were 31 children who participated in both years, the final sample size amounts to a total of $n = 88$.

Characteristics	2015 $n = 73$ (%)	2017 $n = 46$ (%)	Total $n = 88$ (%) θ
Males	35 (48%)	24 (52.2%)	43 (48.9%)
Females	38 (52%)	22 (47.8%)	45 (51.1%)
Age (years), *mean (SD)*	10.3 (1.98)	9.40 (2.25)	9.83 (2.25)
Soil Transmitted Helminthiases (STH) Profile			
Overall STH prevalence	30 (41.1%)	10 (21.7%) ‡‡	34 (38.6%) ‡‡
Ascaris lumbricoides infection	10 (13.7%)	2 (4.3%) ‡‡	10 (11.4%) ‡‡
Trichuris trichiura infection	26 (35.6%)	10 (21.7%) ‡‡	30 (34.1%) ‡‡
Hookworm infection	6 (8.2%)	0 (0%) ‡‡	6 (6.8%) ‡‡
Polyparasitic infections	13 (17.8%)	2 (4.3%)	11 (12.5%)
Awareness of STH	57 (78.1%)	24 (52.2%)	62 (70.5%)
Recalled having STH infection	48 (65.7%)	24 (52.2%) §	54 (71.1%) §
Anti-*Toxocara* Antibody Serology and Eosinophilia			
Positive by TES-ELISA	56 (76.7%)	45 (97.8%)	80 (90.9%)
Confirmed by Western Blot	56 (100%)	43 (95.6%)	78 (97.5%)
Eosinophilia (≥500 eosinophils/µL) *	16 (21.9%)	NA	16 (21.9%) *
Domestic Animal Conditions			
Dog ownership ($n = 88$)	53 (72.6%)	34 (73.9%)	63 (71.6%)
Free-ranging owned dogs	39 (73.5%)	23 (67.6%) +	45 (72.6%) +
Cat ownership ($n = 46$)	NA	24 (52.1%) †	24 (52.1%) †
Free-ranging owned cats	NA	16 (66.7%) †	16 (66.7%) †
Children's Behavior †			
Contact with soil in the village	NA	37 (80.4%)	37 (80.4%)
Contact with soil in school playground	NA	41 (91.1%) ««	41 (91.1%) ««
Geophagia	NA	2 (4.3%)	2 (4.3%)
Onychophagia	NA	11 (23.9%)	11 (23.9%)
Thumb-sucking	NA	4 (8.7%)	4 (8.7%)
Consume undercooked beef	NA	21 (45.6%)	21 (45.6%)
Consume raw fruits/vegetables	NA	35 (79.5%) ◊◊	35 (79.5%) ◊◊

NA: data not collected; * data for 2015 only; † data collected for 2017 participants only; ‡‡ two children did not provide satisfactory stool samples for Kato-Katz examination; § data not recalled for 10 children; + data not recalled for one child; ◊◊ data not recalled for two children; «« data not recalled for one child; θ 31 dual participants counted only once. TES-ELISA: *Toxocara* spp. purified excretory-secretory antigens enzyme-linked immunosorbent assay

Of the seropositive participants, 52.6% (41/78) were males, but neither the univariate analysis nor the logistic regression model identified male sex as statistically significant for seropositivity ($p = 0.09$; OR = 4.43, 95% CI = 0.87–22.42, $p = 0.07$). Due to the high number of children with positive serology (the primary outcome), logistic regression analysis was not possible for most variables. Table 2 shows the results of this analysis for the remaining variables none of which were identified as statistically significant. The results of the dual participants are demonstrated in Table 3. It can be seen that the proportion of seropositive children increased, as 8 of the 31 dual participants seroconverted in the two-year interim (Table 3).

Table 2. Logistic regression analysis of *Toxocara* spp. seropositivity among the studied schoolchildren ($n = 88$).

Variable	Odds Ratio (OR)	95% Confidence Interval (CI)	p Value
Gender (Male)	4.43	0.87–22.42	0.072
Soil Contact	2.19	0.17–27.96	0.547
Onychophagia	0.61	0.04–7.61	0.698
Raw Beef Consumption	–	–	–
Raw Fruit/Vegetable Consumption	4.25	0.23–78.01	0.330
Dog Ownership	1.80	0.46–7.10	0.396
Dog Age ≤ 1 Year	–	–	–
Playground Contact with Soil	–	–	–

(–): Variable omitted from final model.

Table 3. Serological status of "dual participants": schoolchildren who participated in both 2015 and 2017.

Participants	ELISA Positives 2015 n (%)	Western Blot Confirmed 2015 n (%)	ELISA Positives 2017 n (%)	Western Blot Confirmed 2017 n (%)	Seroconverted by 2017 n (%)
Males ($n = 15$)	12 (80%)	12 (80%)	15 (100%)	15 (100%)	3 (20%)
Females ($n = 16$)	9 (56.3%)	9 (56.3%)	15 (93.7%)	14 (87.5%)	5 (31.3%)
Total ($n = 31$)	21 (67.7%)	21 (67.7%)	30 (96.7%)	29 (93.5%)	8 (26%)

3.3. *Toxocara spp. Seropositivity and Eosinophilia*

The eosinophil count performed in 2015 revealed eosinophilia (defined as ≥ 500 eosinophils/μL) in 16 children out of the 73 participants (21.9%). A Mann–Whitney U test was done to see if there was a significant difference in the count of circulating eosinophils in schoolchildren who tested seropositive compared to those seronegative (Table 4). To account for possible confounders, the test was also applied when controlling for individuals with any kind of STH infection and *T. trichiura* specifically. A significant difference was found between both subgroups (Table 4). For those that were found free of any STH infection, *Toxocara*-seropositive children averaged 191.3 eosinophils/μL, compared to 101.2 eosinophils/μL in those who were seronegative ($p = 0.058$). Increased eosinophil levels were also documented for those without trichuriasis ($p = 0.035$) (Table 4).

Table 4. Mann–Whitney U test results comparing geometric mean of circulating eosinophil levels in seropositive vs. seronegative schoolchildren ($n = 73$) †.

Geometric Mean (G-Mean) Value	Western Blot Seropositives (95% CI)	Western Blot Seronegatives (95% CI)	p Value
G-Mean * eosinophils/μL	262.1 (211.7–324.4)	101.2 (59.6–171.9)	0.004
G-Mean eosinophils/μL (without STH)	191.3 (141.7–258.2)	101.2 (59.6–171.9)	0.058
G-Mean eosinophils/μL (without *T. trichiura*)	198.5 (151.2–260.5)	101.2 (59.6–171.9)	0.035

† Eosinophilia data only collected in 2015; * G-Mean: geometric mean.

3.4. *Comparison of Serodiagnostic Techniques*

As an additional step, the performance of the TES-ELISA test used in this study was measured against the Western blot, the current recommended confirmatory test for anti-*Toxocara* antibody detection. The average ELISA sensitivity was 100% (95% CI 95.4–100%) and the average specificity was 80% (95% CI 44.4–97.5%), lower than the 93.7% reported by the manufacturer. With these two parameters, a kappa (κ) statistic was calculated to establish the degree of agreement between the two serodiagnostic tests. In this case, the resulting kappa statistic was $\kappa = 0.87$, an indicator of a strong agreement between the two diagnostic tools. Additionally, the average ELISA's positive and negative predictive value (PPV) were 97.5% (95% CI: 91.3–99.7%) and 100% (95% CI: 63.1–100%), respectively.

3.5. Intestinal Parasitic Infections

Two children provided insufficient or unsatisfactory stool samples for the Kato-Katz technique, so the samples were instead analyzed by direct wet mount. Overall, 34 of 88 (38.6%) children were infected with at least one STH species of which *T. trichiura* was the most prevalent (30/88 or 34.1%). Concurrent parasitoses were observed in 11 (12.5%) participants, highlighting the possibility of potential cross-reacting antibodies (Table 1).

3.6. Identification of *Toxocara* spp. in Soil Samples

Microscopic examination after sucrose concentration of soil samples did not yield any positive results. However, eggs of *T. trichiura* and *A. lumbricoides* were detected with this method in 3 (6%) samples.

In contrast, in the nested PCR-RFLP we identified 3 of the 50 samples (6%) as positive for *Toxocara* spp.; two were identified as *T. canis* and one as *T. cati* DNA. These 3 samples were collected in two of the five collection sites, one of which turned out to be the playground adjacent to the school. These *Toxocara* positive samples were negative for any STH by microscopy after the Sheather's concentration technique.

4. Discussion

Adding to the list of neglected tropical diseases (NTDs) in Honduras, this work documents for the first time, high levels of human exposure to *Toxocara* spp. in the country, and suggests the potential for this infection to be seriously underreported.

To our knowledge, only one clinical case of toxocariasis has been published in Honduras. Puerto-Sanabria et al. [23] described in 2016 a case in a 14-month-old infant with central nervous system involvement. Canine toxocariasis is poorly documented as well, even though the infection is frequently treated at veterinary clinics (Sanchez A, personal observations). Reference to the infection circulating in Honduran puppies is made in a 2002 review paper by Javier and Alger [24]. In addition, through an exhaustive search of Latin American databases and Honduran journals, we were able to find two publications: a study published in the Honduran Medical Journal reporting a toxocariasis prevalence of 3.8% in a sample of 207 dogs (82 owned, 69 from a kennel, and 56 free-roaming) [25], and a conference poster presentation by Valle-Ramirez & collaborators describing *T. canis* infection in 12% of 177 dogs examined [26].

Other than the publications mentioned above, we were not able to find more toxocariasis-related data either published or in the grey literature. Nonetheless, given that canine and human toxocariasis are prevalent in countries with similar climatic and socio-economic characteristics [6], we theorized that this parasitic disease is highly prevalent in Honduras.

The study findings confirmed our hypothesis —at least in the study sample—as we determined an overall seroprevalence of 88.6%. This is a surprisingly high seropositivity, but with the use of a confirmatory test (i.e., Western blot), we are confident that our results are reliable. Such high seroprevalence warrants a clinical investigation as covert toxocariasis would be a serious concern among the studied children [3]. Further, evidence indicates strong links between seropositivity and cognitive and developmental delays [1,4,5,27,28]. To reinforce the plausible link between seropositivity and health effects, we found that after controlling for STH infections, the presence of anti-*Toxocara* antibodies was associated with high levels of eosinophilia. In fact, of 73 children tested in 2015, 16 had high counts of circulating eosinophils and all were seropositive. A difference was observed between the eosinophil geometric means of seropositive children when compared to those of seronegative ones (191.3 eosinophils/μL vs. 101.2 eosinophils/μL, respectively), but this difference did not reach statistical significance ($p = 0.058$).

Many studies have already pointed out eosinophilia as a clinical marker for several helminthic and some protozoal infections [21]. Among helminthic infections, strongyloidiasis is commonly associated with strong eosinophilic reactions, whereas ascariasis and trichuriasis are known to be eosinophilia-inducing, albeit to a lesser degree [29–31]. *A. lumbricoides*, *T. trichiura*, and hookworm infections showed a pattern of endemic transmission among the studied children, with an overall prevalence of 38.6% across the 2-year period. The higher prevalence of trichuriasis is noteworthy—a fact that we have demonstrated in other Honduran communities and that had prompted us to investigate anthelminthic resistance in light of decades of deworming campaigns in the country [32].

In Honduras, strongyloidiasis is not reported frequently, especially in children [12]. Other parasitoses characterized by eosinophilia such as trichinellosis, filariasis, fascioliasis, echinococcosis, schistosomiasis, etc. [21,29,31–36] are not prevalent in the country.

Eosinophilia, on the other hand, has long been recognized as an important biomarker for toxocariasis [37–40]. In the major clinical presentation, visceral larva migrans (VLM) syndrome, eosinophilia is a distinguishable biomarker that can be drastically elevated [37,41]. In other clinical presentations for instance, ocular larva migrans (OLM), covert toxocariasis or neurotoxocariasis, eosinophilia can still be present, but on average, at lower levels than in VLM [20,37,42]. The concurrent findings of eosinophilia and seropositivity among the studied children are consistent with results from other studies [43–46]. Moreover, the combination of eosinophilia and seropositivity among the studied children may suggest the presence of an active infection (i.e., with viable larvae in tissues) [47]. A clinical and laboratory examination of these children could elucidate whether their seropositive status can be linked to covert (inapparent) or common toxocariasis [3].

Gender of the participating children was not identified as a statistically significant risk factor in our study either. It is interesting to note, however, that the proportion of seropositive boys (41/45, 95.35%) was higher than that of girls (37/45, 82.22%), and that the logistic regression analysis identified boys at about 4-fold increased odds of having anti-*Toxocara* antibodies. It is generally speculated that this association is related to boys' increased exposure to infective eggs in the soil from outdoor activities as well as their proclivity to play and have more contact with animals than girls [48,49].

In terms of epidemiological factors associated to seropositivity, we aimed to identify those postulated in the literature (e.g., soil contact, geophagia, dog ownership, raw beef consumption) but unfortunately, the substantial levels of seropositivity within such a small sample prevented us from detecting statistically significant associations, notably between plausible variables such as soil contact, dog ownership, undercooked beef consumption, or geophagia.

In fact, with almost all children (95%) reporting frequent exposure to soil, and almost 90% of them being seropositive, it would have been surprising to detect any statistical association between these two variables. Still, despite the lack of statistical significance, our logistic regression analysis detected that those reporting soil contact were twice as likely to have anti-*Toxocara* spp. antibodies.

We were also unable to identify the consumption of raw fruits or vegetables as a significant risk factor for anti-*Toxocara* spp. antibody presence. Yet, children who affirmed these dietary habits were found to be at four-times greater odds of being seropositive. A great proportion of children who admitted consuming raw fruits/vegetables were found to be seropositive (34/35, 97.14%).

Lastly, in terms of risk factors, even though the association was not significant, most children reporting family dog ownership (57/63) had almost twice the odds of being seropositive compared to their counterparts. This finding may reflect the considerable impact of these canine populations as a source of contamination, especially for children [50–52]. This is particularly true in areas such as the one studied here, where we observed free-ranging dogs running rampant with unrestricted access to public spaces. It would be important to conduct a canine seroepidemiological survey in the community—and in the country at large—to ascertain the size of the dog population and get an overview of the prevailing health issues including zoonotic pathogens such as toxocariasis.

A unique aspect of the present investigation is the testing of the study population in two different years, which allowed for data collection within the same community at two separate time points (2015 and 2017). Moreover, since the second phase of this study (2017) was carried out within the very same school as two years prior, overlap of some participants was inevitable. Initially, 21 of 31 (67.7%)

dual participants tested seropositive via TES-ELISA in 2015. In 2017, this proportion increased to 30 of the 31 (96.7%). Of these 9 seroconverted participants, the confirmatory Western blot identified one as a false positive, leading to the conclusion that 8 children had been exposed to the parasite during the two-year interim. Seroconversion may be attributed to changes in social and recreational behaviors of children as they age. In the two-year study gap, these children could have experienced dietary changes or new/more frequent contact with definitive or paratenic hosts, contaminated environments or fomites, or acquisition or strengthening of unhygienic habits (e.g., geophagia, inadequate handwashing, etc.) [2,18,53]. Some authors suggest that seroconversion is not intrinsically related to behavior changes. They propose that an increase in antibody titers to detectable levels might be due to the cumulative effect of persistent exposure and infection, or to the constant antigenic stimulation elicited by live larvae in tissues [1]. While in the studied population all these scenarios are possible, the fact remains that there is in the community a continuous presence of infectious sources.

Finally, to further investigate potential sources of infection, we integrated into the study an environmental component. Out of the 50 soil samples collected from 5 community sites, 3 samples (6%) from two sites contained *Toxocara* spp. eggs. Two of the three positive samples were collected from the playground adjacent to the school; an unfenced area that is heavily trafficked by children and animals, even outside school hours. In agreement with worldwide literature [54], our data suggest that the playground could be an important source of exposure to *Toxocara* spp. and if so, installing a fence around its perimeter would help mitigate the risk of exposure.

There are some limitations and strengths to this study. An important limitation that prevents generalization is the small sample size restricted to one cohort of schoolchildren. Not only did the study lack statistical power, but a cluster effect most certainly led to capturing a high prevalence phenomenon. Naturally, a small sample size and the extremely high seropositivity observed hindered meaningful statistical analyses. A second caveat worth mentioning pertains to the lack of clinical data from the studied children. Without investigating the potential health implications of a seropositive status, our study can only suggest that the high levels of exposure to *Toxocara* in this community underscore the need for appropriate attention from the health and veterinary sectors. One more limitation entails not including a canine survey. Although this was considered, we could not secure trained personnel to capture free-ranging dogs to obtain blood and stool samples.

Limitations notwithstanding, the study draws strength from the use of both an ELISA and a confirmatory Western blot, which lends reliability to our seroprevalence data. In addition, we were successful in detecting through PCR *Toxocara* spp. eggs in soil samples of 2 out of 5 collection sites. Further, we were able to identify both *T. canis* and *T. cati* in soil samples, opening research possibilities for the study of feline populations as well. A unique strength of the study is having a sub-sample of participants enrolled in both 2015 and 2017. This allowed us to run a nested comparison at two different time points and identify continued seropositivity as well as seroconversion.

In conclusion, we here present the first serological survey on human toxocariasis in Honduras, filling an important knowledge gap not only in the country but in the Central American region. Next steps should include conducting larger epidemiological, veterinary and clinical investigations using a One Health approach. Such data would inform an initial assessment of the burden of this neglected—almost invisible—zoonotic disease.

Author Contributions: Conceptualization, A.S., M.C. and R.M.; methodology, S.A.H., J.A.G., C.A.R., G.M., M.M.R., M.C. and A.S.; formal analysis, S.A.H., J.A.G., G.M., and A.S.; investigation, S.A.H.; J.A.G.; C.A.R.; G.M.; M.M.R.; M.C. and A.S.; resources, A.S., M.C., and R.M.; data curation, S.A.H., and J.A.G.; writing—original draft preparation, A.S., and S.A.H.; writing—review and editing, A.S., S.A.H., G.M., J.A.G. and R.M.; supervision, A.S. and M.C.; project administration, A.S. All authors have read and agreed to the published version of the manuscript.

Acknowledgments: We are grateful to the municipal health authorities for their interest and support, and for making available Tela's Hospitals clinical laboratory for sample analyses. Our gratitude also goes to the school principal and teachers for their decisive support to the study. A special thanks to Sara Ávalos (Universidad Nacional

Autónoma de Honduras) for her valuable participation in the field work, as well as to Anneliese von Eicken and Nick Orrego (Brock University) for assisting with laboratory work.

References

1. Walsh, M.G.; Haseeb, M.A. Reduced cognitive function in children with toxocariasis in a nationally representative sample of the United States. *Int. J. Parasitol.* **2012**, *42*, 1159–1163. [CrossRef]
2. Chen, J.; Liu, Q.; Liu, G.H.; Zheng, W.B.; Hong, S.J.; Sugiyama, H.; Zhu, X.-Q.; Elsheikha, H.M. Toxocariasis: A silent threat with a progressive public health impact. *Infect. Dis. Poverty* **2018**, *7*, 59. [CrossRef]
3. Auer, H.; Walochnik, J. Toxocariasis and the clinical spectrum. *Adv. Parasitol.* **2020**, *109*, 111–130. [CrossRef] [PubMed]
4. Hotez, P.J. Neglected infections of Poverty in the United States and their effects on the brain. *JAMA Psychiatry* **2014**, *71*, 1099–1100. [CrossRef] [PubMed]
5. Tyungu, D.L.; McCormick, D.; Lau, C.L.; Chang, M.; Murphy, J.R.; Hotez, P.J.; Mejia, R.; Pollack, H. *Toxocara* species environmental contamination of public spaces in New York City. *PLoS Negl. Trop. Dis.* **2020**, *14*, e0008249. [CrossRef] [PubMed]
6. Rostami, A.; Riahi, S.M.; Holland, C.V.; Taghipour, A.; Khalili-Fomeshi, M.; Fakhri, Y.; Omrani, V.F.; Hotez, P.J.; Gasser, R.B. Seroprevalence estimates for toxocariasis in people worldwide: A systematic review and meta-analysis. *PLoS Negl. Trop. Dis.* **2019**, *13*, e0007809. [CrossRef]
7. Bolívar-Mejía, A.; Alarcón-Olave, C.; Calvo-Betancourt, L.S.; Paniz-Mondolfi, A.; Delgado, O.; Rodriguez-Morales, A.J. Toxocariasis in the Americas: Burden and disease control. *Curr. Trop. Med. Rep.* **2014**, *1*, 62–68. [CrossRef]
8. Hotez, P.J.; Bottazzi, M.E.; Franco-Paredes, C.; Ault, S.K.; Periago, M.R. The neglected tropical diseases of Latin America and the Caribbean: A review of disease burden and distribution and a roadmap for control and elimination. *PLoS Negl. Trop. Dis.* **2008**, *2*, e300. [CrossRef]
9. Ketzis, J.K.; Lucio-Forster, A. *Toxocara canis* and *Toxocara cati* in domestic dogs and cats in the United States, Mexico, Central America and the Caribbean: A review. *Adv. Parasitol.* **2020**, *109*, 655–714.
10. Ma, G.; Rostami, A.; Wang, T.; Hofmann, A.; Hotez, P.J.; Gasser, R.B. Global and regional seroprevalence estimates for human toxocariasis: A call for action. *Adv. Parasitol.* **2020**, *109*, 275–290. [CrossRef]
11. Sanchez, A.L.; Gabrie, J.A.; Usuanlele, M.T.; Rueda, M.M.; Canales, M.; Gyorkos, T.W. Soil-transmitted helminth infections and nutritional status in school-age children from rural communities in Honduras. *PLoS Negl. Trop. Dis.* **2013**, *7*, e2378. [CrossRef] [PubMed]
12. Torres, R.E.M.; Garcia, D.N.F.; Sandoval, G.A.F.; Santana, A.H.; Singh, P.; Bucheli, S.T.M.; Saboyá, M.; Paz, M.Y. Prevalence and intensity of soil-transmitted helminthiasis, prevalence of malaria and nutritional status of school going children in Honduras. *PLoS Negl. Trop. Dis.* **2014**, *8*, e3248. [CrossRef]
13. Mikaeili, F.; Mathis, A.; Deplazes, P.; Mirhendi, H.; Barazesh, A.; Ebrahimi, S.; Kia, E.B. Differentiation of *Toxocara canis* and *Toxocara cati* based on PCR-RFLP analyses of rDNA-ITS and mitochondrial cox1 and nad1 regions. *Acta Parasitol.* **2017**, *62*, 549–556. [CrossRef] [PubMed]
14. INE—Instituto Nacional de Estadísticas Honduras. Available online: https://www.ine.gob.hn/V3/ (accessed on 21 July 2020).
15. Climate and Average Monthly Weather in Tela, Honduras. Available online: https://weather-and-climate.com/average-monthly-Rainfall-Temperature-Sunshine-fahrenheit,Tela,Honduras (accessed on 21 July 2020).
16. Hotez, P.J.; Wilkins, P.P. Toxocariasis: America's most common neglected infection of poverty and a helminthiasis of global importance? *PLoS Negl. Trop. Dis.* **2009**, *3*, e400. [CrossRef]
17. Mizgajska, H. The role of some environmental factors in the contamination of soil with *Toxocara* spp. and other geohelminth eggs. *Parasitol. Int.* **1997**, *46*, 67–72. [CrossRef]
18. Despommier, D. Toxocariasis: Clinical aspects, epidemiology, medical ecology, and molecular aspects. *Clin. Microbiol. Rev.* **2003**, *16*, 265–272. [CrossRef]
19. Macpherson, C.N. Human behaviour and the epidemiology of parasitic zoonoses. *Int. J. Parasitol.* **2005**, *35*, 1319–1331. [CrossRef]
20. Magnaval, J.F.; Glickman, L.T.; Dorchies, P.; Morassin, B. Highlights of human toxocariasis. *Korean J. Parasitol.* **2001**, *39*, 1–11. [CrossRef]

21. Kovalszki, A.; Weller, P.F. Eosinophilia. *Prim. Care.* **2016**, *43*, 607–617. [CrossRef]
22. McHugh, M.L. Interrater reliability: The kappa statistic. *Biochem. Med. (Zagreb).* **2012**, *22*, 276–282. [CrossRef]
23. Puerto Sanabria, C.R.; Tovar, S. Infección al sistema nervioso por *Toxocara canis* en Hospital Escuela Universitario, Honduras. *Rev. Fac. Cienc. Méd.* **2016**, *13*, 47–51.
24. Javier, C.A.; Alger, J. Larva migrans visceral: Enfoque diagnóstico con énfasis en el inmunodiagnóstico. *Rev. Med. Hond.* **2002**, *70*, 125–126.
25. Kaminsky, R.; Groothousen, C.M.; Zúniga, A.M.; Contreras, M.; Ferrera, A.M.; Henríquez, K.C. Infección por *Toxocara canis* en perros y riesgo de toxocariasis humana, Honduras. *Rev. Med. Hond.* **2014**, *82*, 2–50.
26. Manuel, V.R.; Nelys, H.F.; David, C.P.; Saharai, D.M.Y.; Rubén, R.A. *Prevalencia de Parasitos Intestinales en Caninos de la Ciudad de Catacamas*; Departamento de Olancho: Juticalpa, Honduras, 2016; Volume 167.
27. Ma, G.; Holland, C.V.; Wang, T.; Hofmann, A.; Fan, C.-K.; Maizels, R.M.; Hotez, P.; Gasser, R.B. Human toxocariasis. *Lancet Infect. Dis.* **2018**, *18*, e14–e24. [CrossRef]
28. Holland, C.V.; Hamilton, C.M. The significance of cerebral toxocariasis: A model system for exploring the link between brain involvement, behaviour and the immune response. *J. Exp. Biol.* **2013**, *216 Pt 1*, 78–83. [CrossRef]
29. Mejia, R.; Nutman, T.B. Evaluation and differential diagnosis of marked, persistent eosinophilia. *Semin. Hematol.* **2012**, *49*, 149–159. [CrossRef]
30. Ustianowski, A.; Zumla, A. Eosinophilia in the returning traveler. *Infect. Dis. Clin. N. Am.* **2012**, *26*, 781–789. [CrossRef]
31. Salzer, H.J.; Rolling, T.; Vinnemeier, C.D.; Tannich, E.; Schmiedel, S.; Addo, M.M.; Cramer, J.P. Helminthic infections in returning travelers and migrants with eosinophilia: Diagnostic value of medical history, eosinophil count and IgE. *Travel Med. Infect. Dis.* **2017**, *20*, 49–55. [CrossRef]
32. Matamoros, G.; Rueda, M.M.; Rodríguez, C.; Gabrie, J.; Canales, M.; Fontecha, G.; Sánchez, A. High Endemicity of Soil-transmitted helminths in a population frequently exposed to albendazole but no evidence of antiparasitic resistance. *Trop. Med. Infect. Dis.* **2019**, *4*, 73. [CrossRef]
33. Taylor, M.J.; Hoerauf, A.; Bockarie, M. Lymphatic filariasis and onchocerciasis. *Lancet* **2010**, *376*, 1175–1185. [CrossRef]
34. Esteban, J.; Bargues, M.; Mas-Coma, S. Geographical distribution, diagnosis and treatment of human fascioliasis: A review. *Res. Rev. Parasitol.* **1998**, *58*, 13–42.
35. Brunetti, E.; Kern, P.; Vuitton, D.A. Writing Panel for the W-I. Expert consensus for the diagnosis and treatment of cystic and alveolar echinococcosis in humans. *Acta Trop.* **2010**, *114*, 1–16. [CrossRef] [PubMed]
36. Tang, Z.L.; Huang, Y.; Yu, X.B. Current status and perspectives of *Clonorchis sinensis* and clonorchiasis: Epidemiology, pathogenesis, omics, prevention and control. *Infect. Dis. Poverty.* **2016**, *5*, 71. [CrossRef] [PubMed]
37. Fillaux, J.; Magnaval, J.F. Laboratory diagnosis of human toxocariasis. *Vet. Parasitol.* **2013**, *193*, 327–336. [CrossRef] [PubMed]
38. Pawlowski, Z. Toxocariasis in humans: Clinical expression and treatment dilemma. *J. Helminthol.* **2001**, *75*, 299–305. [CrossRef]
39. Yoon, S.Y.; Baek, S.; Park, S.Y.; Shin, B.; Kwon, H.S.; Cho, Y.S.; Moon, H.-B.; Kim, T.-B. Clinical course and treatment outcomes of toxocariasis-related eosinophilic disorder. *Medicine (Baltimore)* **2018**, *97*, e12361. [CrossRef]
40. Kwon, N.-H.; Oh, M.-J.; Lee, S.P.; Lee, B.-J.; Choi, D.-C. The prevalence and diagnostic value of toxocariasis in unknown eosinophilia. *Ann. Hematol.* **2006**, *85*, 233–238. [CrossRef]
41. Lassmann, B.; Tsigrelis, C.; Virk, A. 33-year-old woman with marked eosinophilia. *Mayo Clin. Proc.* **2007**, *82*, 103–106. [CrossRef]
42. Ikotun, K.; Sowemimo, O.; Chou, C.-M.; Ajenifuja, K.; Chuang, T.-W.; Asaolu, S.; Akinwale, O.; Gyang, V.; Nwafor, T.; Henry, E.; et al. High seroprevalence of *Toxocara* antibodies in pregnant women attending an antenatal clinic at a university hospital in Ile-Ife, Nigeria. *Trans. R. Soc. Trop. Med. Hyg.* **2020**, *114*, 301–307. [CrossRef]
43. Ciarmela, M.L.; Pezzani, B.C.; Minvielle, M.C. Toxocariasis, intestinal parasitoses and eosinophilia in schoolchildren from Argentina. *Curr. Health Sci. J.* **2016**, *42*, 5–11. [CrossRef]

44. Roldan, W.H.; Espinoza, Y.A.; Huapaya, P.E.; Huiza, A.F.; Sevilla, C.R.; Jimenez, S. Frequency of human toxocariasis in a rural population from Cajamarca, Perú determined by DOT-ELISA test. *Rev. Inst. Med. Trop. Sao Paulo.* **2009**, *51*, 67–71. [CrossRef] [PubMed]
45. Martínez, M.; Garcia, H.; Figuera, L.; Gonzalez, V.; Lamas, F.; López, K.; Mijares, V.; Corrales, Y.; Lares, M.; Ferrer, E. Seroprevalence and risk factors of toxocariasis in preschool children in Aragua state, Venezuela. *Trans. R. Soc. Trop. Med. Hyg.* **2015**, *109*, 579–588. [CrossRef]
46. Mendonça, L.R.; Veiga, R.V.; Dattoli, V.C.; Figueiredo, C.A.; Fiaccone, R.; Santos, J.; Cruz, A.A.; Rodrigues, L.C.; Cooper, P.J.; Pontes-De-Carvalho, L.C.; et al. *Toxocara* seropositivity, atopy and wheezing in children living in poor neighbourhoods in urban Latin America. *PLoS Negl. Trop. Dis.* **2012**, *6*, e1886. [CrossRef] [PubMed]
47. Łuzna-Lyskov, A.; Andrzejewska, I.; Lesicka, U.; Szewczyk-Kramska, B.; Luty, T.; Pawlowski, Z. Clinical interpretation of eosinophilia and ELISA values (OD) in toxocarosis. *Acta Parasitol.* **2000**, *45*, 35–39.
48. Roldan, W.; Espinoza, Y.; Atúncar, A.; Ortega, E.; Martinez, A.; Saravia, M. Frequency of eosinophilia and risk factors and their association with *Toxocara* infection in schoolchildren during a health survey in the North of Lima, Peru. *Rev. Inst. Med. Trop. Sao Paulo.* **2008**, *50*, 273–278. [CrossRef]
49. Holland, C.V.; O'Lorcain, P.; Taylor, M.R.; Kelly, A. Sero-epidemiology of toxocariasis in school children. *Parasitology.* **1995**, *110 Pt 5*, 535–545. [CrossRef]
50. Macpherson, C.N. The epidemiology and public health importance of toxocariasis: A zoonosis of global importance. *Int. J. Parasitol.* **2013**, *43*, 999–1008. [CrossRef]
51. Fan, C.K.; Liao, C.W.; Cheng, Y.C. Factors affecting disease manifestation of toxocarosis in humans: Genetics and environment. *Vet. Parasitol.* **2013**, *193*, 342–352. [CrossRef]
52. Overgaauw, P.A.; van Knapen, F. Veterinary and public health aspects of *Toxocara* spp. *Vet. Parasitol.* **2013**, *193*, 398–403. [CrossRef]
53. Correa, C.; Bismarck, C. Toxocariasis: Incidence, prevalence and the time serum remains positive in school children from Campinas, SP, Brazil. *J. Trop. Pediatr.* **2009**, *56*, 215–216. [CrossRef]
54. Fakhri, Y.; Gasser, R.; Rostami, A.; Fan, C.-K.; Ghasemi, S.; Javanian, M.; Bayani, M.; Armoon, B.; Moradi, B. *Toxocara* eggs in public places worldwide—A systematic review and meta-analysis. *Environ. Pollut.* **2018**, *242 Pt B*, 1467–1475. [CrossRef]

5

The Skin—A Common Pathway for Integrating Diagnosis and Management of NTDs

David John Chandler * and Lucinda Claire Fuller

Dermatology Department, Brighton General Hospital, East Sussex BN2 3EW, UK; claire.fuller@nhs.net
* Correspondence: davidchandler1@nhs.net;

Abstract: Many of the neglected tropical diseases (NTDs) have major skin manifestations. These skin-related NTDs or 'skin NTDs' cause significant morbidity and economic hardship in some of the poorest communities worldwide. We draw attention to the collective burden of skin disease and suggest that the skin be used as a platform for the integration of control activities for NTDs. The opportunities for integration are numerous, ranging from diagnosis and disease mapping to mass drug administration and morbidity management. The dermatology community has an important role to play, and will be expected to support research and control activities globally.

Keywords: integration; neglected tropical diseases; disease mapping; mass drug administration; morbidity management

---

1. Introduction

Skin and subcutaneous diseases account for substantial morbidity worldwide, with a high burden of disease in resource-poor tropical regions [1,2]. Neglected tropical diseases (NTDs) are a group of communicable diseases that are present throughout the tropical and subtropical regions of the world, where they affect the poorest and most marginalised communities. The World Health Organization (WHO) portfolio of NTDs comprises a list of 20 diseases that affect more than 2 billion people worldwide [3].

Eighteen of the twenty NTDs on the WHO list have recognised skin manifestations. In some cases, involvement of the skin is the primary manifestation of the disease; examples include Buruli ulcer, leprosy, scabies, and mycetoma. In other cases, skin involvement may be an associated clinical feature, such as the urticarial rash that can occur in schistosomiasis, soil-transmitted helminthiases, and foodborne trematodiases. The only NTDs that do not have skin manifestations are rabies and trachoma. In addition, several other diseases affecting the skin, whilst not prioritised on the WHO list, are recognised as NTDs; examples include cutaneous larva migrans, impetigo and cellulitis, podoconiosis, tropical ulcer, and tungiasis.

These skin-related NTDs or 'skin NTDs' frequently result in physical impairment and disfigurement, which can lead to life-long disability, inability to work, social stigmatisation, and discrimination. Examples of disability include permanent nerve damage and limb deformity in leprosy, advanced lymphoedema and hydrocele in lymphatic filariasis, severe itching and hanging groin in onchocerciasis, and amputation in cases of severe mycetoma. However, the true global burden of many skin NTDs is poorly understood. Data from the Global Burden of Disease Study (GBD) 2013 identified lymphatic filariasis and scabies as the 4th and 5th leading causes of morbidity out of all NTDs, resulting in 2.02 million and 1.71 million years lived with disability (YLD), respectively; however, these estimates are likely to be conservative [1,3,4].

Fungal diseases have been neglected for many years, with very little funding made available for research and control activities [5]. Consequently, high-quality data on the epidemiology and associated morbidity of superficial and deep mycoses do not exist, which makes it difficult to advocate for increased funding. The addition of this disease group to the WHO list of NTDs in 2017 should assist in raising its profile in the global health agenda; the same applies for scabies, which joined the WHO list at the same time.

The impoverishing effects of NTDs are amplified in poor and vulnerable communities; physical labour is often the main source of income, and social protection mechanisms (insurance against ill-health and disability) are not accessible [6]. In rural India, households with a family member affected by leprosy can incur catastrophic health expenditure, mostly as a result of loss of income due to chronic ill-health [7,8]. Significant health expenditure and productivity loss has also been demonstrated for other skin NTDs including podoconiosis and leishmaniasis [9–11].

Historically, disease control activities have operated within vertical programs that were set up to deal with specific priority diseases; however, these were resource intensive and inefficient. Integration offers a cost-effective and efficient approach for tackling groups of related conditions. Skin NTDs are frequently co-endemic in low-resource settings, and many of the available treatments and management strategies are beneficial for more than one condition; the skin has therefore been proposed as a common pathway to enhance the control of these neglected diseases.

From the growing literature on this subject, two key articles are worth highlighting. Engelman et al. discuss in detail many of the opportunities and challenges of integration [12]. In a paper that followed shortly after, an expert panel develop some of these ideas and offer practical advice on how to approach integration of surveillance and management activities for the skin NTDs [13].

The purpose of this review is to provide an update on the subject of skin NTDs and the opportunities for integration. We highlight examples where integration has been successful and draw attention to research questions that remain unanswered.

2. Methodology

We considered all types of publication and study design in our literature search; articles not written in English were excluded. We searched the following databases to July 2018: MEDLINE (from 1946), Embase (from 1947), and Allied & Complementary Medicine (from 1985). Core search terms included but were not limited to 'neglected tropical diseases', 'skin NTDs', 'integration', 'diagnosis', 'disease mapping', 'morbidity management', and 'mass drug administration'. We communicated with researchers active in this field to identify unpublished data and used the bibliographies of articles to expand our search.

3. Integrated Approach to Skin NTDs

An integrated approach to tackling skin NTDs offers many benefits, and the dermatology community has an important role to play in guiding this process. Integration in this context refers to combining activities for two or more diseases at the same time and in the same communities. Integration could be beneficial for several activities, from diagnosis and mapping to treatment and education, and these are discussed in more detail below.

4. Diagnosis

Skin disease is very common in resource-poor regions. Individuals frequently have more than one skin NTD, in addition to other, much more common skin conditions. Reliable diagnostic tests do not exist for many NTDs; therefore, diagnosis is based on clinical examination.

Clinical signs of skin NTDs are diverse; however, the diagnostic process can be simplified with the use of syndrome-based assessment tools. WHO have produced a training guide titled 'Recognising neglected tropical diseases through changes on the skin', which is intended to support front-line health workers without specialist knowledge of dermatology to detect skin changes suggestive of an underlying NTD [14]. Four major skin changes are identified: lumps, ulcers, swollen limbs, and patches. For each skin change there is a diagnostic flow-chart which guides the user towards a likely diagnosis and a decision on treatment or further assessment (referral).

The success of training health workers to identify skin NTDs has been demonstrated at the community level previously. Limited training of primary health care workers in Mali, focusing on leprosy and common skin diseases, resulted in significant improvements in diagnostic accuracy, appropriateness of referrals, and ability to correctly examine neurological (sensory) function, 12–18 months after the training was completed [15]. Traditional healers and those practising alternative systems of medicine are widely available in many African countries and throughout India, particularly in the rural communities, where they are easy to access and often a preferred source of treatment for health problems including leprosy [16]. Several studies have shown that it is both feasible and cost-effective to recruit traditional healers and train them to detect the signs of leprosy and refer suspected cases to specialist leprosy services [17–19]. Enhancing new case detection and avoiding delays to treatment are important goals of leprosy control. However, a recent article by Darlong et al. conducted in West Bengal, India, highlights delays to diagnosis in children with multibacillary leprosy, resulting in a significant number of cases of grade 2 disability at presentation [20]. All of the affected children in the study had leprosy-specific symptoms for more than 6 months before diagnosis, many of which involved visible skin changes such as ulceration or a skin patch. Strategies are needed to increase detection of these cases, including educational interventions that encourage earlier presentation to health services.

Integration of control activities for skin NTDs might offer further benefit by providing an operational framework through which other common (non-NTD) skin conditions can be detected and treated; however, the challenge this will provide should not be underestimated, and health workers in this setting should receive training in general dermatology. For example, it is important to appreciate that a hypopigmented skin patch has several causes, many of which are much more likely than leprosy, such as pityriasis versicolor, pityriasis alba, and achromic naevus. The importance of this particular point has been highlighted recently by several authors [21,22]. In a survey of skin NTDs, involving more than 13,000 schoolchildren aged 5 to 15 in Côte d'Ivoire, West Africa, the overall prevalence of skin disease was 25.6% [21]. Superficial mycoses were by far the most common diagnoses, and the majority of children were diagnosed with 2 or more skin conditions. Of 986 children examined by a dermatologist, the skin NTDs detected included one case of leprosy and 36 cases of scabies. Barogui and colleagues report similar findings from their experience of integrated control activities against Buruli ulcer, leprosy, and yaws in Benin, West Africa [22]. Trained health workers and community health volunteers identified 1106 patients with skin disease. Skin NTDs included only 15 cases of Buruli ulcer and 3 cases of leprosy. There were 185 suspected cases of yaws; however, these all tested negative using the point-of-care Dual Path Platform (DPP) syphilis assay.

An integrated approach to diagnosis offers the opportunity to detect multiple conditions in a single encounter. Vertical disease programs have a narrow focus and do not necessarily allow for detection and treatment of other important co-existent skin conditions. The majority of skin disease is accounted for by a few common conditions; these include bacterial skin infections (impetigo, boils), superficial mycoses, non-infective conditions such as eczema, and traumatic lesions. Algorithms for detecting and managing these skin conditions have been validated and applied in various settings and these could be applied in future integration efforts [23,24]. It would be appropriate and realistic for community-based health workers with limited dermatological training to focus on identifying and managing these common skin conditions for which relatively simple and effective treatments are available.

5. Disease Mapping and Surveillance

High-quality epidemiological data are lacking for many skin NTDs, and it is important for the success of integrated control efforts that this is addressed early. Disease mapping and identification of geographic areas of co-endemicity are important to determine disease burden and direct further research and control strategies. This step must take place before integrated management and control programmes can be planned and resources allocated. Consensus criteria for diagnosis of skin NTDs should be used, such as those available for podoconiosis [25] and, more recently, scabies [26].

Disease mapping refers to the collection of georeferenced data used to visualise the distribution and prevalence of a disease in space and time [27]. Maps are developed using a geographical information system (GIS) which allows storage, analysis, and presentation of spatial data. The African Programme for Onchocerciasis Control (APOC) was one of the earliest GIS-based mapping initiatives and has been used throughout Africa to identify priority areas for community treatment with ivermectin; APOC has also been used to map the distribution of *Loa loa* and identify areas of high prevalence where there is an increased risk of developing serious adverse events following treatment with ivermectin [28].

Integration of mapping and surveillance activities could be better suited to certain diseases, particularly those that share demographic and geographic preferences. Diseases causing lymphoedema provide a good example of where integration is suitable and where integrated mapping has been successful. Lymphoedema in the tropics has two main causes—lymphatic filariasis (LF), which is caused by infection with a parasitic nematode, predominantly *Wuchereria bancrofti*, and podoconiosis, which is caused by prolonged contact with irritant red clay soils derived from volcanic deposits.

Sime and colleagues describe their experience of the first integrated mapping of LF and podoconiosis, which captured almost 130,000 people from 1315 communities across 659 districts of Ethiopia during a 3-month period [29]. LF cases were identified by taking a blood sample and testing for circulating *Wuchereria bancrofti* antigen using an immunochromatographic card test (ICT). Podoconiosis was diagnosed clinically by excluding other causes of lymphoedema such as rheumatic heart disease, leprosy, and onchocerciasis. Smartphones were used for data collection; data were entered in real time and geographic coordinates were captured using an inbuilt geographic positioning system (GPS) function. The authors reported that using an integrated process was cost-effective and enabled rapid mapping of a larger geographical area than would otherwise have been achieved by using an individual disease survey. Recently, an integrated mapping exercise was conducted in Ethiopia, in 20 districts co-endemic for LF and podoconiosis, to identify all cases of lymphoedema [30]. More than 26,000 cases of lymphoedema and/or hydrocele were identified, and the majority of cases (>95%) had leg lymphoedema only, which could be due to LF or podoconiosis. These results will inform the planning and implementation of morbidity management and disability prevention (MMDP) services which are equally beneficial in both LF and podoconiosis.

Integrated mapping is more cost-effective than disease-specific mapping and allows for more precise mapping of co-endemic diseases and related conditions. In the Solomon Islands, Mason et al. conducted a cross-sectional study to assess the prevalence of scabies and impetigo [31], recruiting more than 1900 patients to the study; this was achieved by integrating data collection with an existing epidemiological study investigating clinical and serological markers of yaws [32].

6. Treatment

The last two decades have seen significant achievements in the control of a number of important tropical infections, including significant reductions in the prevalence of diseases such as lymphatic filariasis, guinea worm, and leprosy [33,34]. The successes of energetic vertical programmes are acknowledged; however, resource constraints have led to an increasing emphasis on integrating control activities.

Many of the opportunities for integrated treatment of skin NTDs exist for conditions that are suitable for control using mass drug administration (MDA), and, in particular, those that exhibit significant geographical overlap. Of note, seven of the most prevalent and debilitating NTDs have been the target of control efforts using integrated MDA; these include lymphatic filariasis, onchocerciasis, schistosomiasis, trachoma, and the three major soil-transmitted helminth infections (ascariasis, trichuriasis, and hookworm infection) [35]. Partnership between public and private organisations, multinational drug companies, and national ministries of health enabled the distribution of 'rapid-impact' packages of drugs throughout Africa, providing treatment for all seven of the NTDs at low cost. Ivermectin is highly effective at killing microfilariae in lymphatic filariasis and onchocerciasis, and was one of the drugs included in the rapid-impact package. Mostly due to drug company donations, it was possible to achieve a unit cost of US$0.40 per person annually, and in some cases even lower [35]. Data from the Global Burden of Disease (GBD) Study 2016 have shown considerable reductions in disease prevalence and burden (measured in DALYs) for six of the seven NTDs targeted by 'rapid-impact' integrated MDA over the last decade [36].

Ivermectin is widely recognised as a broad-spectrum antiparasitic drug, capable of killing parasites both inside and outside the body. It is particularly useful for the control of several skin NTDs. It is the treatment of choice for strongyloidiasis, and it is highly effective against scabies, pediculosis capitis, and cutaneous larva migrans [37,38]. Collateral benefits of ivermectin MDA have been observed in various settings, for example, in the lymphatic filariasis and onchocerciasis control programmes, where it was responsible for reducing the prevalence of tungiasis and scabies [38–40]. Ivermectin is also an effective treatment for gnathostomiasis and soil-transmitted helminthiasis. Improving access to low-cost generic ivermectin and broadening the licensed indications for use are some of the challenges to be addressed in order to realise the full public health potential of this drug. Studies of ivermectin MDA for scabies control have shown that the drug has a very good safety profile [41]. Although robust safety data in pregnant women and children under 5 years of age are lacking, the few published studies have failed to identify any difference in birth defects or developmental status in children born to women inadvertently treated with ivermectin during pregnancy [42–44]. Monitoring of existing ivermectin MDA programmes for safety outcomes will add to our understanding.

Moxidectin is a second-generation macrocyclic lactone related to ivermectin. It has demonstrated superior efficacy over ivermectin for the treatment of onchocerciasis [45], and recently received FDA approval (June 2018) for patients 12 years of age and older. In addition, moxidectin looks promising as a treatment for scabies. It has enhanced bioavailability (half-life of over 20 days, compared with 14 h for ivermectin) and better skin retention, meaning that a single-dose regimen may be possible [46]. Moxidectin is superior to ivermectin against the scabies mite in vitro [47]; however, clinical studies are required in order to establish suitable doses and evaluate efficacy in cases of scabies.

Integrated treatment programs can be particularly advantageous for diseases that can be treated using a single medication, as this removes the possibility of drug interactions and adverse safety events that may arise from coadministration of multiple drugs. For example, both yaws and trachoma can be targeted by mass administration of azithromycin, although the recommended doses for each are different—20 mg/kg for trachoma, and 30 mg/kg for yaws. However, a study conducted in the Solomon Islands showed that the lower dose (20 mg/kg) was effective against yaws; no active cases of yaws were identified following a single round of treatment using the lower dose in a previously endemic population [32]. This supports the argument for merging and simplifying treatment algorithms where possible and integrating mass treatment of these conditions.

On the other hand, mass treatment using more than one drug has the benefit of targeting a greater number of diseases and therefore delivering a greater impact to the health of the affected population. The effectiveness of ivermectin against highly symptomatic skin diseases such as scabies is an important factor in promoting adherence with further rounds of treatment in MDA programmes [48]; administering ivermectin together with other drugs against co-endemic skin NTDs would likely have a positive effect on overall compliance. Ivermectin and albendazole can be administered together safely, and there is evidence that they can be combined safely with other medications including azithromycin, praziquantel, and diethylcarbamazine (DEC) [49–51].

7. Morbidity Management

All of the skin NTDs have the potential to cause chronic ill-health and long-term disability, even after successful treatment of the underlying cause. The patient with treated lepromatous leprosy may have disabling limb deformity and experience recurrent and prolonged episodes of immune-mediated inflammation (erythema nodosum leprosum or type 2 leprosy reaction) for many years after treatment. The patient with treated lymphatic filariasis may suffer with debilitating lymphoedema and repeated episodes of ill-health due to acute dermatolymphangioadenitis (ADLA). The dermatology community can support these patients through interventions that focus on achieving healthy skin and preventing chronic disease complications.

The burden of disease resulting from chronic complications of skin NTDs is poorly understood, and more data are needed to support political advocacy and fundraising. Efforts are being made to address this, for example, through the development of a toolkit for monitoring morbidity and disability across multiple NTDs [52]. The prototype toolkit was validated in Northeast Brazil in patients with Chagas' disease (American trypanosomiasis), leishmaniasis, leprosy, and schistosomiasis, where it was well accepted.

Community dermatology is the branch of dermatology that addresses skin health at the population level, and this is perhaps most relevant in the poorest communities where the burden of skin disease is high and skin NTDs are prevalent [53,54]. It focuses on providing low-cost interventions for the most common skin diseases, and includes strategies for managing wounds and lymphoedema that are applicable to many skin NTDs.

Simple hygiene-based interventions, typically involving daily washing of affected limbs with soap and water, are known to be effective for the management of lymphoedema in LF-endemic areas, resulting in a reduced incidence of ADLA [55]. Recent data have shown that a low-cost lymphoedema self-care package is effective in reducing the frequency and duration of ADLA in podoconiosis [56]. In this study, the package of care included instructions for foot hygiene, skin care, bandaging, exercises, and use of socks and shoes, and this was reinforced by trained members of the local community at regular monthly meetings. Patients in the treatment group experienced 4.5 fewer episodes of ADLA per person-year compared with the control group who received no intervention.

Lymphatic filariasis (LF) and podoconiosis benefit from a very similar management, and in countries where there is a high burden of both diseases, it is sensible that morbidity management activities should be integrated in order to reduce programme costs and expand coverage. Deribe and colleagues describe the successful integration of these services in Ethiopia [57], where more than 500 government-employed health workers from 24 districts were trained by lymphoedema experts on integrated morbidity management and disability prevention for LF and podoconiosis. Trained health workers follow a management algorithm and deliver a defined package of care to patients, similar to that described earlier [56], focusing on daily hygiene measures, use of emollients to restore skin function, leg elevation, exercise, use of socks and shoes, and bandaging if required. Water, sanitation, and hygiene (WASH) interventions are important for the control of other major NTDs, including trachoma, soil-transmitted helminths, and schistosomiasis [58–60], highlighting further possibilities for integrated activities particularly where diseases are co-endemic.

Self-help group interventions are beneficial in many areas of medicine, and could be a useful approach to improve health behaviours for the management of morbidity associated with skin NTDs, with the potential for empowering 'expert patients' to take a lead role. For example, women's groups practising participatory learning and action (PLA) on preventive and care-seeking behaviours are a cost-effective strategy to improve maternal and neonatal survival in low-resource settings [61]. The potential benefits for the skin NTDs are numerous, and range from improved self-care behaviours in the management of lymphoedema to earlier presentation and treatment-seeking in new cases of leprosy in children. A recent study conducted in Nepal showed that the integration of self-care for filarial lymphoedema into existing community leprosy self-help groups was feasible, and attitudes towards integration were positive [62]. Opportunities were identified for LF-affected participants to increase their knowledge of self-care and access to health services.

Stigma and social isolation are a major problem for many NTDs, not least those that have highly visible skin manifestations. The severe stigmatisation of persons affected by leprosy is well described; however, this disability extends to several other skin NTDs including lymphatic filariasis, podoconiosis, Buruli ulcer, onchocerciasis, and leishmaniasis, with similar health-related and psychosocial consequences [63]. Importantly, the reasons for stigmatisation across the different NTDs are remarkably similar; these include appearance, fear of contagion, being a burden to the family, and the inability to fulfil gender roles. It has been suggested, therefore, that integrated approaches to reduce stigmatisation may be feasible and more efficient than disease-specific interventions.

Integrated morbidity management services will also offer an opportunity to promote skin health more broadly. The GBD 2013 data on skin diseases show that dermatitis accounts for the largest global burden, with high DALY rates in many regions of the world, but particularly in central sub-Saharan Africa. The ability to recognise a failing epidermis and prescribe an emollient would be beneficial for many patients, including those with dermatitis and those affected by many of the skin NTDs.

8. Conclusions and Future Directions

The grouping together of NTDs that affect the skin draws attention to the significant burden of skin disease that occurs almost exclusively in impoverished populations in the developing world. The concept of skin NTDs is useful for a number of reasons. It facilitates the integration of control activities, from diagnostic processes to community mass drug administration. It creates a strong argument for funding for research and control activities, considering the collective burden of disease. Finally, it places the dermatology community in a strong position to help in the fight against NTDs. Dermatologists can contribute through developing appropriate clinical guidelines, training health workers, coordinating research, and guiding the design and implementation of control activities. This in turn will foster better research relationships internationally and strengthen the fields of tropical and global health dermatology. There is a growing body of literature describing experiences of integration in a variety of settings, offering explanations behind the successes and failures, and it will be important going forward to learn from these experiences. Integrated fieldwork activities, from disease mapping to mass treatment, must be well planned and supported by relevant political bodies and funding agencies. The integrated control of skin NTDs, led by the dermatology community, has the potential to strengthen health systems in resource-poor settings and improve skin health for millions of the world's most disadvantaged people.

Author Contributions: D.J.C. and L.C.F. contributed equally to all aspects of this work.

References

1. Karimkhani, C.; Dellavalle, R.P.; Coffeng, L.E.; Flohr, C.; Hay, R.J.; Langan, S.M.; Nsoesie, E.O.; Ferrari, A.J.; Erskine, H.E.; Silverberg, J.I.; et al. Global skin disease morbidity and mortality: An update from the Global Burden of Disease Study 2013. *JAMA Dermatol.* **2017**, *153*, 406–412. [CrossRef] [PubMed]
2. Clucas, D.B.; Carville, K.S.; Connors, C.; Currie, B.J.; Carapetis, J.R.; Andrews, R.M. Disease burden and health-care clinic attendances for young children in remote Aboriginal communities of northern Australia. *Bull. World Health Organ.* **2008**, *86*, 275–281. [PubMed]
3. Herricks, J.R.; Hotez, P.J.; Wanga, V.; Coffeng, L.E.; Haagsma, J.A.; Basáñez, M.G.; Buckle, G.; Budke, C.M.; Carabin, H.; Fèvre, E.M.; et al. The Global Burden of Disease Study 2013: What does it mean for the NTDs? *PLoS Negl. Trop. Dis.* **2017**, *11*, e0005424. [CrossRef] [PubMed]
4. Hay, R.J.; Johns, N.E.; Williams, H.C.; Bolliger, I.W.; Dellavalle, R.P.; Margolis, D.J.; Marks, R.; Naldi, L.; Weinstock, M.A.; Wulf, S.K.; et al. The Global Burden of Skin Disease in 2010: An analysis of the prevalence and impact of skin conditions. *J. Investig. Dermatol.* **2014**, *134*, 1527–1534. [CrossRef] [PubMed]
5. Rodrigues, M.L.; Albuquerque, P.C. Searching for a change: The need for increased support for public health and research on fungal diseases. *PLoS Negl. Trop. Dis.* **2018**, *12*, e0006479. [CrossRef] [PubMed]

6. Houweling, T.A.J.; Karim-Kos, H.E.; Kulik, M.C.; Stolk, W.A.; Haagsma, J.A.; Lenk, E.J.; Richardus, J.H.; de Vlas, S.J.; et al. Socioeconomic inequalities in neglected tropical diseases: A systematic review. *PLoS Negl. Trop. Dis.* **2016**, *10*, e0004546. [CrossRef] [PubMed]
7. Chandler, D.J.; Hansen, K.S.; Mahato, B.; Darlong, J.; John, A.; Lockwood, D.N.J. Household costs of leprosy reactions (ENL) in rural India. *PLoS Negl. Trop. Dis.* **2015**, *9*, e0003431. [CrossRef] [PubMed]
8. Tiwari, A.; Suryawanshi, P.; Raikwar, A.; Arif, M.; Richardus, J.H. Household expenditure on leprosy outpatient services in the Indian Health System: A comparative study. *PLoS Negl. Trop. Dis.* **2018**, *12*, e0006181. [CrossRef] [PubMed]
9. Tembei, A.M.; Kengne-Ouaffo, J.A.; Ngoh, E.A.; John, B.; Nji, T.M.; Deribe, K.; Enyong, P.; Nkuo-Akenji, T.; Davey, G.; Wanji, S. A comparative analysis of economic cost of podoconiosis and leprosy on affected households in the northwest region of Cameroon. *Am. J. Trop. Med. Hyg.* **2018**, *98*, 1075–1081. [CrossRef] [PubMed]
10. Uranw, S.; Meheus, F.; Baltussen, R.; Rijal, S.; Boelaert, M. The household costs of visceral leishmaniasis care in south-eastern Nepal. *PLoS Negl. Trop. Dis.* **2013**, *7*, e2062. [CrossRef] [PubMed]
11. Lenk, E.J.; Redekop, W.K.; Luyendijk, M.; Rijnsburger, A.J.; Severens, J.L. Productivity loss related to neglected tropical diseases eligible for preventive chemotherapy: A systematic literature review. *PLoS Negl. Trop. Dis.* **2016**, *10*, 1–19. [CrossRef] [PubMed]
12. Engelman, D.; Fuller, L.C.; Solomon, A.W.; McCarthy, J.S.; Hay, R.J.; Lammie, P.J.; Steer, A.C. Opportunities for integrated control of neglected tropical diseases that affect the skin. *Trends Parasitol.* **2016**, *32*, 843–854. [CrossRef] [PubMed]
13. Mitjà, O.; Marks, M.; Bertran, L.; Kollie, K.; Argaw, D.; Fahal, A.H.; Fitzpatrick, C.; Fuller, L.C.; Izquierdo, B.G.; Hay, R.; et al. Integrated control and management of neglected tropical skin diseases. *PLoS Negl. Trop. Dis.* **2017**, *11*, e0005136. [CrossRef] [PubMed]
14. Department of Control of Neglected Tropical Diseases. *Recognizing Neglected Tropical Diseases Through Changes on the Skin: A Training Guide for Front-Line Health Workers*; WHO: Geneva, Switzerland, 2018.
15. Faye, O.; Hay, R.J.; Ryan, T.J.; Keita, S.; Traoré, A.K.; Mahé, A. A public health approach for leprosy detection based on a very short term-training of primary health care workers in basic dermatology. *Lepr. Rev.* **2007**, *78*, 11–16. [PubMed]
16. Chandler, D. Integrated care and leprosy in India: A role for indian systems of medicine and traditional health practice in the eradication of leprosy. *Curr. Sci.* **2016**, *111*, 351–355. [CrossRef]
17. Oswald, I.H. Are traditional healers the solution to the failures of primary health care in rural Nepal? *Soc. Sci. Med.* **1983**, *17*, 255–257. [CrossRef]
18. Kaur, P.; Sharma, U.C.; Pandey, S.S.; Gurmohan, S. Leprosy care through traditional healers. *Lepr. Rev.* **1984**, *55*, 57–61. [CrossRef] [PubMed]
19. Ezenduka, C.; Post, E.; John, S.; Suraj, A.; Namadi, A.; Onwujekwe, O. Cost-effectiveness analysis of three leprosy case detection methods in northern Nigeria. *PLoS Negl. Trop. Dis.* **2012**, *6*, e1818. [CrossRef] [PubMed]
20. Darlong, J.; Govindharaj, P.; Darlong, F.; Mahato, N. A study of untreated leprosy affected children reporting with grade 2 disability at a referral centre in West Bengal, India. *Lepr. Rev.* **2017**, *88*, 298–305.
21. Yotsu, R.R.; Kouadio, K.; Vagamon, B.; N'guessan, K.; Akpa, A.J.; Yao, A.; Aké, J.; Abbet, A.R.; Tchamba, A.A.; Bedimo, R.; et al. Skin disease prevalence study in schoolchildren in rural Côte d'Ivoire: Implications for integration of neglected skin diseases (Skin NTDs). *PLoS Negl. Trop. Dis.* **2018**, *12*, e0006489. [CrossRef] [PubMed]
22. Barogui, Y.T.; Diez, G.; Anagonou, E.; Johnson, R.C.; Gomido, I.C.; Amoukpo, H.; Bachirou, Z.S.; Houezo, J.G.; Saizonou, R.; Sopoh, G.E.; et al. Integrated approach in the control and management of skin neglected tropical diseases in Lalo, Benin. *PLoS Negl. Trop. Dis.* **2018**, *12*, e0006584. [CrossRef] [PubMed]
23. Mahé, A.; Faye, O.; N'Diaye, H.T.; Ly, F.; Konaré, H.; Kéita, S.; Traoré, A.K.; Hay, R. Definition of an algorithm for the management of common skin diseases at primary health care level in sub-Saharan Africa. *Trans. R. Soc. Trop. Med. Hyg.* **2005**, *99*, 39–47. [CrossRef] [PubMed]
24. Steer, A.C.; Tikoduadua, L.V.; Manalac, E.M.; Colquhoun, S.; Carapetis, J.R.; Maclennan, C. Validation of an integrated management of childhood illness algorithm for managing common skin conditions in Fiji. *Bull. World Health Organ.* **2009**, *87*, 173–179. [CrossRef] [PubMed]

25. Deribe, K.; Wanji, S.; Shafi, O.; Tukahebwa, M.E.; Umulisa, I.; Molyneux, D.H.; Davey, G. The feasibility of eliminating podoconiosis. *Bull. World Health Organ.* **2015**, *93*, 712–718. [CrossRef] [PubMed]
26. Engelman, D.; Fuller, L.C.; Steer, A.C.; International Alliance for the Control of Scabies Delphi Panel. Consensus criteria for the diagnosis of scabies: A delphi study of international experts. *PLoS Negl. Trop. Dis.* **2018**, *12*, e0006549. [CrossRef] [PubMed]
27. Brooker, S.J.; Smith, J.L. Mapping neglected tropical diseases: A global view. *Community Eye Heal.* **2013**, *26*, 32.
28. Noma, M.; Nwoke, B.E.B.; Nutall, I.; Tambala, P.A.; Enyong, P.; Namsenmo, A.; Remme, J.; Amazigo, U.V.; Kale, O.O.; Sékétéli, A. Rapid epidemiological mapping of onchocerciasis (REMO): Its application by the African Programme for Onchocerciasis Control (APOC). *Ann. Trop. Med. Parasitol.* **2002**, *96*, S29–S39. [CrossRef] [PubMed]
29. Sime, H.; Deribe, K.; Assefa, A.; Newport, M.J.; Enquselassie, F.; Gebretsadik, A.; Kebede, A.; Hailu, A.; Shafi, O.; Aseffa, A.; et al. Integrated mapping of lymphatic filariasis and podoconiosis: Lessons learnt from Ethiopia. *Parasit. Vectors* **2014**, *7*, 397. [CrossRef] [PubMed]
30. Kebede, B.; Martindale, S.; Mengistu, B.; Kebede, B.; Mengiste, A.; H/Kiros, F.; Tamiru, A.; Davey, G.; Kelly-Hope, L.A.; Mackenzie, C.D. Integrated morbidity mapping of lymphatic filariasis and podoconiosis cases in 20 co-endemic districts of Ethiopia. *PLoS Negl. Trop. Dis.* **2018**, *12*, e0006491. [CrossRef] [PubMed]
31. Mason, D.S.; Marks, M.; Sokana, O.; Solomon, A.W.; Mabey, D.C.; Romani, L.; Kaldor, J.; Steer, A.C.; Engelman, D. The prevalence of scabies and impetigo in the Solomon Islands: A population-based survey. *PLoS Negl. Trop. Dis.* **2016**, *10*, e0004803. [CrossRef] [PubMed]
32. Marks, M.; Vahi, V.; Sokana, O.; Chi, K.H.; Puiahi, E.; Kilua, G.; Pillay, A.; Dalipanda, T.; Bottomley, C.; Solomon, A.W.; et al. Impact of community mass treatment with azithromycin for trachoma elimination on the prevalence of yaws. *PLoS Negl. Trop. Dis.* **2015**, *9*, e0003988. [CrossRef] [PubMed]
33. Molyneux, D.H. 'Neglected' diseases but unrecognised successes—Challenges and opportunities for infectious disease control. *Lancet* **2004**, *364*, 380–383. [CrossRef]
34. Hotez, P.J.; Remme, J.H.F.; Buss, P.; Alleyne, G.; Morel, C.; Breman, J.G. Combating tropical infectious diseases: Report of the Disease Control Priorities in Developing Countries Project. *Clin. Infect. Dis.* **2004**, *38*, 871–988. [CrossRef] [PubMed]
35. Molyneux, D.H.; Hotez, P.J.; Fenwick, A. 'Rapid-impact interventions': How a policy of integrated control for Africa's neglected tropical diseases could benefit the poor. *PLoS Med.* **2005**, *2*, e336. [CrossRef] [PubMed]
36. Hotez, P.J.; Fenwick, A.; Ray, S.E.; Hay, S.I.; Molyneux, D.H. 'Rapid impact' 10 years after: The first 'decade' (2006-2016) of integrated neglected tropical disease control. *PLoS Negl. Trop. Dis.* **2018**, *12*, e0006137. [CrossRef] [PubMed]
37. Omura, S.; Crump, A. Ivermectin: Panacea for resource-poor communities? *Trends Parasitol.* **2014**, *30*, 445–455. [CrossRef] [PubMed]
38. Heukelbach, J.; Winter, B.; Wilcke, T.; Muehlen, M.; Albrecht, S.; de Oliveira, F.A.S.; Kerr-Pontes, L.R.; Liesenfeld, O.; Feldmeier, H. Selective mass treatment with ivermectin to control intestinal helminthiases and parasitic skin diseases in a severely affected population. *Bull. World Health Organ.* **2004**, *82*, 563–571. [PubMed]
39. Ottesen, E.A.; Hooper, P.J.; Bradley, M.; Biswas, G. The Global Programme to Eliminate Lymphatic Filariasis: Health impact after 8 years. *PLoS Negl. Trop. Dis.* **2008**, *2*, e317. [CrossRef] [PubMed]
40. Krotneva, S.P.; Coffeng, L.E.; Noma, M.; Zouré, H.G.M.; Bakoné, L.; Amazigo, U.V.; de Vlas, S.J.; Stolk, W.A. African Program for Onchocerciasis Control 1995–2010: Impact of annual ivermectin mass treatment on off-target infectious diseases. *PLoS Negl. Trop. Dis.* **2015**, *9*, e0004051. [CrossRef] [PubMed]
41. Romani, L.; Whitfeld, M.J.; Koroivueta, J.; Kama, M.; Wand, H.; Tikoduadua, L.; Tuicakau, M.; Koroi, A.; Andrews, R.; Kaldor, J.M.; et al. Mass drug administration for scabies control in a population with endemic disease. *N. Engl. J. Med.* **2015**, *373*, 2305–2313. [CrossRef] [PubMed]
42. Pacqué, M.; Muñoz, B.; Poetschke, G.; Foose, J.; Greene, B.M.; Taylor, H.R. Pregnancy outcome after inadvertent ivermectin treatment during community-based distribution. *Lancet* **1990**, *336*, 1486–1489. [CrossRef]
43. Gyapong, J.O.; Chinbuah, M.A.; Gyapong, M. Inadvertent exposure of pregnant women to ivermectin and albendazole during mass drug administration for lymphatic filariasis. *Trop. Med. Int. Health* **2003**, *8*, 1093–1101. [CrossRef] [PubMed]

44. Ndyomugyenyi, R.; Kabatereine, N.; Olsen, A.; Magnussen, P. Efficacy of ivermectin and albendazole alone and in combination for treatment of soil-transmitted helminths in pregnancy and adverse events: A randomized open label controlled intervention trial in Masindi District, Western Uganda. *Am. J. Trop. Med. Hyg.* **2008**, *79*, 856–863. [CrossRef] [PubMed]
45. Opoku, N.O.; Bakajika, D.K.; Kanza, E.M.; Howard, H.; Mambandu, G.L.; Nyathirombo, A.; Nigo, M.M.; Kasonia, K.; Masembe, S.L.; Mumbere, M.; et al. Single dose moxidectin versus ivermectin for *Onchocerca volvulus* infection in Ghana, Liberia, and the Democratic Republic of the Congo: A randomised, controlled, double-blind phase 3 trial. *Lancet* **2018**. [CrossRef]
46. Korth-Bradley, J.M.; Parks, V.; Patat, A.; Matschke, K.; Mayer, P.; Fleckenstein, L. Relative bioavailability of liquid and tablet formulations of the antiparasitic moxidectin. *Clin. Pharmacol. Drug Dev.* **2012**, *1*, 32–37. [CrossRef] [PubMed]
47. Mounsey, K.E.; Walton, S.F.; Innes, A.; Cash-Deans, S.; McCarthy, J.S. In vitro efficacy of moxidectin versus ivermectin against *Sarcoptes scabiei*. *Antimicrob. Agents Chemother.* **2017**, *61*, e00381. [CrossRef] [PubMed]
48. Ndyomugyenyi, R.; Byamungu, A.; Korugyendo, R. Perceptions on onchocerciasis and ivermectin treatment in rural communities in Uganda: Implications for long-term compliance. *Int. Health* **2009**, *1*, 163–168. [CrossRef] [PubMed]
49. Coulibaly, Y.I.; Dicko, I.; Keita, M.; Keita, M.M.; Doumbia, M.; Daou, A.; Haidara, F.C.; Sankare, M.H.; Horton, J.; Whately-Smith, C.; et al. A cluster randomized study of the safety of integrated treatment of trachoma and lymphatic filariasis in children and adults in Sikasso, Mali. *PLoS Negl. Trop. Dis.* **2013**, *7*, e2221. [CrossRef] [PubMed]
50. Mohammed, K.A.; Haji, H.J.; Gabrielli, A.F.; Mubila, L.; Biswas, G.; Chitsulo, L.; Bradley, M.H.; Engels, D.; Savioli, L.; Molyneux, D.H. Triple co-administration of ivermectin, albendazole and praziquantel in Zanzibar: A safety study. *PLoS Negl. Trop. Dis.* **2008**, *2*, e171. [CrossRef] [PubMed]
51. Thomsen, E.K.; Sanuku, N.; Baea, M.; Satofan, S.; Maki, E.; Lombore, B.; Schmidt, M.S.; Siba, P.M.; Weil, G.J.; Kazura, J.W.; et al. Efficacy, safety, and pharmacokinetics of coadministered diethylcarbamazine, albendazole, and ivermectin for treatment of bancroftian filariasis. *Clin. Infect. Dis.* **2016**, *62*, 334–341. [CrossRef] [PubMed]
52. Van 't Noordende, A.T.; Kuiper, H.; Ramos, A.N.; Mieras, L.F.; Barbosa, J.C.; Pessoa, S.M.F.; Souza, E.A.; Fernandes, T.A.; Hinders, D.C.; Praciano, M.M.; et al. Towards a toolkit for cross-neglected tropical disease morbidity and disability assessment. *Int. Health* **2016**, *8*, i71–81. [CrossRef] [PubMed]
53. Ryan, T.J. The International Society of Dermatology's Task Force for Skin Care for All: Community dermatology. *Int. J. Dermatol.* **2011**, *50*, 548–551. [CrossRef] [PubMed]
54. Kaur, P.; Singh, G. Community dermatology in India. *Int. J. Dermatol.* **1995**, *34*, 322. [CrossRef] [PubMed]
55. Stocks, M.E.; Freeman, M.C.; Addiss, D.G. The effect of hygiene-based lymphedema management in lymphatic filariasis-endemic areas: A systematic review and meta-analysis. *PLoS Negl. Trop. Dis.* **2015**, *9*, e0004171. [CrossRef] [PubMed]
56. Negussie, H.; Molla, M.; Ngari, M.; Berkley, J.A.; Kivaya, E.; Njuguna, P.; Fegan, G.; Tamiru, A.; Kelemework, A.; Lang, T.; et al. Lymphoedema management to prevent acute dermatolymphangioadenitis in podoconiosis in northern Ethiopia (GoLBeT): A pragmatic randomised controlled trial. *Lancet Glob. Heal.* **2018**, *6*, e795–803. [CrossRef]
57. Deribe, K.; Kebede, B.; Tamiru, M.; Mengistu, B.; Kebede, F.; Martindale, S.; Sime, H.; Mulugeta, A.; Kebede, B.; Sileshi, M.; et al. Integrated morbidity management for lymphatic filariasis and podoconiosis, Ethiopia. *Bull. World Health Organ.* **2017**, *95*, 652–656. [CrossRef] [PubMed]
58. Stocks, M.E.; Ogden, S.; Haddad, D.; Addiss, D.G.; McGuire, C.; Freeman, M.C. Effect of water, sanitation, and hygiene on the prevention of trachoma: A Systematic review and meta-analysis. *PLoS Med.* **2014**, *11*, e1001605. [CrossRef] [PubMed]
59. Strunz, E.C.; Addiss, D.G.; Stocks, M.E.; Ogden, S.; Utzinger, J.; Freeman, M.C. Water, sanitation, hygiene, and soil-transmitted helminth infection: A systematic review and meta-analysis. *PLoS Med.* **2014**, *11*, e1001620. [CrossRef] [PubMed]
60. Grimes, J.E.T.; Croll, D.; Harrison, W.E.; Utzinger, J.; Freeman, M.C.; Templeton, M.R. The relationship between water, sanitation and schistosomiasis: A systematic review and meta-analysis. *PLoS Negl. Trop. Dis.* **2014**, *8*, e3296. [CrossRef] [PubMed]

61. Seward, N.; Neuman, M.; Colbourn, T.; Osrin, D.; Lewycka, S.; Azad, K.; Costello, A.; Das, S.; Fottrell, E.; Kuddus, A.; et al. Effects of women's groups practising participatory learning and action on preventive and care-seeking behaviours to reduce neonatal mortality: A meta-analysis of cluster-randomised trials. *PLoS Med.* **2017**, *14*, e1002467. [CrossRef] [PubMed]
62. Pryce, J.; Mableson, H.E.; Choudhary, R.; Pandey, B.D.; Aley, D.; Betts, H.; Mackenzie, C.D.; Kelly-Hope, L.A.; Cross, H. Assessing the feasibility of integration of self-care for filarial lymphoedema into existing community leprosy self-help groups in Nepal. *BMC Public Health* **2018**, *18*, 201. [CrossRef] [PubMed]
63. Hofstraat, K.; van Brakel, W.H. Social Stigma Towards Neglected Tropical Diseases: A systematic review. *Int. Health* **2016**, *8*, i53–i70. [CrossRef] [PubMed]

6

Poverty, Dietary Intake, Intestinal Parasites and Nutritional Status among School-Age Children in the Rural Philippines

Allen G. Ross [1,*], Keren Papier [2], Ruby Luceres-Catubig [3], Thao N. Chau [4], Marianette T. Inobaya [1,3] and Shu-Kay Ng [1]

1. Menzies Health Institute Queensland, Griffith University, Gold Coast, QLD 4222, Australia; net_inobaya@yahoo.com (M.T.I.); s.ng@griffith.edu.au (S.-K.N.)
2. National Centre for Epidemiology & Population Health, Australian National University, Canberra, ACT 2601, Australia; keren.papier@anu.edu.au
3. Department of Health, Research Institute for Tropical Medicine, Muntinlupa 1781, Metro Manila, Philippines; ruby.luceres@yahoo.com
4. Discipline of Public Health, School of Health Sciences, Flinders University, Adelaide, SA 5001, Australia; tnpchau@gmail.com

* Correspondence: a.ross@griffith.edu.au;

Abstract: Intestinal helminths are endemic throughout the Philippines; however, there is limited evidence with respect to their prevalence, intensity, and impact on children's nutritional status. A cross-sectional survey was carried out on 693 children from five rural villages in Northern Samar, the Philippines. Data on dietary intake, nutritional status, and intestinal parasites were collected. Infection with *Schistosoma japonicum*, *Ascaris lumbricoides*, *Trichuris trichiura*, and hookworm was evident in 20.1, 54.4, 71.4, and 25.3% of the children. The majority (84.7%) was infected with one or more helminth species, with about one-quarter of the sample (24.7%) infected with three or more. About half (49.2%, $n = 341$) of the children were stunted and 27.8% ($n = 193$) were wasted. A lower prevalence of normal height-for-age (48.3%) appeared in those with polyparasitism, while the prevalence of stunted children increased with infection (46.7% monoparasitism and 51.7% polyparasitism). There was a decreasing trend between infection intensity and the mean values of HAZ and BAZ identified for *T. trichiura* or hookworm infections. Stunted children were more likely to be male (AOR = 1.58; 95% CI: 1.05–2.39; $p = 0.028$), older in age (10–14 years) (AOR = 1.93; 95% CI: 1.29–2.88; $p = 0.001$), and living in poorer households with palm leaves/nipa roof (AOR = 1.85; 95% CI: 1.14–3.01; $p = 0.013$). Intestinal parasitic treatment needs to be combined with nutrient supplements and health education in order to interrupt the parasite life cycle and achieve sustainable control.

Keywords: childhood; malnutrition; intestinal parasites; nutritional status; poverty

---

1. Introduction

More than a third of the world's population is infected with soil-transmitted helminths (STH), mainly in the developing nations of Asia, Africa, and Latin America [1]. STHs are intestinal parasitic nematode worms causing human disease. They are the most common of the 17 major neglected tropical diseases (NTDs) and the most widespread and disabling chronic infections globally [2]. *Ascaris lumbricoides* is the most prevalent STH with an estimated one billion infections; and *Trichuris trichiura* and hookworms (*Necator americanus* and *Ancylostoma duodenale*) each infect approximately 600–800 million [1]. STHs are a significant public health concern in the Philippines, particularly among school-aged children who, if infected, suffer from profound physical deficits, including anaemia and malnutrition, stunted growth, reduced fitness, and cognitive delays [2–8]. Sixteen out of 17 regions in the Philippines are endemic for STHs with a prevalence of $\geq$50% [9]. A nationwide survey performed over 10 years found the prevalence in children aged 2–14 years was 50–90%; and up to 30% of the 22 million children in the Philippines were infected with more than one of the three STH species [10,11].

The cornerstone of intestinal parasitic control is recurrent mass drug administration (MDA) with benzimidazole anthelmintics (e.g., 400 mg albendazole) that are cheap, safe, and effective. The current WHO strategy is to continually treat pre-school and school-age children, women of childbearing age, and adults at high risk, once or twice per year, depending on prevalence [8,9]. This is partially effective in achieving morbidity control; however, it does not prevent re-infection. A number of studies have shown that once treatment is stopped, prevalence returns to pre-treatment levels within 12–18 months [2,7–11]. Therefore, interventions that prevent re-infection and boost immunity (e.g., the use of micro/macronutrient supplements) are required to augment chemotherapy as part of an integrated approach. The global target is to eliminate morbidity due to soil-transmitted helminthiases in children by 2020 [8]. This will only be achieved by regularly treating at least 75% of the children in endemic areas (an estimated 873 million), who are free from malnutrition [8,9].

Nutritional deficiencies and infectious diseases can negatively impact the nutritional status of children and adolescents [12,13]. Intestinal helminth worm infections can damage a child's internal mucosa, leading to impaired digestion and poor absorption of nutrients [14]. Deficiencies in macro- and micronutrient intakes during childhood can impair both physical and cognitive growth as well as increase the risk of mortality [15]. Moreover, inadequate intake of selected micronutrients can cause immune deficiency and increase susceptibility to infection [16]. The micronutrients vitamin A, vitamin B_{12}, vitamin C, β-carotene, riboflavin, zinc, selenium, and iron all have immune-modulating functions, enabling them to influence the course of an infection [16]. Laboratory studies have shown that vitamin A deficiency can reduce schistosome (human blood fluke)-specific antibody responses, suggesting a possible link between vitamin A deficiency and susceptibility to schistosomiasis [12]. Deficiency of some nutrients may reduce the host's immune function, impairing the body's resistance to infectious diseases and increasing susceptibility to intestinal parasites [17]. Once present, parasitic infections can promote the further loss of nutrients, leading to reduced growth and poor nutritional status as part of a vicious cycle [18]. Children aged 5–14 years suffer from the highest burden of infectious disease [19], partly due to their increased behavioural risk, frequent outdoor exposure, and poor personal hygiene [20].

Intestinal helminths are endemic throughout the Philippines and efforts are underway to decrease their burden. However, there is limited evidence with regards to their prevalence, intensity and their impact on children's nutritional status. The purpose of this study was to examine the relationship between poverty, dietary intake, intestinal parasites, and childhood nutritional status in the rural Philippines.

2. Material and Methods

2.1. Study Population

A cross-sectional survey was conducted in 2013 on 693 children from five rural villages in Palapag [21], Northern Samar, the Philippines. Villagers there are typically poor rice farmers, with over 50% of the population living below the poverty line. Water, sanitation, and hygiene conditions are most often rudimentary. Most households typically have 6–10 children per family and the prevalence rates of parasitic diseases, acute respiratory infections, diarrhoeal diseases, and other communicable diseases, are high [22].

2.2. Study Procedures

Individuals were asked, over the course of a week, to provide two stool specimens from which six Kato–Katz thick smears were prepared on microscope slides. These slides were examined under a light microscope by experienced laboratory technicians who counted the number of STH and *Schistosoma japonicum* (SJ) eggs per slide. For quality control, 10% of slides were randomly selected and re-examined by a senior microscopist at the Research Institute for Tropical Medicine, Manila. Individual and head of household questionnaires were completed to collect the following information: occupation, level of education, home and land ownership, number of animals owned and raising practices, animal waste disposal practices, pasturing of animals, sanitation, and housing characteristics (roofing, wall, and floor materials). For wealth status, participants were classified as wealthy if their house had a cement floor, a galvanized roof, cement walls, and a tile/marble floor. Participants were classified as poor if they had a house with a nipa (palm) roof and a soil floor, and without cement walls. All other participants were classified as having a moderate wealth status.

2.3. Nutritional Assessment

Anthropometric measurements of height and weight were collected using standard procedures [23]. Weight was measured using a portable digital scale to the nearest 0.1 kg. Height was assessed to the nearest 0.1 cm using a tape measure. The Z values for weight-for-height (WAZ) (children aged <10 years only), body mass index (BMI)—for-age (BAZ), and height-for-age (HAZ) were calculated according to World Health Organization (WHO) guidelines using the new WHO growth standards [24,25]. Weight-for-height is considered an inappropriate indicator for monitoring child growth beyond the age of 10 due to its inability to distinguish between relative height and body mass. Therefore, BMI-for-age was used to assess thinness/wasting for children aged ≥10 and for adolescents. Based on the Z values, the children were categorized as 'thin/wasted' (BAZ < −2 and/or WAZ < −2) and 'stunted' (HAZ < −2). Children with Z values > −2 for BAZ, WAZ, and HAZ were categorized as 'normal'.

2.4. Dietary Intake Data

Dietary intake information was elicited using a 24-h recall method. Three qualified nutritionists together with 10 field nurses collected the data. Household food utensils were used to assist study participants quantify food portions and liquids consumed. In order to estimate food weights, macro- and micronutrient intakes were calculated for each child using food composition tables developed by the Food and Nutrition Research Institute [26]. These tables contained data on 17 food components of 1541 foods commonly consumed in the Philippines. Dietary intake data was evaluated against the national Filipino recommended energy and nutrient intake (RENI) values by age and sex [27].

2.5. Statistical Analysis

Data were double-entered into FoxPro (version 6.0), crosschecked, and subsequently analysed using STATA SE version 13.0 software (StataCorp LP, College Station, TX, USA). All variables including sex, age group, and endemic setting were explored individually by Chi-square statistics. Infection intensity was explored with the Student *t*-test and Kruskal–Wallis test. The standard error (SE) of each estimate was converted to a variance; all variances were summed to provide an overall variance, SE, and 95% confidence interval (CI). The Chi-square test and the Student *t*-test were used to explore associations of a participant's demographic and socio-economic characteristics and the likelihood of having *S. japonicum*, any STH, and any helminth infection. Significant demographic and socio-economic factors were entered into the mixed-effect logistic regression analysis to obtain the final model for predicting stunting. Random barangay (village) and household effects were included in the model to account for the correlation among observations within each barangay and household, respectively. Adaptive Gaussian quadrature with 10 points was adopted to approximate the log likelihood for all levels of both random effects in the mixed model. Factors that were not significantly relevant (cut-off for significance = 0.05) were removed in a stepwise backward regression elimination procedure.

2.6. Study Oversight

Ethical consent for the study was obtained from the ethics review boards of the Department of Health in the Philippines (IRB # 2012-13-0) and Griffith University, Australia. Written informed consent was obtained from the parents/legal guardians. All questionnaires were translated into the local dialect and back-translated into English. Individuals found positive for a STH or *S. japonicum* were treated according to the Department of Health clinical guidelines.

3. Results

3.1. Demographic, Household, and Nutritional Characteristics and Prevalence of Infection

A cross-sectional survey was carried out on 693 children, of whom 53% were male. A total of 41.7% of the study population was aged between 6–9 years with the remainder between 10–14 years. The majority of children (56%) lived in a house with a roof made from either palm leaves or nipa, an indirect indicator of lower socioeconomic status. Infection with *S. japonicum*, *Ascaris lumbricoides*, *Trichuris trichiura*, and hookworm was evident in 20.1, 54.4, 71.4, and 25.3% of the 667 children sampled for intestinal parasites. The majority of the children (84.7%) was infected with one or more helminth species, with about one-quarter of the study sample (24.7%) infected with three or more different worm species.

The demographic, household, and nutritional characteristics of the study sample are presented in Table 1. About half (49.2%, $n = 341$) of the study sample were stunted and 27.8% ($n = 193$) were thin. Both mean HAZ and BAZ scores were below world standard (−2.0 SD and −1.3 SD from world mean, respectively). SJ infection occurred more often for males (64.2%, $p = 0.003$) and higher age group (70.2%, $p = 0.002$). Children with *S. japonicum* infection also had lower BAZ scores (−1.603, $p = 0.039$). Children with any STH infection were more likely to be of higher age group (60.5%, $p = 0.019$) or living in houses with palm leaves/nipa roofs (57.5%, $p = 0.040$). There was no significant difference for the nutrition indicators between children with and without any STH infection. Age group and roof material were the only factors that differentiated the three children groups of non-infected, monoparasitism, and polyparasitism (proportion of polyparasitism was higher for the higher age group, $p = 0.018$, and for those with house roof materials of palm leaves or nipa, $p = 0.021$).

3.2. Demographic, Household, and Nutritional Characteristics and Intensity of Infection

Table 2 presents the demographic, household, and nutritional characteristics of the study sample, by intensity of infection. Significant results were found between negative, light, and moderate/heavy SJ infection. Males ($p = 0.01$) and older children ($p = 0.009$) were more likely to have *S. japonicum* infection. For *A. lumbricoides* infections, children in the household without toilets ($p = 0.009$) or without galvanized iron/cement roof ($p < 0.001$) were more likely to have moderate or heavy infections. These factors have the same impact for *T. trichiura* infections. Children in households without toilets ($p < 0.001$) or galvanized iron/cement roof ($p = 0.038$) were more likely to have moderate or heavy infections. Moreover, children with moderate or heavy *T. trichiura* infections had a significantly higher mean levels of vitamin C intake, compared to those with light infections ($p = 0.038$). Finally, children with light hookworm infections were more likely to be male (62.1% versus 49.4%, $p = 0.004$), to be stunted (61.5% versus 44.8%, $p < 0.001$), and had a higher proportion of households without toilets (25.7% versus 17.9%, $p = 0.028$), and lower mean HAZ Z-scores (−2.14 versus −1.92, $p = 0.014$) and BAZ Z-scores (−1.61 versus −1.37, $p = 0.013$).

Table 1. Demographic, household, and nutritional characteristics of the study sample (n = 693) according to *Schistosoma japonicum* (SJ) and/or soil-transmitted helminth (STH) infections.

Characteristic	All Children (n = 693)	Positive for SJ Infection (n = 134)		Positive for any STH Infection (n = 552)		Non-Infected (n = 102)	Monoparasitism (n = 184)	Polyparasitism (n = 381)	p Value [b]
			p value [a]		p value [a]				
Gender									
Male	365 (52.7%)	86 (64.2%)	0.003 *	294 (53.3%)	0.470	49 (48.0%)	90 (48.9%)	212 (55.6%)	0.195
Female	328 (47.3%)	48 (35.8%)		258 (46.7%)		53 (52%)	94 (51.1%)	169 (44.4%)	
Age group									
6–9	289 (41.7%)	40 (29.9%)	0.002 *	218 (39.5%)	0.019 *	55 (53.9%)	76 (41.3%)	146 (38.3%)	0.018 *
10–14	404 (58.3%)	94 (70.2%)		334 (60.5%)		47 (46.1%)	108 (58.7%)	235 (61.7%)	
Toilet									
Yes	547 (80.0%)	108 (81.2%)	0.726	434 (79.6%)	0.492	84 (83.2%)	149 (81.9%)	295 (78.5%)	0.451
No	137 (20.0%)	25 (18.8%)		111 (20.4%)		17 (16.8%)	33 (18.1%)	81 (21.5%)	
Own home									
Yes	620 (90.4%)	121 (91.0%)	0.965	497 (90.9%)	0.671	92 (91.1%)	170 (92.4%)	340 (90.4%)	0.746
No	66 (9.6%)	12 (9.0%)		50 (9.1%)		9 (8.9%)	14 (7.6%)	36 (9.6%)	
Roof material									
Palm leaves/nipa	380 (56.1%)	72 (54.1%)	0.692	312 (57.5%)	0.040 *	44 (44.9%)	97 (53.0%)	223 (59.8%)	0.021 *
Galvanized iron/cement	298 (43.9%)	61 (45.9%)		231 (42.5%)		54 (55.1%)	86 (47.0%)	150 (40.2%)	
Height for age									
Normal	352 (50.8%)	60 (44.8%)	0.108	274 (49.6%)	0.130	58 (56.9%)	98 (53.3%)	184 (48.3%)	0.235
Stunted	341 (49.2%)	74 (55.2%)		278 (50.4%)		44 (43.1%)	86 (46.7%)	197 (51.7%)	
BMI for age									
Normal	500 (72.2%)	89 (66.4%)	0.103	399 (72.4%)	0.667	71 (69.6%)	133 (72.3%)	276 (72.6%)	0.831
Thin	193 (27.8%)	45 (33.6%)		152 (27.6%)		31 (30.4%)	51 (27.7%)	104 (27.4%)	
Mean HAZ score	−1.985 (0.973)	−2.091 (0.976)	0.131	1.999 (0.986)	0.196	−1.85 (0.92)	−1.98 (1.04)	−2.01 (0.96)	0.360
Mean BAZ score	−1.285 (3.961)	−1.603 (1.099)	0.039 *	−1.448 (1.082)	0.412	−1.39 (1)	−1.34 (1.14)	−1.49 (1.05)	0.291
Mean energy (kj)	7512 (3078)	7371 (2737)	0.577	7463 (3166)	0.531	7528 (2538)	7489 (2663)	7486 (3382)	0.992
Mean protein (g)	55.3 (52.3)	52.8 (20.8)	0.304	55.48 (57.80)	0.765	54.51 (20.13)	51.35 (18.45)	57.46 (68.38)	0.435
Mean total fat (g)	36.7 (31.6)	35.6 (22.8)	0.654	36.50 (34.04)	0.911	35.95 (17.61)	37.33 (21.74)	36.18 (38.17)	0.908
Mean carbohydrate (g)	310.7 (119.7)	307.4 (124.1)	0.764	308.0 (117.2)	0.313	314.6 (121.3)	311.9 (122.7)	308.1 (116.3)	0.864
Mean water (g)	1997 (699)	2016 (661)	0.614	2016 (661.246	0.614	1989 (674)	1956 (736)	2006 (681)	0.725
Mean thiamin (g)	0.663 (1.33)	0.578 (0.292)	0.121	0.671 (1.480)	0.611	0.63 (0.33)	0.61 (0.33)	0.70 (1.77)	0.713
Mean riboflavin (mg)	0.583 (0.617)	0.532 (0.303)	0.108	0.586 (0.679)	0.769	0.59 (0.29)	0.54 (0.30)	0.60 (0.79)	0.571
Mean niacin (mg)	17.1 (10.9)	16.5 (8.5)	0.473	0.487 (11.448)	0.803	17.06 (8.77)	15.87 (7.21)	17.53 (12.84)	0.242
Mean vitamin C (mg)	36.0 (52.1)	30.4 (44.7)	0.110	36.62 (52.12)	0.645	33.94 (56.45)	39.62 (55.43)	35.13 (49.91)	0.569

Data are count (%) for categorical variables and mean (standard deviation) for continuous variables. [a] Test differences between participants with positive infection vs negative infection (using either t-test or Chi-square test). [b] Test differences among participants without infection, monoparasitism, and polyparasitism (2–4 infections of SJ or any STH) (using either t-test or Chi-square test). * Significance at the 0.05 level.

Table 2. Demographic, household, and nutritional characteristics of the study sample according to intensity of infection.

Characteristic	*Schistosoma japonicum* [a]			*A. lumbricoides* [b]			*T. trichiura* [c]			Hookworms [d]	
	Negative (n = 533)	Light (n = 124)	Mod-Heay (n = 10)	Negative (n = 304)	Light (n = 241)	Mod-Heavy (n = 122)	Negative (n = 191)	Light (n = 392)	Mod-Heavy (n = 84)	Negative (n = 498)	Light (n = 169)
Gender [a,d]											
Male	265 (49.7%)	79 (63.7%)	7 (70.0%)	161 (53.0%)	131 (54.4%)	59 (48.4%)	99 (51.8%)	202 (51.5%)	50 (59.5%)	246 (49.4%)	105 (62.1%)
Female	268 (50.3%)	45 (36.3%)	3 (30.0%)	143 (47.0%)	110 (45.6%)	63 (51.6%)	92 (48.2%)	190 (48.5%)	34 (40.5%)	252 (50.6%)	64 (37.9%)
Age group [a]											
6–9	237 (44.5%)	37 (29.8%)	3 (30.0%)	128 (42.1%)	98 (40.7%)	51 (41.8%)	91 (47.6%)	151 (38.5%)	35 (41.7%)	211 (42.4%)	66 (39.1%)
10–14	296 (55.5%)	87 (70.2%)	7 (70.0%)	176 (57.9%)	143 (59.3%)	71 (58.2%)	100 (52.4%)	241 (61.5%)	49 (58.3%)	287 (57.6%)	103 (60.9%)
Toilet [b,c,d]											
Yes	420 (79.9%)	99 (80.5%)	9 (90.0%)	253 (84.1%)	190 (79.8%)	85 (70.8%)	153 (81.0%)	325 (83.6%)	50 (61.7%)	404 (82.1%)	124 (74.3%)
No	106 (20.1%)	24 (19.5%)	1 (10.0%)	48 (15.9%)	48 (20.2%)	35 (29.2%)	36 (19.0%)	64 (16.4%)	31 (38.3%)	88 (17.9%)	43 (25.7%)
Own home											
Yes	481 (91.1%)	113 (91.9%)	8 (80.0%)	278 (92.1%)	217 (90.8%)	107 (89.2%)	175 (92.1%)	353 (90.8%)	74 (90.2%)	452 (91.5%)	150 (89.8%)
No	47 (8.9%)	10 (8.1%)	2 (20.0%)	24 (7.9%)	22 (9.2%)	13 (10.8%)	15 (7.9%)	36 (9.2%)	8 (9.8%)	42 (8.5%)	17 (10.2%)
Roof material [b,c]											
Palm leaves/nipa	292 (56.1%)	67 (54.5%)	5 (50.0%)	142 (47.5%)	137 (57.8%)	85 (72.0%)	95 (51.1%)	214 (55.2%)	55 (68.8%)	264 (54.2%)	100 (59.9%)
Galvanized iron/cement	229 (43.9%)	56 (45.5%)	5 (50.0%)	157 (52.5%)	100 (42.2%)	33 (28.0%)	91 (48.9%)	174 (44.8%)	25 (31.2%)	223 (45.8%)	67 (40.1%)
Height for age [d]											
Normal	280 (52.5%)	56 (45.2%)	4 (40.0%)	160 (52.6%)	125 (51.9%)	55 (45.1%)	106 (55.5%)	196 (50.0%)	38 (45.2%)	275 (55.2%)	65 (38.5%)
Stunted	253 (47.5%)	68 (54.8%)	6 (60.0%)	144 (47.4%)	116 (48.1%)	67 (54.9%)	85 (44.5%)	196 (50.0%)	46 (54.8%)	223 (44.8%)	104 (61.5%)
BMI for age											
Normal	391 (73.5%)	83 (66.9%)	6 (60.0%)	212 (69.7%)	176 (73.3%)	92 (75.4%)	136 (71.2%)	284 (72.6%)	60 (71.4%)	363 (72.9%)	117 (69.6%)
Thin	141 (26.5%)	41 (33.1%)	4 (40.0%)	92 (30.3%)	64 (26.7%)	30 (24.6%)	55 (28.8%)	107 (27.4%)	24 (28.6%)	135 (27.1%)	51 (30.4%)
Mean HAZ score [d]	−1.95 (1.0)	−2.09 (1.0)	−2.05 (1.0)	−1.98 (1.0)	−1.94 (0.9)	−2.05 (1.0)	−1.86 (1.0)	−2.00 (1.0)	−2.15 (1.0)	−1.92 (1.0)	−2.14 (0.9)
Mean BAZ score [d]	−1.39 (1.1)	−1.61 (1.1)	−1.56 (1.4)	−1.45 (1.1)	−1.47 (1.1)	−1.32 (0.9)	−1.35 (1.1)	−1.45 (1.1)	−1.54 (0.8)	−1.37 (1.1)	−1.61 (1.1)
Mean energy (kj)	7349 (2792)	7643 (2015)	7990 (3178)	7536 (2544)	7628 (3890)	7122 (2372)	7632 (2811)	7472 (3308)	7279 (2477)	7483 (3105)	7523 (2993)
Mean protein (g)	55.97 (58.6)	52.32 (20.8)	58.29 (20.7)	52.86 (19.0)	60.29 (84.6)	51.67 (20.1)	54.14 (20.7)	55.90 (67.2)	55.34 (21.3)	54.93 (54.8)	56.48 (48.3)
Mean totalfat (g)	36.68 (33.7)	35.80 (23.0)	32.93 (21.4)	36.57 (19.5)	38.59 (46.7)	31.99 (15.6)	38.76 (22.7)	36.65 (37.4)	30.36 (16.6)	36.73 (32.4)	35.67 (29.8)
Mean carbohydrate (g)	310.9 (117)	306.1 (126)	324.3 (99.3)	315.0 (120)	308.4 (120)	301.6 (113)	314.6 (128)	307.9 (114)	310.8 (119)	309.3 (119)	312.6 (119)
Mean water (g)	1982 (704)	2005 (672)	2158 (519)	1992 (681)	1984 (711)	1994 (705)	2005 (693)	1973 (690)	2028 (728)	1976 (694)	2028 (700)
Mean thiamin (g)	0.69 (1.51)	0.58 (0.30)	0.54 (0.22)	0.60 (0.29)	0.80 (2.22)	0.57 (0.26)	0.65 (0.38)	0.69 (1.74)	0.57 (0.24)	0.67 (1.39)	0.65 (1.24)
Mean riboflavin (mg)	0.60 (0.69)	0.53 (0.31)	0.51 (0.25)	0.54 (0.27)	0.64 (0.98)	0.57 (0.29)	0.59 (0.32)	0.57 (0.78)	0.61 (0.29)	0.58 (0.64)	0.60 (0.58)
Mean niacin (mg)	17.13 (11.5)	16.18 (8.1)	20.34 (12.3)	16.33 (7.8)	17.88 (15.0)	16.93 (7.8)	16.81 (8.4)	16.79 (12.4)	18.40 (8.7)	16.76 (11.1)	17.70 (10.8)
Mean vitamin C [c] (mg)	37.65 (54.2)	29.76 (44.0)	38.24 (55.0)	37.55 (55.4)	35.66 (49.1)	33.83 (51.8)	36.12 (53.2)	33.37 (47.3)	49.51 (69.7)	36.01 (51.2)	36.71 (56.2)

Data are count (%) for categorical variables and mean (standard deviation) for continuous variables. [a] Significant difference between negative, light, and moderate/heavy SJ infection in gender ($p = 0.01$) and age group ($p = 0.009$). [b] Significant difference between negative, light, and moderate/heavy *A. lumbricoides* infection in the proportions of owning toilet ($p = 0.009$) and galvanized iron/cement roof material ($p < 0.001$). [c] Significant difference between negative, light, and moderate/heavy *T. trichiura* infection in the proportions of owning toilet ($p < 0.001$) and galvanized iron/cement roof material ($p = 0.028$), and the mean level of vitamin C ($p = 0.038$). [d] Significant difference between negative and light hookworms infection in gender ($p = 0.004$), the proportions of owning toilet ($p = 0.028$) and stunted children ($p < 0.001$), and the mean levels of the HAZ Z-score ($p = 0.014$) and the BAZ Z-score ($p = 0.013$).

As depicted in Figure 1, a decreasing trend between infection intensity and the mean values of HAZ and BAZ was identified for *T. trichiura* or hookworm infections (that is, the heavier the intensity, the lower the HAZ and BAZ mean values). For SJ or *A. lumbricoides* infections, the trend was not so obvious.

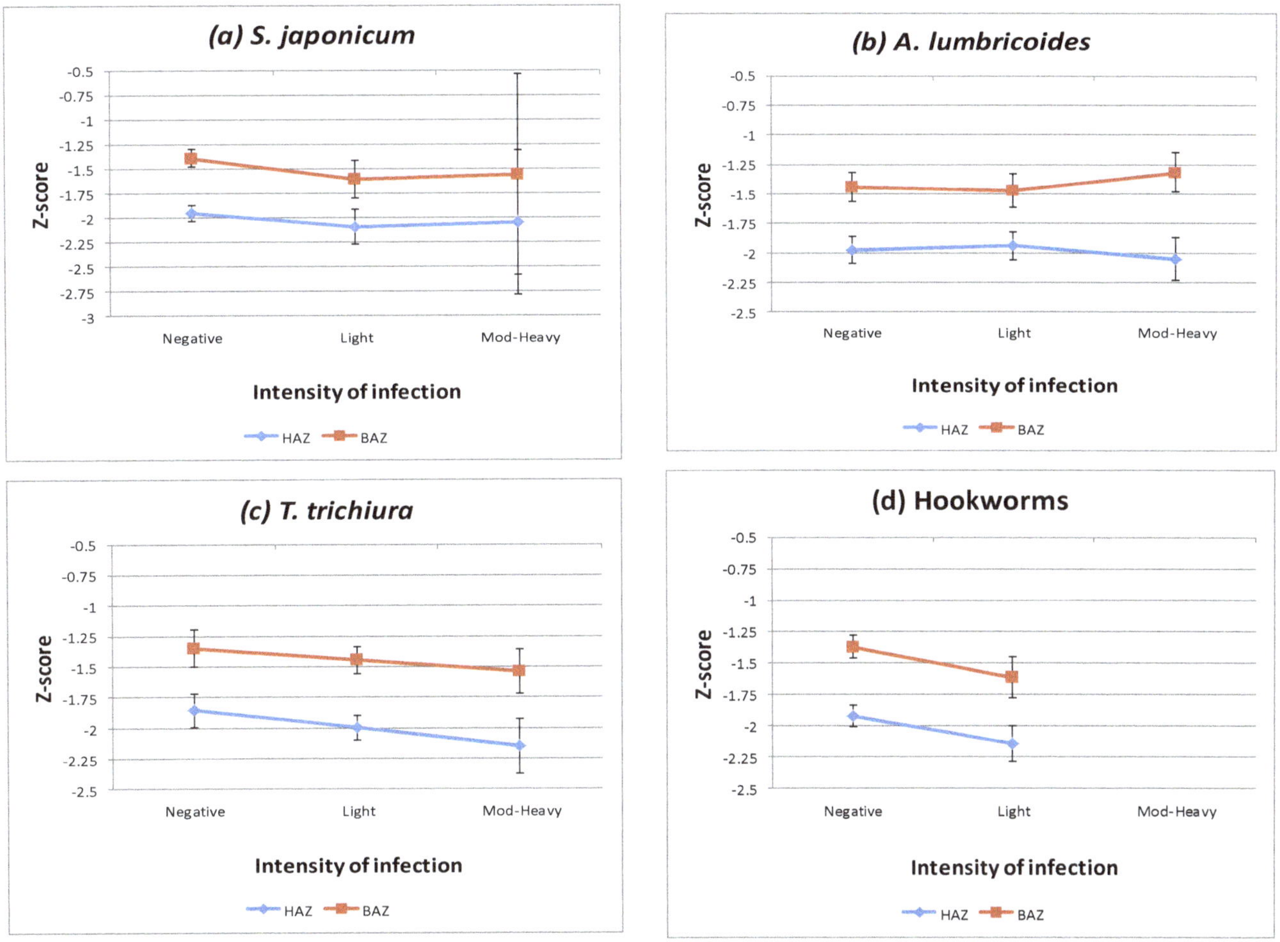

Figure 1. Plots of Z-scores for the anthropometric indicators versus (**a**) *Schistosoma japonicum*; (**b**) *T. trichiura*; (**c**) *A. lumbricoides*; (**d**) hookworms infection. Note HAZ: height for age Z-score; BAZ: BMI for age Z-score. Mod-Heavy: infections of moderate to heavy intensity.

3.3. Demographic, Socioeconomic Factors and Stunting

Table 3 displays the mixed-effect logistic regression model for stunting. Compared to children with normal height for age, stunted children were more likely to be male (AOR = 1.58; 95% CI: 1.05–2.39; $p = 0.028$), older in the age group of 10–14 (AOR = 1.93; 95% CI: 1.29–2.88; $p = 0.001$), and living in poorer households with palm leaves/nipa roofs (AOR = 1.85; 95% CI: 1.14–3.01; $p = 0.013$). All nutrition factors were not significantly associated with stunting. Variation among the predicted barangay-specific random effects for stunting was not statistically significant. However, there is significant household-specific random effects (estimated variance: 1.82, $p < 0.001$) in the probability of stunting, indicating that unknown household effects other than the identified household risk factor (roof materials) exist.

Table 3. Mixed-effect logistic regression analysis of the relationship between stunting with demographic and socio-economic variables.

Variable	Height for Age		Stunting Versus Normal	
	Normal (n = 352)	Stunted (n = 341)	Adjusted OR (95% CI)	p-Value
Gender				
Male	172 (48.9%)	193 (56.6%)	1.58 (1.05–2.39)	0.028
Female	180 (51.1%)	148 (43.4%)	Reference	
Age group				
6–9	167 (47.4%)	122 (35.8%)	Reference	
10–14	185 (52.6%)	219 (64.2%)	1.93 (1.29–2.88)	0.001
Roof material				
Palm leaves/nipa	173 (50.0%)	207 (62.4%)	1.85 (1.14–3.01)	0.013
Galvanized iron/cement	173 (50.0%)	125 (37.6%)	Reference	
Barangay variance			0.10 (0.01–1.25)	
Household variance			1.82 (0.91–3.64)	

4. Discussion

The current WHO strategy for intestinal helminths in children is to continually treat pre-school and school-age children at high risk once or twice per year depending on prevalence [8]. This is effective in achieving morbidity control; however, it does not prevent re-infection. Our study area has participated in national control efforts for over two decades yet the prevalence of helminth infection remains stubbornly high due largely to poverty and malnutrition. In our study, we found that approximately 85% of the rural children were infected with one or more helminth infections. *T. trichiura* infections (71.4%) were found to be more prevalent than *A. lumbricoides* (54.4%) infections. Moreover, about half (49%) of the study sample were stunted and almost a third (28%) were wasted. Stunted children were more likely to be male, older in age (10–14 years), and living in poorer households with palm leaves/nipa roofs.

In the mixed-effect logistic regression model for stunting all of the nutrition factors (i.e., grams) were found not to be significantly associated with stunting. However, we previously found a significant association between the coinfection of all four helminthiases and low intakes of energy, thiamine, and riboflavin among children, when the recommended energy and nutrient intake (RENI) for total calories was examined [21]. Thiamine and riboflavin deficiencies are common in Northern Samar, where dairy and meat intakes are low and mostly rice-based meals are consumed [21]. Iron deficiency has been associated with impairments in both adaptive and innate immunity and with lowering the body's resistance to infectious diseases [21]. Poor nutrient intake may increase susceptibility to parasitic diseases and together they negatively affect the nutritional status of children and adolescents [21].

We believe that a deworming program must be coupled with a nutrition program at the primary school level. Children are presently eating 1–2 meals per day at home and this is insufficient to meet their macro or micronutrient requirements. An additional meal at school appears to be of paramount importance for those severely malnourished. In order to address this problem the Philippine government has initiated the school-based feeding program called '*Gulayan sa Paaralan*', which has been successfully piloted in approximately one percent of schools. However, to date it has not been formally evaluated in a clinical trial.

An appropriate eight-week micronutrient weaning period of 'ready-to-use therapeutic foods' (RUTF), with demonstrated immune-modulating functions—including iron, zinc, calcium, vitamin A, B and C, n-3 and n-6 fatty acids—also needs to be considered following the macronutrient school intervention. In a recent pilot study conducted at the Philippine General Hospital, the researchers created their modified version of RUTF from commercially-available ingredients including milk, sugar, coconut oil, and peanut butter [28]. A total of 100 children (aged 18 months to 10 years) was randomized to either a RUTF group, who received the supplement, and a control group, who did not [28]. The treatment group received RUTF on weekdays for five weeks. Changes in weight, height, and arm circumference were recorded for five weeks and two weeks after supplementation. Results of the study showed that RUTF was an effective, safe, and acceptable alternative supplement for children with mild to severe malnutrition [28].

Annual or biannual albendazole treatment (i.e., 400 mg) needs to be combined with macro/micronutrient supplements, WASH, and health education in order to interrupt the life cycles of STH diseases, prevent reinfection, and achieve sustainable control. A well-nourished population, with an intact immune system, has a better chance of warding off future parasitic infection. Simply providing drugs to malnourished populations, which is a common practice in the global control of STHs, is not the answer. Both poverty and malnutrition must be addressed if future MDA programs for NTDs are to have a lasting impact.

Acknowledgments: We thank the Australian National Health and Medical Research Council for providing financial support for this research in the Philippines.

Author Contributions: A.G.R. and K.P. conceived and designed the experiments; A.G.R., K.P. and R.L.-C. performed the field studies; S.-K.N, T.N.C. and M.T.I. analyzed and interpreted the data; all authors contributed to writing the paper.

References

1. Bethony, J.; Brooker, S.; Albonico, M.; Geiger, S.M.; Loukas, A.; Diemert, D.; Hotez, P.J. Soil-transmitted helminth infections: Ascariasis, trichuriasis, and hookworm. *Lancet* **2006**, *367*, 1521–1532. [CrossRef]
2. Hotez, P.J. Mass drug administration and integrated control for the world's high-prevalence neglected tropical diseases. *Clin. Pharmacol. Ther.* **2009**, *85*, 659–664. [CrossRef] [PubMed]
3. Brooker, S.; Hotez, P.J.; Bundy, D.A. Hookworm-related anaemia among pregnant women: A systematic review. *PLoS Negl. Trop. Dis.* **2008**, *2*, e291. [CrossRef] [PubMed]
4. Miguel, E.A.; Kremer, M. Worms: Identifying impacts on education and health in the presence of treatment externalities. *Econometrica* **2004**, *72*, 159–217. [CrossRef]
5. Sakti, H.; Nokes, C.; Hertanto, W.S.; Hendratno, S.; Hall, A.; Bundy, D.A. Evidence for an association between hookworm infection and cognitive function in Indonesia school children. *Trop. Med. Int. Health* **1999**, *4*, 322–334. [CrossRef] [PubMed]
6. Nokes, C.; Grantham-McGregor, S.M.; Sawyer, A.W.; Cooper, E.S.; Robinson, B.A.; Bundy, D.A. Moderate to heavy infections of *Trichuris trichiura* affect cognitive function in Jamaican school children. *Parasitology* **1992**, *104*, 539–547. [CrossRef] [PubMed]
7. Hotez, P. Hookworm and poverty. *Ann. N. Y. Acad. Sci.* **2008**, *1136*, 38–44. [CrossRef] [PubMed]
8. World Health Organization (WHO). *Deworming for Health and Development*; Report of the Third Global Meeting of the Partners for Parasite Control; World Health Organization: Geneva, Switzerland, 2005.
9. World Health Organization (WHO). *Priority Communicable Diseases: Health in Asian and the Pacific*; Chapter 7; World Health Organization: Geneva, Switzerland, 2008.
10. Belizario, V.Y., Jr.; de Leon, W.U.; Lumampao, Y.F.; Anastacio, M.B.; Tai, C.M. Sentinel surveillance of soil-transmitted helminthiases in selected local government units in the Philippines. *Asia Pac. J. Public Health* **2009**, *21*, 26. [CrossRef] [PubMed]
11. Easton, A. Intestinal worms impair child health in the Philippines. *BMJ* **1999**, *318*, 214. [CrossRef] [PubMed]
12. Reilly, L.; Nausch, N.; Midzi, N.; Mduluza, T.; Mutapi, F. Association between micronutrients (vitamin A, D, iron) and schistosome-specific cytokine responses in Zimbabweans exposed to *Schistosoma haematobium*. *J. Parasitol. Res.* **2012**, *2012*, 128628. [CrossRef] [PubMed]
13. Zhou, H.; Ohtsuka, R.; He, Y.; Yuan, L.; Yamauchi, T.; Sleigh, A.C. Impact of parasitic infections and dietary intake on child growth in the schistosomiasis-endemic Dongting Lake Region, China. *Am. J. Trop. Med. Hyg.* **2005**, *72*, 534–539. [PubMed]
14. Hesham, M.S.; Edariah, A.B.; Norhayati, M. Intestinal parasitic infections and micronutrient deficiency: A review. *Med. J. Malaysia* **2004**, *59*, 284–293. [PubMed]

15. Katona, P.; Katona-Apte, J. The interaction between nutrition and infection. *Clin. Infect. Dis.* **2008**, *46*, 1582–1588. [CrossRef] [PubMed]
16. Cunningham-Rundles, S.; McNeeley, D.F.; Moon, A. Mechanisms of nutrient modulation of the immune response. *J. Allergy Clin. Immunol.* **2005**, *115*, 1119–1128. [CrossRef] [PubMed]
17. Nga, T.T.; Winichagoon, P.; Dijkhuizen, M.A.; Khan, N.C.; Wasantwisut, E.; Wieringa, F.T. Decreased parasite load and improved cognitive outcomes caused by deworming and consumption of multi-micronutrient fortified biscuits in rural Vietnamese schoolchildren. *Am. J. Trop. Med. Hyg.* **2011**, *85*, 333–340. [CrossRef] [PubMed]
18. Amare, B.; Ali, J.; Moges, B.; Yismaw, G.; Belyhun, Y.; Gebretsadik, S.; Woldeyohannes, D.; Tafess, K.; Abate, E.; Endris, M.; et al. Nutritional status, intestinal parasite infection and allergy among school children in northwest Ethiopia. *BMC Pediatr.* **2013**, *13*, 7. [CrossRef] [PubMed]
19. Sanza, M.; Totanes, F.I.; Chua, P.L.; Belizario, V.Y., Jr. Monitoring the impact of a mebendazole mass drug administration initiative for soil transmitted helminthiasis (STH) control in the Western Visayas region of the Philippines from 2007 through 2011. *Acta Trop.* **2013**, *127*, 112–117. [CrossRef] [PubMed]
20. Belizario, V.Y., Jr.; Totanes, F.I.; de Leon, W.U.; Lumampao, Y.F.; Ciro, R.N. Soil transmitted helminth and other intestinal parasitic infections among school children in indigenous people communities in Davao del Norte, Philippines. *Acta Trop.* **2011**, *120* (Suppl. S1), S12–S18. [CrossRef] [PubMed]
21. Papier, K.; Williams, G.M.; Frauk, A.; Olveda, R.M.; McManus, D.P.; Harn, D.A.; Li, Y.S.; Gray, D.J.; Chau, T.N.P.; Ross, A.G. Chronic malnutrition and parasitic helminth interations. *Clin. Infect. Dis.* **2014**, *59*, 234–243. [CrossRef] [PubMed]
22. Ross, A.G.; Olveda, R.M.; Chy, D.; Olveda, D.U.; Li, Y.; Harn, D.A.; Gray, D.J.; McManus, D.P.; Tallo, V.; Chau, T.N.; et al. Can mass drug administration lead to the sustainable control of schistosomiasis? *J. Infect. Dis.* **2015**, *211*, 283–289. [CrossRef] [PubMed]
23. Gibson, R.S. *Principles of Nutritional Assessment*, 2nd ed.; Oxford University Press: New York, NY, USA, 2005.
24. World Health Organization (WHO). *WHO AnthroPlus for Personal Computers Manual: Software for Assessing Growth of the World's Children and Adolescent*; World Health Organization: Geneva, Switzerland, 2009.
25. World Health Organization (WHO). *WHO AnthroPlus Software: Software for Assessing Growth and Development of the World's Children*; World Health Organization: Geneva, Switzerland, 2007.
26. Philippine Statistics Authority. National Statistical Coordination Board, Department of Science and Technology: Taguig, Philippines, 1997; p. 163.
27. Food and Nutrition Research Institute. *Recommended Energy and Nutrient Intakes*; Department of Science and Technology: Taguig, Metro Manila, Philippines, 2002; p. 423.
28. Laylo-Navarr, C.; Limos, E. A randomized controlled trial on the efficacy and safety of a modified ready to use therapeutic food among malnourished children. *Acta Med. Philipp.* **2011**, *45*, 29–33.

7

The Mite-Gallery Unit: A New Concept for Describing Scabies through Entodermoscopy

Gaetano Scanni

MD Dermatologist, Dipartimento di Medicina dei Servizi ASL Bari, Via Vico Traversa 11, 70127 Bari, Italy; gaetano.scanni@alice.it

Abstract: Scabies has always represented a diagnostic challenge for dermatologists, especially in subclinical cases or in atypical ones due to the coexistence of other diseases. Fortunately, dermatoscopy has enabled easier and faster in situ diagnosis. The aim of this study is to examine old and new dermatoscopic signs that *Sarcoptes scabiei* produces on the skin during its whole life cycle through *entodermoscopy* (dermatoscopy with an entomological focus) which, unlike traditional optical microscope examination, allows the local micro-environment to be preserved intact. Patients were enrolled during outbreaks of scabies from hospitals or nursing homes for the elderly in Bari (Italy). The study was performed applying both immersion and polarized dry dermatoscopy. The systematic use of dermatoscopy highlighted the morphological complexity of the *Sarcoptes* tunnel that had been described previously as a simple unitary structure. On the contrary, it is possible to distinguish three separate segments of the burrow that introduce a new anatomo-functional concept called the Mite-Gallery Unit (MGU). This approach, based on the mite life cycle and local skin turnover (the latter usually being ignored), allows the dermatologist to recognize not only *Sarcoptes* using the gallery, but also new descriptors including tunnels without *Sarcoptes*, those with acari alone, and those with associated signs of inflammation. The diagnosis of scabies using optical microscopy until recently has always involved demonstrating the mite and its products outside the human body (on a glass slide) without taking into account exactly what happens within the epidermis. Entodermoscopy is a term used to encapsulate both the presence of the parasite, the usual target of microscopy, and the changes produced in the superficial layers of the epidermis in situ. Thus, the scabies tunnel or burrow can be shown to be composed of three parts, the Head, Body, and Tail, in which different events affecting both mite and host develop. The Mite-Gallery Unit provides a new anatomical and functional explanation of scabies because it provides a more comprehensive in vivo and in situ dermatoscopic diagnosis. In this respect, dermatoscopy takes into account the behavior of the mite in addition to its interaction with its habitat, the human skin.

Keywords: Mite-Gallery Unit (MGU); Entodermoscopy (EDS); Dry Dermatoscopy (d-DS); Wet Dermatoscopy (w-DS); Enhanced Dermatoscopy (e-DS)

---

1. Introduction

Diagnosis of scabies, even in the presence of objective and subjective epidemiological evidence, requires the detection of mites and their products. In clinical variants or in forms complicated by co-morbidities (diabetes, senile pruritus, neurological syndromes) or side effects of therapy (cortisone, acaricides), the detection of mites is absolutely essential for diagnosis because other clinical clues are unreliable or misleading [1]. The purpose of this article is to demonstrate that, by using entodermoscopy, it is possible to obtain direct and indirect evidence which may improve diagnostic reliability in both ordinary and atypical cases of scabies.

2. Materials and Methods

Two types of dermatoscope were used. The Delta 20 (Heine Optotechnik GmbH & Co. KG Kientalstraße 7, 82211 Herrsching, Germany) uses a glass plate and mineral oil at the skin interface in a mode that will be referred to as wet dermatoscopy (w-DS). The DermLite Pro II (Dermlite, 3Gen, San Juan Capistrano, CA, USA) is a dermatoscope without plate and liquid as it uses a polarized light that blocks the reflections from the epidermis; a side button allows the operator to switch alternately between polarized and normal light. This mode of observation will be referred to as dry dermatoscopy (d-DS). Pictures were obtained using two compact digital cameras: a Minolta G850 (5 Mp 3× optical, Minolta Corp., Osaka, Japan) for the Delta 20 (w-DS) and a Sony W70 (7 Mp 3× optical, Sony Corp., Tokyo, Japan) for the Dermlite (d-DS). The method using a dermatoscope with a digital camera is commonly referred to as digital dermatoscopy. The clinical observations herein are based on 63 patients examined in nursing homes for the elderly or public hospitals in the city of Bari (Italy) during contained outbreaks of scabies over the period 2011–2014.

Photographic documentation was generated after receiving patients' informed consent.

Entodermoscopy as a Diagnostic Tool

Entodermoscopy is a neologism proposed in 2006 by Scanni and Bonifazi for the dermoscopic diagnosis of ectoparasitosis [2], subsequently extended to superficial skin infections by Zalaudek et al. [3]. Entodermoscopy is not only a new term, but, importantly, it represents a different approach to the observation of the relationship between host and parasite for which a deeper knowledge of microbiology, entomology, and behaviour is required. Epiluminescence microscopy can be compared to traditional microscopic examination in which the instrument is resting on the patient to look directly at the skin. Consequently, the mite and its burrow can be observed in situ and in vivo, two conditions that together allow the observer to preserve the local microhabitat which is disassembled by more traditional methods (e.g., optical microscopy). As a tool, entodermoscopy has two major requirements. First, it requires magnifications higher than 10×, which can be achieved in digital dermatoscopy by extending the camera's optical zoom (generally about 3–5×) and in post-production by examining the image (jpg file) in full format. Thanks to the combination of these two steps (maximum optical zoom + full-frame jpg file), sufficient detail is obtained to capture all the features of the tunnel in a mode that can be referred to as enhanced digital dermatoscopy (e-DS). This approach can help the dermatologist when videodermatoscopy is not available. Digital zoom is generally avoided because artifacts (pixelation/noise) are incompatible with a true and reliable image. The second requirement of entodermoscopy is the type of illumination and mode of contact between instrument and skin. The differences between wet contact and dry non-contact dermatoscopy in the case of melanocytic lesions are already known [4]. In the case of parasitosis, polarized dermatoscopes offer the advantage of leaving the microhabitat intact without the need to wet or crush the field of observation. This option is essential with, for example, pathogens such as lice or ticks.

In addition, the alternate switching from normal to polarized light allows a quick comparison between skin texture and structures below it, respectively, as well as the insect's cuticle and internal organs, accurately completing the morphological and topographical reconstruction. The new findings described in this article derive from the comparative use of different dermatoscopes and light sources.

3. Results

In health facilities where scabies has already been diagnosed and treated, the main objective is often to understand if persistent itching is caused by the side effects of acaricides (e.g., benzyl benzoate), pre-existing co-morbidities, failure of therapy, or re-infestation. Since direct examination is not always sufficient to resolve these questions and optical microscopy is time consuming, any other instrumental help, including dermatoscopy, is worthy of attention and investigation. The methodical use of dermatoscopes has led to the introduction of a list of eight points, some already known and others previously undescribed, as an innovative morphological/functional key.

3.1. Definition of the Mite-Gallery Unit (MGU)

Generally, the burrow of scabies is described as a linear formation a few millimeters in length that has always been considered a unitary structure (Figure 1).

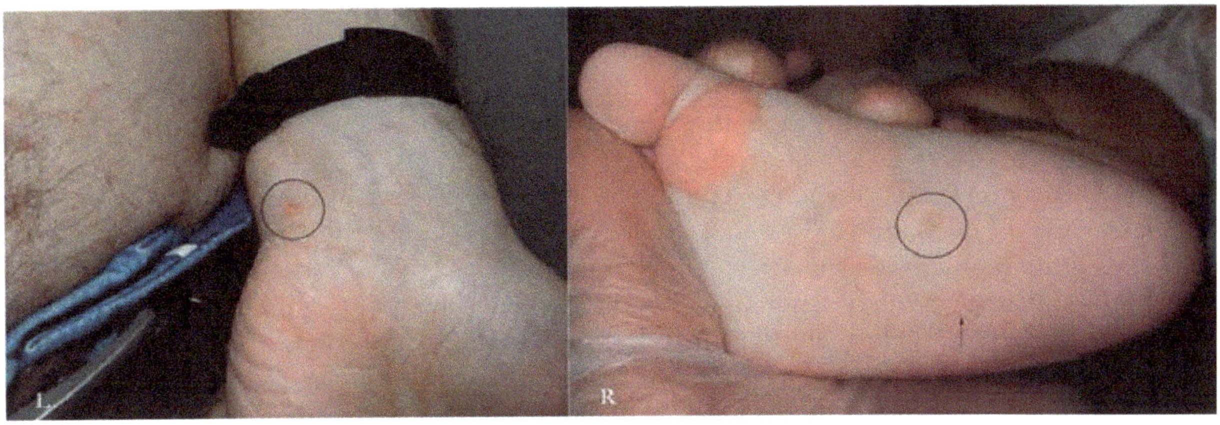

Figure 1. Objective examination of scabies in adults (L) and children (R).

An intact burrow is a whitish, slightly raised linear structure with a tortuous path a few millimeters long set against a variably erythematous background (circles, L-R). The appearance is pathognomonic. However, scratching that partially or completely destroys it can change its macroscopic and dermatoscopic appearance (arrow, R).

Dermatoscopy reveals different *anatomical and functional* sections determined by both the mite life cycle and host epidermal turnover usually not taken into consideration but, none the less, able to affect the morphology of the tunnel itself. The gallery can be divided into three contiguous segments—Head, Body, and Tail—that together provide a new set of diagnostic markers called the Mite-Gallery Unit (MGU) (Figure 2).

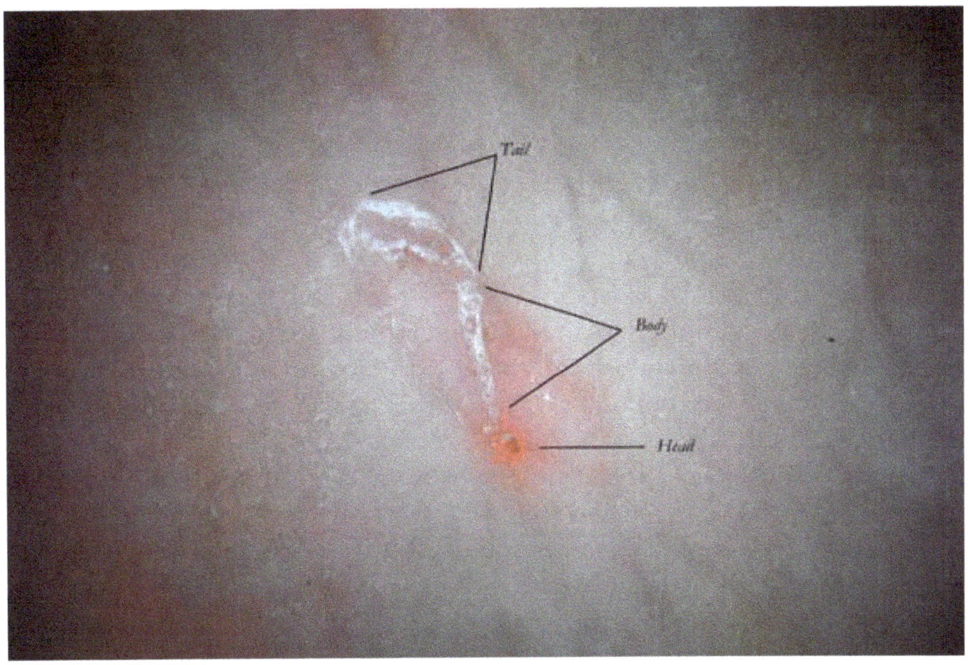

Figure 2. The Mite-Gallery Unit (MGU) in non-polarized dry dermatoscopy (d-DS).

The Mite-Gallery Unit (MGU) structure can be divided into three parts: the *Head* hosting the mite; the *Body*, which represents what is clinically defined as the burrow containing the eggs and feces of the parasite; and the *Tail* at the end of the tunnel, which provides an incomplete structure as it is without a roof but is made of keratin collarettes, visible only in d-DS. Erythema may be present in the background around and immediately behind the mite.

The dermatoscopic observation should preferably be conducted at magnifications between 10 and 30× with different results depending on whether a liquid interface (wet dermatoscopy) or dry skin surface free from the compression of the plate (dry dermatoscopy) are used.

The MGU Head houses the mite which is visible due to its refractile area located anteriorly between the buccal apparatus (*gnatosoma*) and the second pair of legs. It appears as a dark "V" formation with the vertex that indicates the point of progression of the tunnel towards the healthy skin. In this segment, the roof of the tunnel is intact.

The MGU Body represents the longest part of the entire tunnel and appears white if observed with wet dermatoscopy. In this segment, the roof of the tunnel is no longer intact because it is interrupted by holes at roughly regular intervals.

The MGU Tail is the terminal segment of the tunnel even if the roof is completely absent. This part can only be identified in dry dermatoscopy as this is able to define the edges of the tunnel in the form of small desquamatory collarettes. In w-DS the liquid medium prevents these from being visible, which explains why in previous studies this morphological variation was not reported.

The first description of the tunnel compared its appearance to that of a jet plane with delta wings followed by a white trail as a result of observation under wet dermatoscopy [5]. The observation of this phenomenon, however, was not accompanied by any functional interpretation. Entodermoscopy by studying the microstructure of the three components of the tunnel explains the "jet trail" effect as the interaction between the liquid interface and air contained in the tunnel that, due to the pressure of the dermatoscope, emerges from the small holes of the roof, forming a strip of small reflective bubbles under the optical plate.

In fact, if dry dermatoscopy is used, the white trail is no longer visible and only a tunnel can be observed whose roof is interrupted by several openings from which air escapes if compressed (Figure 3).

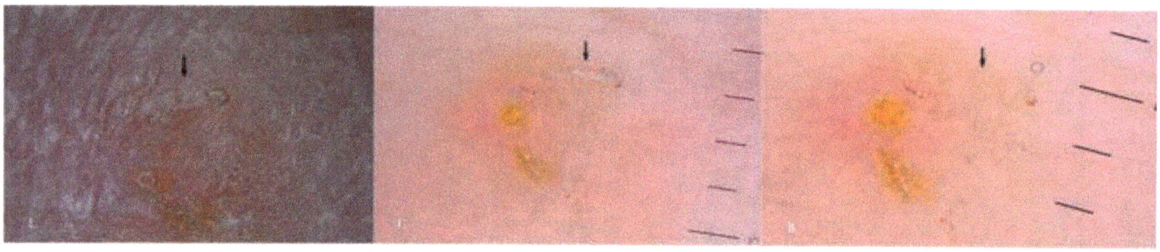

Figure 3. Dry dermatoscopy vs. wet dermatoscopy (w-DS) of the same Mite-Gallery Unit.

When viewed using d-DS, the roof of the tunnel appears to be interrupted by several holes that allow air to exit (L). The first description of an MGU resembling a white jet trail was due to trapped air between the tunnel and the glass plate used in the w-DS (C). Under continued pressure, this picture disappears as all of air bubbles are pushed away and the liquid medium passes inside (R). Beneath there is a collection of serum that reflects the LEDs of the dermatoscope (L).

Another consequence of these holes, not previously described in the literature, is that the microbubble trail is by no means a persistent sign as it disappears when MGU observation is repeated several times or for excessive time in the wet modality. After the first contact with the dermatoscope, all the air inside the tunnel will be largely dispersed on the surface and replaced by the interface fluid; this makes the roof indistinguishable from the surrounding skin (Figure 3 R). In this situation, the tunnel body can only be recognized because of the head that houses the *Sarcoptes*, reducing the local diagnostic sensitivity which relies on the tunnel's refractability. Therefore, in order to obtain good photographic documentation in w-DS of an intact MGU, it is necessary to keep the microbubbles under the plate without breaking off skin contact and to avoid repeating the viewing session. However, if air leakage decreases the dermatoscopic sensitivity as regards the external structure of the MGU, it provides ideal conditions to better observe the internal components of the tunnel (local diagnostic specificity).

3.2. Content of the Gallery and Other Markers of the Mite

Thanks to the higher magnifications (e-DS) and to the fact that the roof of the tunnel in w-DS becomes transparent when liquid medium is inside, it is possible to distinguish, with sufficient clarity, the eggs of the *Sarcoptes* located behind the mite. The oval eggs are grouped at a short distance from each other with a major axis that is generally at right angles to that of the MGU, which also allows the edges of the embryo inside to be glimpsed, if enlarged further. In this part of the gallery there are also the parasite's feces derived by the digestion of keratin and cellular fluids; under the optical microscope, feces usually appear as dark refractile dots (stercoraceous bullets), whereas under dermatoscopy, they appear as small white-gray spheres (Figure 4).

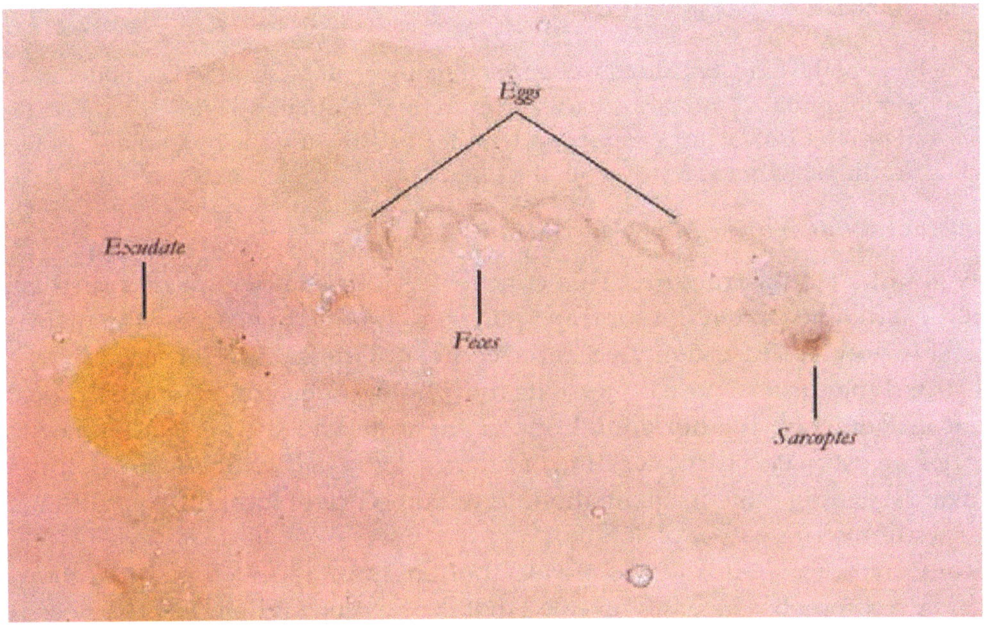

Figure 4. Content of the gallery. An MGU in enhanced wet dermatoscopy mode.

The absence of bubbles and the penetration of the liquid film into the tunnel makes the roof transparent and allows one to glimpse the row of eggs, which is otherwise not easily visible. The white dots are the feces of the mite. A seropurulent exudate is located to the left.

If the examiner is interested in studying the inside of the tunnel, he/she must use wet dermatoscopy and make sure that all the air in the tunnel is extruded, pushing the dermatoscope plate several times onto the skin to ensure entry of the liquid medium.

It is commonly thought that the only visible part of the mite in w-DS is the front end, in the shape of a "V" which corresponds to the *gnatosoma* and the first pair of legs. But enhanced dermatoscopy allows the identification of novel structures on the body of the *Sarcoptes scabiei* that, under conditions of optimal magnification, show some visible refraction. These are mechano-sensory structures [6] located on the back of the mite called "bristles" (*spine-like type*) whose thicker bases (*sockets*) appear under a dermatoscope as fine brown dots (*ladybird sign*). This feature, not yet reported in the literature, is a good example of convergence between dermatoscopy and entomology. Even the body of the mite, which is usually transparent, can be distinguished by the slight opalescence of its cuticle under enhanced wet dermatoscopy (Figure 5).

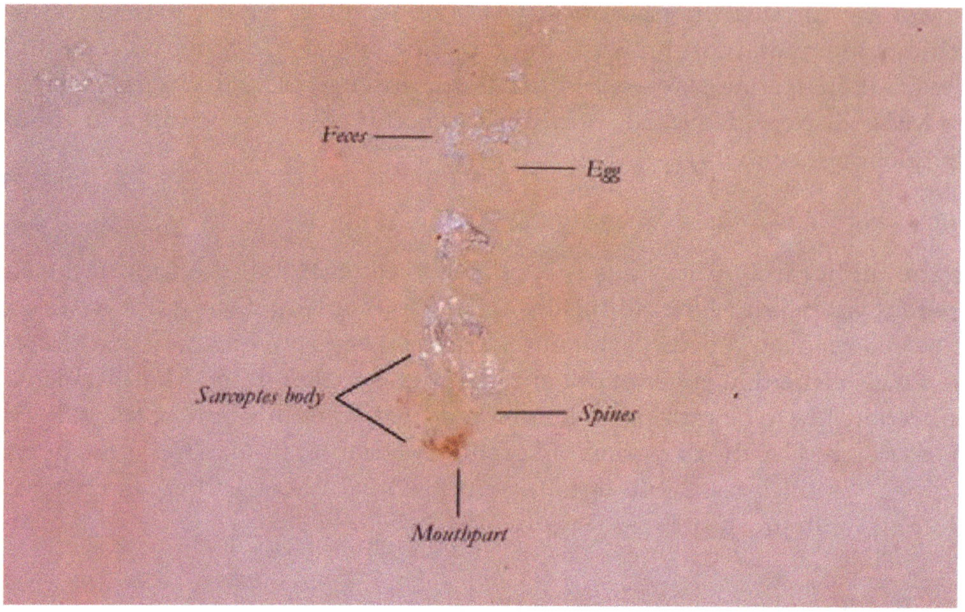

Figure 5. The Body of the mite. Enhanced wet dermatoscopy of an MGU in w-DS mode. In addition to refraction of its anterior part, *Sarcoptes scabiei* shows an opalescent body with several scattered dark dots (*ladybird sign*). These structures correspond to the "bristles" on the body that enable, amongst other things, the adherence of the mite within the tunnel.

3.3. Spatio-Temporal Evolution of the Mite-Gallery Unit

The MGU is not a static structure. This concept is not usually explored further because it is irrelevant to clinical diagnosis. On the contrary, patterns change if we access the microscopic details that are appreciable only in situ and in vivo in the context of the entodermoscopy.

The MGU is a dynamic structure because its morphology derives from a reciprocal interference of two different movements: the horizontal one of the mite and the vertical one of the epidermis. The epidermis has an estimated turnover time of around 45 days [7] during which the cellular layers are pushed upwards, ending with desquamation. In the presence of local inflammation (e.g., psoriasis) the upwards growth rate is greatly accelerated.

Histologically, the scabies burrow was always thought to be allocated in the *stratum corneum* even though confocal microscopy has recently revealed that the *Sarcoptes* mite is located closer to the *stratum spinosum* [8].

The integrity of the tunnel is therefore subordinate to the mite's ability to maintain the same height in the epidermis to resist the tangential (rubbing) and elastic (contraction and distension) forces that act on the skin during the natural movements of the human body. The mite must out of necessity compensate for the direction of growth of the epidermis [9] in order to protected itself, but especially to ensure that the eggs can hatch just inside the tunnel. It follows that the tunnel represents two different time sequences depending on the point being observed, with the head being the newest part and the tail the initial and oldest part.

Therefore, as a dynamic structure the gallery moves closer to the skin surface with the passing of time and is at its most superficial at the tail where the roof becomes thin enough to collapse under the effect of the forces acting on it [10]. For this reason, near the tail there is no longer an intact tunnel but, rather, the borders of its base as collarettes visible only with dry dermatoscopy. Entodermoscopy, through linking the local factors of the host to the biology of the parasite, highlights an anatomic and functional difference of the MGU not previously appreciated under conditions of ordinary optical microscopy which cannot provide a detailed view of the mite's whole microenvironment. Dermatoscopy instead reveals that the MGU is a dynamic entity in terms of both space (elongation phase) and time (maturation phase).

The collapsed roof is the result of an autonomous phenomenon and cannot be attributed to the scratching by the host as that would also destroy the other parts of the gallery rather than a very small part of it (the tail). This is further confirmed by the fact that the skin immediately around and adjacent to the tail remains intact (Figure 2).

3.4. MGU Perforated Roof

As mentioned above, the roof of the MGU body is interrupted by holes (Figure 6). At the moment, the reason for these openings has not been precisely identified [11]. It is possible that they represent the exit sites for the larvae to leave the tunnel, but other explanations cannot be ruled out. The possibility exists that the *Sarcoptes* mite itself pierces the roof to guarantee exchange of air and humidity necessary for hatching the eggs. Another possibility is that the tunnel intercepts the ostia of the sweat glands by separating them from the rest of the duct. In any case, these holes cause the strip of microbubbles under the plate used in wet dermatoscopy to show the pathognomonic appearance of a "jet trail" [5].

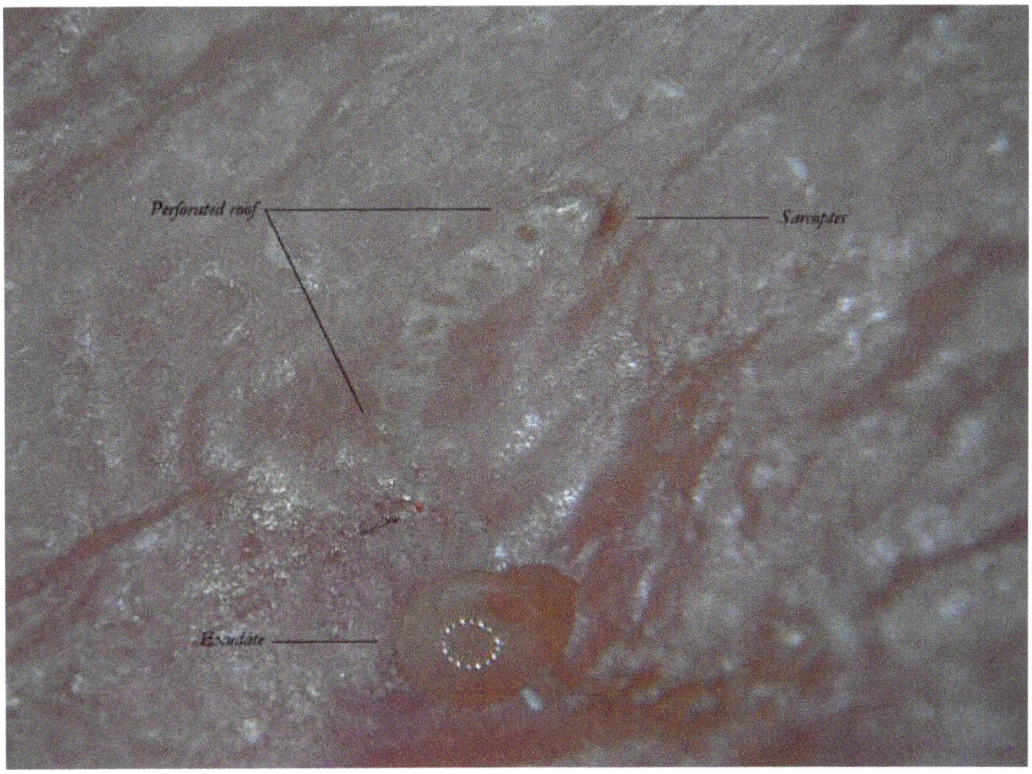

Figure 6. Enhanced dermatoscopy of the MGU's roof in non-polarized dry mode (d-DS). The body of the gallery is not completely intact due to numerous holes which give it a riddled aspect. From these openings the larvae of the *Sarcoptes* are believed to exit. On the right, one can see the reflective front part of the mite. At the bottom, dermatoscope LEDs are reflected on the serous exudate.

3.5. Moulting and Coupling Pockets

The greater part of the MGU consists of the tunnel body where the most important events of the mite life cycle take place. In this segment, eggs are collected and hatch. After about four days, these eggs produce six-legged larvae morphologically similar to a miniature adult [12]. The larvae must undergo two more moults to the eight legged stage (proto/trito nymph) before becoming an adult; this process appears to take place mainly outside the mother tunnel in small niches, called "moulting pockets", dug in order to provide limited shelter. Only when fully developed and after fertilization does the female mite dig a new definitive tunnel as it is known in temperate climates [13].

The moulting pockets, well known to entomologists, present as small dimples in the most superficial layer of the *stratum corneum*; in these, the larvae remain attached, maturing into nymphs and then into the adult [12].

Mating is also performed in a pocket in which the adult female is found by a male whose track is lost afterwards. Normally, these niches are not described in dermatological textbooks because they have no diagnostic relevance and are of dimensions invisible to the naked eye. However, their significance increases if we return to dermatoscopic examination in which they appear as an incomplete MGU composed only of a head without a body and a tail (Figure 7), regardless of the dermatoscope used. The preferred mode of observation is still the d-DS with normal or polarized light.

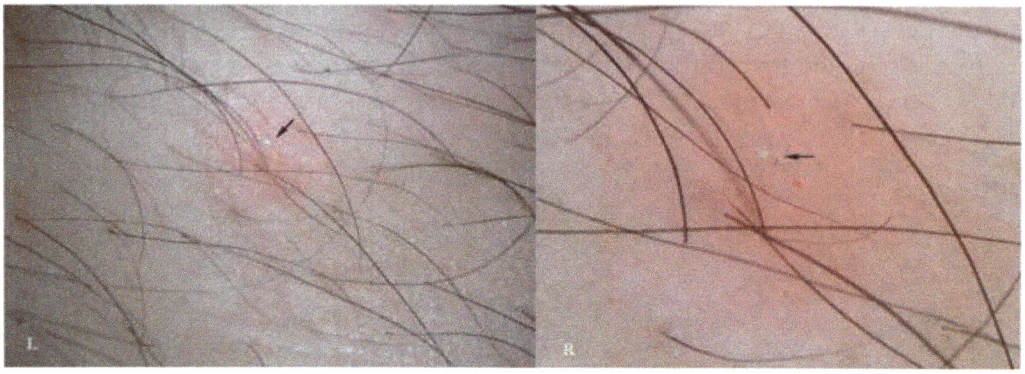

Figure 7. Moulting pocket in dry dermatoscopy with non-polarized (L) and polarized light (R). In this structure the complete Mite-Gallery Unit does not develop because the mite remains stationary until the moulting process is completed or mating happens. There is instead only a small whitish raised area (arrows, L-R), corresponding to the whole body of the *Sarcoptes*, behind which a real tunnel is not visible (R). Around the pocket, an area of erythema with blurred borders is easily recognizable.

According to another report, the immature forms, besides digging a niche or pocket from scratch, can also take refuge in the openings of hair follicles [14]. A rash of pseudo-folliculitis is traditionally considered to be a secondary, non-specific symptom in the course of scabies (Figure 8). Assuming that the juvenile mite may shelter in human follicles, too, then the erythematous change associated with them may be regarded as a new "specific" sign. At the moment, personal observations and those of other authors have not been able to identify any traces of immature forms as features of in vivo refraction in these forms are unknown. It is possible that under higher magnification (>200×) these forms may become appreciable if present and visible.

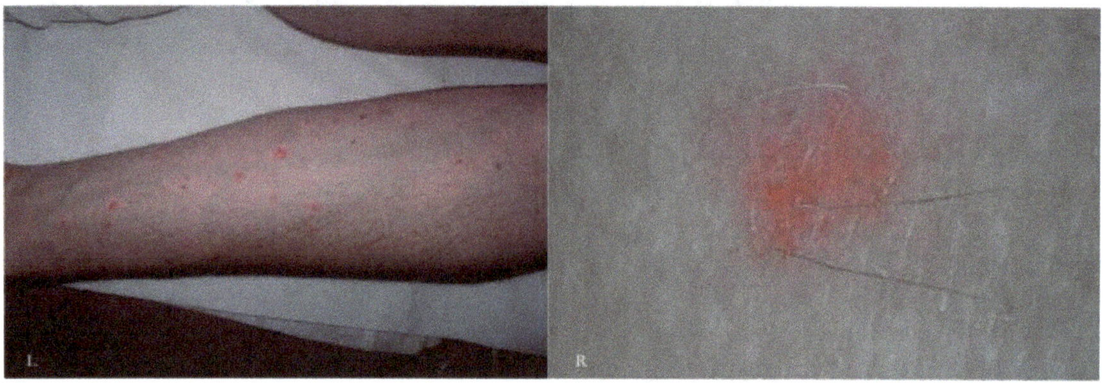

Figure 8. Scabies pseudo-follicular exanthema observed in non-polarized dry dermatoscopy. Folliculitis-like lesions (L) are commonly considered to be a non-specific sign of scabies (L). In dermatoscopy, only a peri-ostial erythematous halo is appreciated with some pinpoint-like vessels inside it (R). There are no signs of a complete or atypical MGU.

3.6. *Inflammatory Response Induced By the MGU*

In a primary infestation, the host's immunity to scabies develops after about four weeks. If we consider only the skin around the MGU, using dermatoscopy we can distinguish different types of response over time and depending on the anatomical sites involved. Generally, there is erythema around the head of the gallery where the mite is located or along the entire length of the MGU.

A vesicular or free exudate appears when the spongiotic inflammatory process [15] reaches the skin surface. If an infection coexists, this phenomenon is more pronounced. Where the skin is thicker, as on the palm of the hand and on the wrist, the exudate remains trapped in the superficial epidermis, forming semitransparent (*dyshidrotic-like*) circular areas [16] that, over time, become superficial as yellowish desquamations (Figure 9). The mite, the feces, and the eggs activate a different humoral and cellular immune response, probably depending on the time of exposure to the antigens that gradually accumulate over the course of the infestation. This reflects the life cycle of the mite.

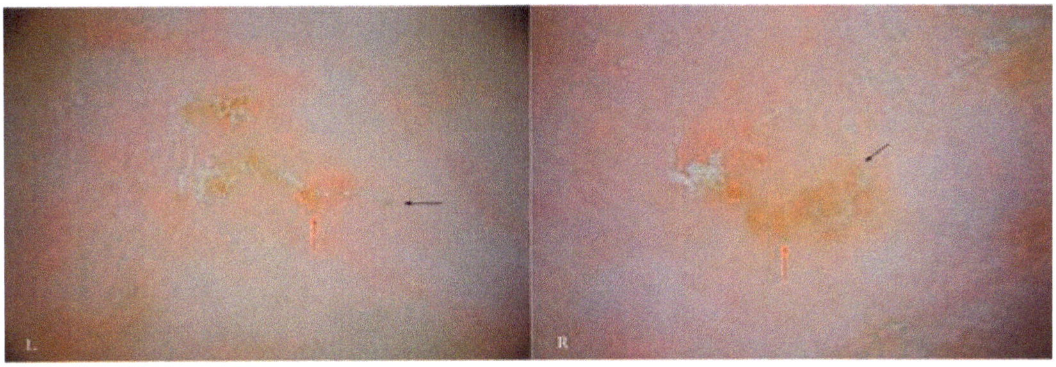

Figure 9. Inflammatory response to an MGU observed under polarized light dry dermatoscopy of a hand lesion. Next to the mite (black arrows, L-R) the skin is normal, while in the central part of the gallery an erythematous halo (red arrow, L) is evident. Immediately behind the mite, inflammation can also occur in microvesicles trapped in the epidermis (red arrow, R). The tail of the gallery is characterized by keratin collarettes.

In other cases, the inflammatory response may be nodular as in the buttocks, genital, and flexural regions. This phenomenon, known for its resistant pruritic symptoms, is interpreted as the effect of cell-mediated hyperreactivity to mite antigens [17] even if scrapings for mites are generally negative. Dermatoscopy, however, can identify the parasite, especially in the initial phases of the formation of nodules compared to the older lesions (Figure 10). Serial dermatoscopic observations could clarify the exact progression of the host's local immune response, probably stimulated by deeper penetration of antigens (intradermal) in areas undergoing physical pressure.

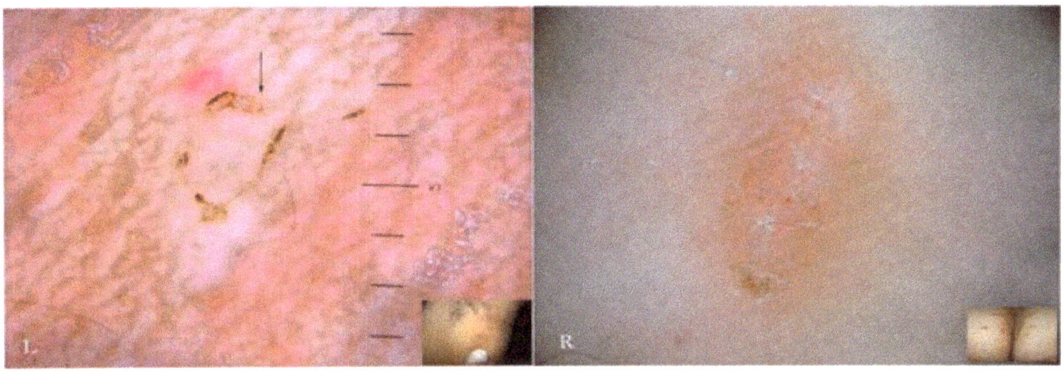

Figure 10. Nodular scabies observed in wet (L) and dry polarized light (R) dermatoscopy. A mite is easily recognizable in one of the axillary (insert) papules of a subject of African ethnicity (arrow, L). A buttock (insert) nodule present for a few weeks appears uninhabited instead (R).

3.7. Morphological Variants of the MGU

The linear MGU is not the only expression of the mite in the host skin–parasite interaction. There are forms of "atypical MGUs" in which only the head of the gallery is recognizable but not the body because it is partly or completely replaced by erosions or polycyclic scales (Figures 11 and 12). These morphological variants develop in areas where local exudative or hyperkeratotic inflammatory reactions have occurred; this fact must be kept in mind because, although they appear clinically to be secondary lesions, this can be excluded by the dermatoscopic examination. The preferred mode of observation is dry dermatoscopy because it is more sensitive to the surface texture. In fact, as it misses the tunnel, wet dermatoscopy would not show any trail of bubbles and the wet scales could become slightly refractive.

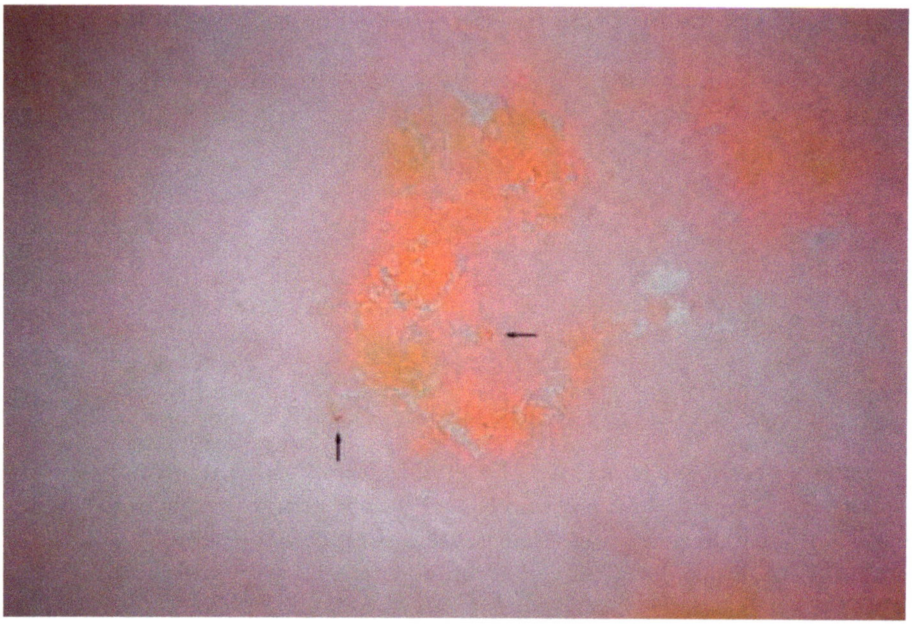

Figure 11. Dry dermatoscopy with polarized light of an atypical MGU. Two mites (arrows) can be recognized behind which there is no tunnel but an erythematous area with polycyclic borders.

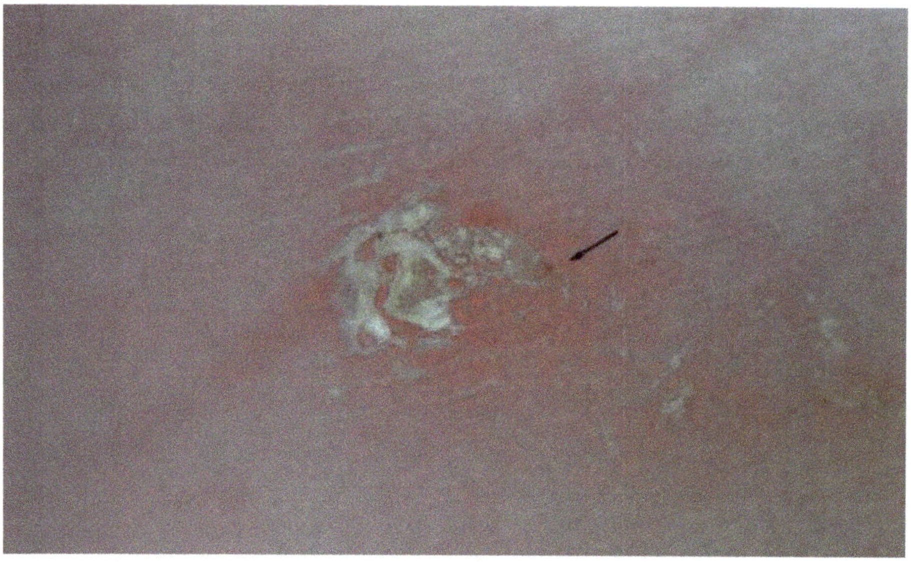

Figure 12. Dry dermatoscopy with non-polarized light of an atypical MGU. The refractive part of the mite (arrow) is evident, behind which there is an aggregate of scales rather than an ordinary gallery.

3.8. MGU Evolution at the End of the Mite Life Cycle or After Therapy

When the formation of new parts of the tunnel ceases, due to therapy or termination of the mite's life cycle, after a few days, all the MGUs will be remodeled and replaced only by traces in the form of polycyclic keratinised outlines appearing like a "*ghost gallery*". Post-inflammatory phenomena and local superinfection can also contribute to their formation. Detection of phantom galleries might be useful in assessing scabies when the therapeutic outcome is uncertain, or in the absence of active MGUs, to confirm the success of a therapy, itching being a subjectively variable criterion (Figure 13).

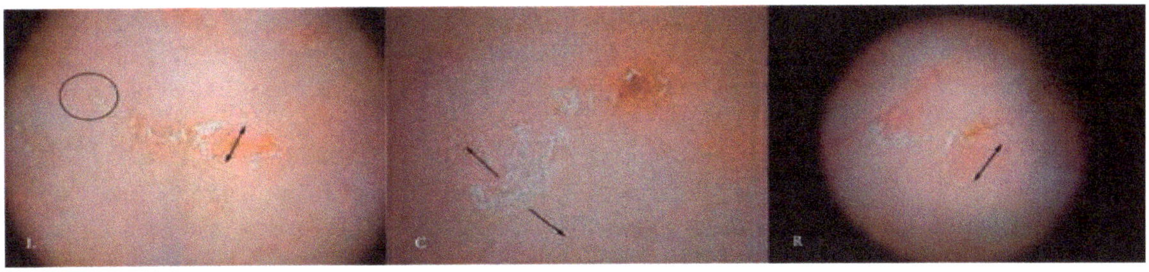

Figure 13. Evolution of an MGU towards a "ghost gallery" under polarized dry dermatoscopy. Three different examples. A mature MGU ends with a tail made up of keratinised collarettes that progressively move away from each other (black arrow, L). *Sarcoptes* is identifiable in the front part of the burrow (circle, L). When the mite is at the end of its life cycle or after therapy, the other parts of the tunnel undergo the normal processes of remodelling of the skin (C), forming the thin and polycyclic keratinic edges of a ghost gallery (C/R).

4. Discussion and Conclusions

Since dermatoscopy provides the description of the only pathognomonic sign of scabies (the burrow) as "delta wing plane + jet trail" [5], dermatologists have tried to replace the traditional scraping test with a faster dermatoscopic diagnosis which is more patient friendly [18].

The mite together with its tunnel is an important high diagnostic feature, but the global diagnostic sensitivity remains low because burrows, during clinical examination, are visible in only about 20% of patients [19]. In this article, the effect of *Sarcoptes* on and within the skin is described as an anatomical and functional entity, that is dynamic in both space and time. This is called the Mite-Gallery Unit (MGU), which consists of a head, body, and tail that take on a definable role in the production of the earlier and later dermatoscopic semeiotics of the insect's life cycle.

This setting allows us to add new diagnostic descriptors in which *Sarcoptes* can be recognized in exudative, hyperkeratotic, and nodular lesions clinically considered to be non-specific but which, on the contrary, are useful sites for dermatoscopic examination.

To detect these signs, it is necessary to use both dry polarized and wet dermatoscopy helped by specific maneuvers to make the outside and inside of the tunnel visible (local diagnostic specificity).

Thanks to entodermoscopy, two other parts of the mite (spines and body cuticle) can be identified, making the diagnosis more reliable even when the *acarus* is not associated with a visible tunnel. The juvenile forms hitherto excluded from the diagnosis can be detected in superficial epidermal *pockets* whose pathological effects are still unknown. Considering human skin turnover is an integral element in the diagnosis it is possible to follow the fate of the MGU even when, at the end of its life cycle, the mite no longer forms new parts of the tunnel but a "phantom" imprint remains nonetheless.

No traditional microscopic examination has ever produced a detailed anatomical and functional description of the tunnel such as the one obtained via entodermoscopy. The principles and rationale of entodermoscopy are very close to a behavioural approach as they involve the study of the acari, while taking care not to modify the local habitat—something that is a feature of traditional optical microscope examinations in scabies and other ectoparasitoses.

A new instrument (*entodermoscope*) with higher magnification (>200×), different light source options (normal/polarized/tangential), and micromanipulators operating in the field of examination could add valuable information as yet unknown. Meanwhile, entodermoscopy provides a new vision of the host–parasite relationship which will benefit diagnosis and as seems likely, in the future, our understanding of transmission and the assessment of innovative preventive or therapeutic strategies.

References

1. Richey, H.K.; Fenske, N.A.; Cohen, L.E. Scabies: Diagnosis and management. *Hosp. Pract.* **1986**, *21*, 124. [CrossRef]
2. Scanni, G.; Bonifazi, E. Viability of the head louse eggs in pediculosis capitis. A dermoscopy study. *Eur. J. Pediat. Dermatol.* **2006**, *16*, 201–204.
3. Zalaudek, I.; Giacomel, J.; Cabo, H.; Di Stefani, A.; Ferrara, G.; Hofmann-Wellenhof, R.; Malvehy, J.; Puig, S.; Stolz, W.; Argenziano, G. Entodermoscopy: A new tool for diagnosing skin infections and infestations. *Dermatology* **2008**, *216*, 14–23. [CrossRef] [PubMed]
4. Benvenuto-Andrade, C.; Dusza, S.W.; Agero, A.L.; Scope, A.; Rajadhyaksha, M.; Halpern, A.C.; Marghoob, A.A. Differences between polarized light dermoscopy and immersion contact dermoscopy for the evaluation of skin lesions. *Arch. Dermatol.* **2007**, *143*, 329–338. [CrossRef] [PubMed]
5. Argenziano, G.; Fabbrocini, G.; Delfino, M. Epiluminescence microscopy. A new approach to in vivo detection of Sarcoptes scabiei. *Arch. Dermatol.* **1997**, *133*, 751–753. [CrossRef] [PubMed]
6. Yoshimura, H.; Ohigashi, T.; Uesugi, M.; Uesugi, K.; Higashikawa, T.; Nakamura, R.; Mori, Y.; Shinohara, K. Sarcoptes scabiei var. hominis: Three-dimensional structure of a female imago and crusted scabies lesions by X-ray micro-CT. *Exp. Parasitol.* **2009**, *122*, 268–272. [CrossRef] [PubMed]
7. Weinstein, G.D.; McCullough, J.L.; Ross, P. Cell Proliferation in Normal Epidermis. *J. Investig. Dermatol.* **1984**, *82*, 623–628. [CrossRef] [PubMed]
8. Levi, A.; Mumcuoglu, K.Y.; Ingber, A.; Enk, C.D. Detection of living Sarcoptes scabiei larvae by reflectance mode confocal microscopy in the skin of a patient with crusted scabies. *J. Biomed. Opt.* **2012**, *17*, 060503. [CrossRef] [PubMed]
9. Arlian, L.G.; Morgan, M.S. A review of Sarcoptes scabiei: Past, present and future. *Parasites Vectors* **2017**, *10*, 297. [CrossRef] [PubMed]
10. Mellanby, K. *Biology of the Parasite in: Scabies*; Oxford University Press: London, UK, 1943; Chapter 2; p. 9.
11. Fimiani, M.; Mazzatenta, C.; Alessandrini, C.; Paccagnini, E.; Andreassi, L. The behaviour of Sarcoptes scabiei var. hominis in human skin: An ultrastructural study. *J. Submicrosc. Cytol. Pathol.* **1997**, *29*, 105–113. [PubMed]
12. Arlian, L.G. Biology, host relations, and epidemiology of Sarcoptes scabiei. *Annu. Rev. Entomol.* **1989**, *34*, 139–161. [CrossRef] [PubMed]
13. Meinking, T.L. Infestations. *Curr. Probl. Dermatol.* **1999**, *11*, 106–107. [CrossRef]
14. Varma, M.R.G. Ticks and mites. In *Medical Insects and Arachnids*; Lane, R.P., Crosskey, R.W., Eds.; Springer: Dordrecht, The Netherlands, 1993; pp. 597–658.
15. Falk, E.S.; Eide, T.J. Histologic and clinical findings in human scabies. *Int. J. Dermatol.* **1981**, *20*, 600–605. [CrossRef] [PubMed]
16. Lyell, A. Diagnosis and treatment of scabies. *Br. Med. J.* **1967**, *2*, 223–225. [CrossRef] [PubMed]
17. Bauer, J.; Blum, A.; Sönnichsen, K.; Metzler, G.; Rassner, G.; Garbe, C. Nodular scabies detected by computed dermatoscopy. *Dermatology* **2001**, *203*, 190–191. [CrossRef] [PubMed]
18. Dupuy, A.; Dehen, L.; Bourrat, E.; Lacroix, C.; Benderdouche, M.; Dubertret, L.; Morel, P.; Feuilhade de Chauvin, M.; Petit, A. Accuracy of standard dermoscopy for diagnosing scabies. *J. Am. Acad. Dermatol.* **2007**, *56*, 53–62. [CrossRef] [PubMed]
19. Hewitt, K.A.; Nalabanda, A.; Cassell, J.A. Scabies outbreaks in residential care homes: Factors associated with late recognition, burden and impact. A mixed methods study in England. *Epidemiol. Infect.* **2015**, *143*, 1542–1551. [CrossRef] [PubMed]

8

Advances in the Treatment of Yaws

Michael Marks

Clinical Research Department, London School of Hygiene & Tropical Medicine, Keppel Street, London WC1E 7HT, UK; michael.marks@lshtm.ac.uk;

Abstract: Yaws is one of the three endemic treponematoses and is recognised by the World Health Organization as a neglected tropical disease. Yaws is currently reported in 15 countries in the Pacific, South-East Asia, West and Central Africa, predominantly affects children, and results in destructive lesions of the skin and soft tissues. For most of the twentieth century penicillin-based treatment was the standard of care and resistance to penicillin has still not been described. Recently, oral azithromycin has been shown to be an effective treatment for yaws, facilitating renewed yaws eradication efforts. Resistance to azithromycin is an emerging threat and close surveillance will be required as yaws eradication efforts are scaled up globally.

Keywords: yaws; *Treponema pallidum*

---

1. Introduction

Yaws, caused by *Treponema pallidum* subsp. *pertenue*, is one of the three endemic treponematoses (along with *T.p.* subsp. *endemicum*, the causative agent of bejel, and *T. carateum*, the causative agent of pinta) and is recognised by the World Health Organization as a neglected tropical disease (NTD) [1,2]. The disease predominantly affects children and results in destructive lesions of the skin and soft tissues. Yaws is still found in Africa, South-East Asia and the Pacific. *T.p.* subsp. *pertenue* is closely related to *T.p.* subsp. *pallidum*, the causative agent of syphilis [3] but neither sexual nor mother-to-child transmission of yaws is believed to occur [2].

2. Epidemiology

Yaws is currently reported in 15 countries in the Pacific, South-East Asia, West and Central Africa [4–9]. Currently the most cases are reported in Papua New Guinea, the Solomon Islands and Ghana and all have reported in excess of 15,000 cases in recent years. In the mid-twentieth century, yaws was endemic in South America and the Caribbean, but control programmes in the mid-twentieth century (see below) are believed to have eliminated yaws from the majority of countries in the region [10,11]. India interrupted transmission in 2004 and declared elimination in 2006 [12] following a sustained programme that began in 1996.

Yaws is restricted to warm and humid environments [13]. Transmission is skin to skin contact from active infectious lesions [14]. Early studies had suggested that flies may play a role in transmission but there is no definitive proof that this occurs [14–16]. The majority of active infections cases occur in children aged under 15 years. Closely-related treponemal infections have been identified in primate populations, but zoonotic transmission to humans has not been established [17,18].

3. Clinical Features

As with other treponemal infections, yaws is characterized by a multi-stage disease process predominantly involving skin, bones and cartilage.

The initial stage of primary yaws is the development of an erythematous lesion that occurs at the site of inoculation after an incubation period of 9–90 days [14,19]. These lesions may break down forming an ulcerated plaque over a period of 1–2 weeks. Primary lesions occur most frequently on the lower limbs or buttocks [13,20], whilst genital lesions are extremely uncommon. If patients are left untreated then primary lesions will heal spontaneously, with scarring, over a period of 3–6 months [21].

Without treatment individuals will progress to secondary yaws. Secondary yaws predominantly involves the skin and bones [20,22]. As with secondary syphilis, both generalised lymphadenopathy and constitutional symptoms, including fever and malaise, are frequently reported in patients with secondary yaws [19]. A wide-range of skin manifestations occur in secondary yaws including macular lesions and hyperkeratotic lesions on the palms and soles ('crab yaws') [14,19,20]. Osteoperiostitis, affecting the fingers (resulting in dactylitis) or long bones (forearm, fibula, tibula) is the most common bony manifestation of secondary yaws. Following treatment of early yaws (primary or secondary) skin lesions usually resolve within 2–4 weeks and bone pain may start to resolve in as little as 48 h [23].

In the absence of treatment of early yaws, patients go on to develop latent infection. During this clinical stage of disease patients have reactive serology but no clinical evidence of infection. Relapse from latent to active disease can occur for a period of up to 5–10 years and serve as a source of onward transmission. Previously up to 10% of patients were reported to develop the late-stage manifestations of tertiary yaws, but this is now much less commonly reported [19]. Tertiary disease may manifest as gummatous nodules resulting in tissue necrosis, a destructive osteitis which can cause destruction of the maxilla (gangosa), or bowing of the shins (sabre shin), or a hypertrophic periostitis causing exostosis of the paranasal maxilla (gondou).

Clinical diagnosis is supported by serological testing. Diagnostic testing combines a treponemal assay (such as the *Treponema pallidum* particle agglutination assay) and a non-treponemal assay (such as the rapid plasma regain assay). Treponemal tests are more specific but remain positive for life. The titre of non-treponemal assays rises following infection and falls following treatment. A four-fold fall in titre (e.g., from 1:16 to 1:4) is considered consistent with serological cure. Newer point-of-care treponemal and non-treponemal assays have increasingly taken on the role of traditional lab-based assays [24,25].

An important recent discovery has been the finding that *Haemophilus ducreyi* may cause ulcerative skin lesions similar to those seen in patients with early yaws [26,27]. *H. ducreyi* may cause lesions in both patients who have non-reactive and reactive serological tests for yaws, which complicates assessment of patients with suspected active yaws as serological point of care tests cannot be used to accurately provide a definitive diagnosis. When molecular tests are used, a large proportion of patients suspected to have active early yaws are found in fact to have latent yaws (reactive serological tests) and a different cause for the current skin lesion.

4. Penicillin-Based Treatment

Early studies conducted in Haiti demonstrated that penicillin-based treatments were highly efficacious in the treatment of yaws [23] and penicillin-based therapy was subsequently adopted as the standard of care worldwide for all endemic treponematoses [14]. Different penicillin-based regimes are effective for the treatment of yaws, but long-acting intramuscular benzathine benzylpenicillin was the most commonly used regimen. Lower doses were used than those recommended for the treatment of venereal syphilis (1.2 million units for the treatment of adults and 0.6 million units for the treatment of children) [14]. Although there have been rare reports of 'treatment failure' with penicillin-based therapy, the inability to distinguish treatment failure from reinfection makes these data extremely difficult to interpret, especially in highly endemic settings [28]. As with syphilis, no evidence of penicillin resistance has developed in yaws despite it being the first-line treatment for more than 50 years.

During the mid-twentieth century, successful treatment campaigns were conducted targeting yaws and the other endemic treponematoses [29]. In 1949, the World Health Assembly passed a resolution supporting efforts for the control and elimination of the endemic treponematoses, including yaws. WHO and UNICEF led a global effort between 1952 and 1964, based on penicillin treatment. At the time, the recommended strategy varied, based on the prevalence of active yaws in the community (Table 1). Although not ultimately successful in achieving eradication, the programme did significantly reduce the global prevalence of yaws by as much as 98% [30]. Following these efforts, the incidence of the disease rebounded in a number of countries in the 1970s, ultimately leading to a further World Health Assembly resolution in 1978, which resulted in some countries renewing control efforts [29].

Table 1. Historical strategy for the eradication of yaws: 1952–1964.

Prevalence of Clinically Active Yaws	Treatment Strategy
Hyperendemic: above 10%	Benzathine benzylpenicillin to the whole community (total mass treatment)
Mesoendemic: 5–10%	Treat all active cases, all children under 15 and all contacts of infectious cases (juvenile mass treatment)
Hypoendemic: under 5%	Treat all active cases and all household and other contacts (selective mass treatment)

5. Azithromycin-Based Treatment

Despite its efficacy, treatment with penicillin remains challenging in many settings. Injectable penicillin requires access to a secure cold chain and trained staff to administer therapy, both of which are not always available in the remote locations where yaws is found. Treatment also carried a small but important risk of anaphylaxis. Supplies of benzathine benzylpenicillin have also been insecure in recent years [31], with implications for reliable access to treatment.

Azithromycin, an oral macrolide antibiotic, had previously been demonstrated to be effective in the treatment of syphilis [32] with cure rates equivalent to those of benzathine benzylpenicillin. Given the high degree of genetic homology between syphilis and yaws, azithromycin was an attractive option for study as an alternative treatment for yaws. In a landmark study conducted in Papua New Guinea, patients with early (primary and secondary) yaws were randomised to receive treatment with either a single dose of intramuscular benzathine benzylpenicillin or a single, oral dose of azithromycin. Azithromycin was shown to be non-inferior to benzathine benzylpenicillin with a cure rate greater than 95% in both arms [33]. Subsequently, a study conducted in Ghana also confirmed the non-inferiority of azithromycin compared to benzathine benzylpenicillin [34].

These initial studies all enrolled patients with early active yaws and used a dose of 30 mg/kg (max. 2 g). Two outstanding questions were whether azithromycin was effective for the treatment of latent infection and whether the lower dose of azithromycin used for the treatment of trachoma (20 mg/kg—max. 1 g) was also efficacious in the treatment of yaws. In a longitudinal cohort study in Papua New Guinea, treatment with azithromycin was demonstrated to have a cure rate for patients with latent yaws equivalent to the cure rate of patients with active yaws [35]. The efficacy of the low versus standard dose azithromycin was compared in a randomised control trial in patients with both early active and latent yaws, conducted in Papua New Guinea and Ghana. The clinical cure rate was equivalent in both low and standard dose arms. The serological cure rate in patients with active yaws was slightly lower in the low-dose arm. In patients with latent yaws the serological cure rate was equivalent with both doses of azithromycin [36]. Taken together with observational data, this suggests that low-dose azithromycin is also effective in the treatment of yaws, although the 30 mg/kg dose remains the standard of care.

Unlike with penicillin, resistance to azithromycin is well described in *T. pallidum*. Resistance is mediated by one of two mutations in the 23s rDNA and can be detected by specific molecular tests [37–41]. In the context of large scale azithromycin-based treatment programmes (see below), treatment failure and genotypic resistance to azithromycin has now also been described in yaws [42].

6. Community Treatment with Azithromycin

Azithromycin has been widely distributed at the community level for the treatment of trachoma [43] and the WHO recommends mass drug administration (MDA) of azithromycin for the elimination of trachoma as a public health problem as part of the SAFE (Surgery, Antibiotics, Facial cleanliness and Environmental improvement) strategy [44]. MDA of azithromycin has been shown to be safe and indeed there is considerable evidence that MDA may result in significant off-target benefits including reductions in child mortality [45].

Taken together, the evidence of the safety of MDA with azithromycin and the efficacy of azithromycin for the treatment of yaws provide the rationale behind the revised WHO strategy for the eradication of yaws (the Morges strategy). This strategy emphasises MDA of azithromycin in communities where yaws is endemic. Following an initial round of MDA (referred to as total community treatment—TCT) it may be appropriate to conduct further MDA or to switch to a strategy of treating active cases and their contacts (total targeted treatment—TTT) [46]. No clear evidence currently exists to guide the decision regarding when to switch between TCT and TTT, but modelling studies suggest that TCT is a preferable strategy because it ensures a higher coverage of latent yaws cases [47,48].

Initial assessments of the efficacy of azithromycin MDA were conducted in both the Pacific and West Africa. In a study in the Solomon Islands, communities received a single round of MDA of azithromycin (conducted for the elimination of trachoma as a public health problem) at a dose of 20 mg/kg (max. 1g) and were followed up at 6 and 18 months following MDA [49–51]. A significant reduction in the prevalence of both active and latent yaws was seen at both 6 and 18 months following MDA. In Ghana, MDA with azithromycin (30 mg/kg, max. 2 g) was conducted in a single district and follow-up conducted at 12 months. As in the Solomon Islands, a significant reduction in both active and latent yaws was documented [52].

The most comprehensive evaluation of the WHO Morges strategy was conducted in Lihir, Papua New Guinea [53]. In this study of more than 15,000 individuals, an initial round of mass treatment was undertaken, followed by six-monthly rounds of surveillance and treatment of new cases and their contacts. In keeping with the studies discussed above, this study demonstrated a marked reduction in the prevalence of both active and latent yaws. Despite this initial success, interruption of transmission was not achieved [42]. Ongoing transmission was driven both by cases imported from outside the study site and cases arising in individuals missed during the initial mass treatment phase of the study. Thirty-six months into the study, a single case of treatment failure was detected. The patient had been treated at 30 months with azithromycin but at month 36 had clinical evidence of progression and serological evidence of treatment failure. Subsequent molecular testing confirmed genotypic azithromycin resistance in this case. Alongside the index case, several contacts were detected at month 36 and month 42 of the study with azithromycin-resistant yaws. Although subsequent treatment with benzathine benzylpenicillin was used to successfully ring-fence the outbreak, these data highlight the risk of emerging azithromycin resistance threatening yaws eradication efforts [42].

7. Conclusions

There has been considerable progress in the treatment of yaws in the last decade. Azithromycin has emerged as an effective and easily deliverable oral treatment option that can be used to treat both individual cases and during community MDA. The emergence of azithromycin resistance highlights the need for ongoing surveillance to support yaws eradication efforts globally. Further studies are needed to better define the optimum MDA strategy including the number of rounds and population coverage required to interrupt the transmission of yaws.

References

1. Marks, M.; Solomon, A.W.; Mabey, D.C. Endemic treponemal diseases. *Trans. R. Soc. Trop. Med. Hyg.* **2014**, *108*, 601–607. [CrossRef] [PubMed]
2. Mitjà, O.; Asiedu, K.; Mabey, D. Yaws. *Lancet* **2013**, *381*, 763–773. [CrossRef]
3. Cejková, D.; Zobaníková, M.; Chen, L.; Pospíšilová, P.; Strouhal, M.; Qin, M.; Mikalová, L.; Norris, S.J.; Muzny, D.M.; Gibbs, R.A.; et al. Whole genome sequences of three *Treponema pallidum* ssp. *pertenue* strains: Yaws and syphilis treponemes differ in less than 0.2% of the genome sequence. *PLoS Negl. Trop. Dis.* **2012**, *6*, e1471.
4. Agadzi, V.K.; Aboagye-Atta, Y.; Nelson, J.W.; Perine, P.L.; Hopkins, D.R. Resurgence of yaws in Ghana. *Lancet* **1983**, *2*, 389–390. [CrossRef]
5. Asiedu, K. The return of yaws. *Bull. World Health Organ.* **2008**, *86*, 507–508. [PubMed]
6. Tharmaphornpilas, P.; Srivanichakorn, S.; Phraesrisakul, N. Recurrence of yaws outbreak in Thailand, 1990. *Southeast Asian J. Trop. Med. Public Health* **1994**, *25*, 152–156. [PubMed]
7. Fegan, D.; Glennon, M.; Macbride-Stewart, G.; Moore, T. Yaws in the Solomon Islands. *J. Trop. Med. Hyg.* **1990**, *93*, 52–57. [PubMed]
8. Fegan, D.; Glennon, M.J.; Thami, Y.; Pakoa, G. Resurgence of yaws in Tanna, Vanuatu: Time for a new approach? *Trop. Doct.* **2010**, *40*, 68–69. [CrossRef] [PubMed]
9. Manning, L.A.; Ogle, G.D. Yaws in the periurban settlements of Port Moresby, Papua New Guinea. *Papua New Guinea Med. J.* **2002**, *45*, 206–212.
10. John, R.K.S. Yaws in the Americas. *Rev. Infect. Dis.* **1985**, *7*, S266–S272. [CrossRef]
11. Scolnik, D.; Aronson, L.; Lovinsky, R.; Toledano, K.; Glazier, R.; Eisenstadt, J.; Eisenberg, P.; Wilcox, L.; Rowsell, R.; Sliverman, M. Efficacy of a targeted, oral penicillin-based yaws control program among children living in rural South America. *Clin. Infect. Dis.* **2003**, *36*, 1232–1238. [CrossRef] [PubMed]
12. Bora, D.; Dhariwal, A.C.; Lal, S. Yaws and its eradication in India—A brief review. *J. Commun. Dis.* **2005**, *37*, 1–11. [PubMed]
13. Hackett, C.J. Extent and nature of the yaws problem in Africa. *Bull. World Health Organ.* **1953**, *8*, 127–182.
14. Perine, P.L.; Hopkins, D.R.; Niemel, P.L.A.; St.-John, R.; Causse, G.; Antal, G.M. *Handbook of Endemic Treponematoses: Yaws, Endemic Syphilis and Pinta*; World Health Organization: Geneva, Switzerland, 1984; Available online: http://apps.who.int/iris/handle/10665/37178?locale=en (accessed on 2 May 2013).
15. Houinei, W.; Godornes, C.; Kapa, A.; Knauf, S.; Mooring, E.Q.; González-Beiras, C.; Watup, R.; Paru, R.; Advent, P.; Bieb, S.; et al. *Haemophilus ducreyi* DNA is detectable on the skin of asymptomatic children, flies and fomites in villages of Papua New Guinea. *PLoS Negl. Trop. Dis.* **2017**, *11*, e0004958. [CrossRef] [PubMed]
16. Knauf, S.; Raphael, J.; Mitjà, O.; Lejora, I.A.V.; Chuma, I.S.; Batamuzi, E.K.; Keyyu, J.D.; Fyumagwa, R.; Lüert, S.; Godornes, C.; et al. Isolation of *Treponema* DNA from necrophagous flies in a natural ecosystem. *EBioMedicine* **2016**, *11*, 85–90. [CrossRef] [PubMed]
17. Harper, K.N.; Fyumagwa, R.D.; Hoare, R.; Wambura, P.N.; Coppenhaver, D.H.; Sapolsky, R.M.; Alberts, S.C.; Tung, J.; Rogers, J.; Kilewo, M.; et al. *Treponema pallidum* infection in the wild baboons of East Africa: Distribution and genetic characterization of the strains responsible. *PLoS ONE* **2012**, *7*, e50882. [CrossRef] [PubMed]

18. Knauf, S.; Liu, H.; Harper, K.N. Treponemal infection in nonhuman primates as possible reservoir for human yaws. *Emerg. Infect. Dis.* **2013**, *19*, 2058–2060. [CrossRef] [PubMed]
19. Koff, A.B.; Rosen, T. Nonvenereal treponematoses: Yaws, endemic syphilis, and pinta. *J. Am. Acad. Dermatol.* **1993**, *29*, 519–535. [CrossRef]
20. Mitjà, O.; Hays, R.; Lelngei, F.; Laban, N.; Ipai, A.; Pakarui, S.; Bassat, Q. Challenges in recognition and diagnosis of yaws in children in Papua New Guinea. *Am. J. Trop. Med. Hyg.* **2011**, *85*, 113–116. [CrossRef] [PubMed]
21. Sehgal, V.N. Leg ulcers caused by yaws and endemic syphilis. *Clin. Dermatol.* **1990**, *8*, 166–174. [CrossRef]
22. Mitjà, O.; Hays, R.; Ipai, A.; Wau, B.; Bassat, Q. Osteoperiostitis in early yaws: Case series and literature review. *Clin. Infect. Dis.* **2011**, *52*, 771–774. [CrossRef] [PubMed]
23. Rein, C.R. Treatment of yaws in the Haitian peasant. *J. Natl. Med. Assoc.* **1949**, *41*, 60–65. [PubMed]
24. Marks, M.; Goncalves, A.; Vahi, V.; Sakana, O.; Puiahi, E.; Zhang, Z.; Dalipanda, T.; Bottomley, C.; Mabey, D.; Solomin, A.W. Evaluation of a rapid diagnostic test for yaws infection in a community surveillance setting. *PLoS Negl. Trop. Dis.* **2014**, *8*, e3156. [CrossRef] [PubMed]
25. Ayove, T.; Houniei, W.; Wangnapi, R.; Bieb, S.V.; Kazadi, W.; Luke, L.N.; Manineng, C.; Moses, P.; Paru, R.; Esfandiari, J.; et al. Sensitivity and specificity of a rapid point-of-care test for active yaws: A comparative study. *Lancet Glob. Health* **2014**, *2*, e415–e421. [CrossRef]
26. Marks, M.; Chi, K.H.; Vahi, V.; Pillay, N.; Sokana, O.; Pavluck, A.; Mabey, D.C.; Chen, C.Y.; Solomon, A.W. *Haemophilus ducreyi* associated with skin ulcers among children, Solomon Islands. *Emerg. Infect. Dis.* **2014**, *20*, 1705–1707. [CrossRef] [PubMed]
27. Mitjà, O.; Lukehart, S.A.; Pokowas, G.; Moses, P.; Kapa, A.; Godones, C.; Robson, J.; Cherian, S.; Houinei, W.; Kazadi, W.; et al. *Haemophilus ducreyi* as a cause of skin ulcers in children from a yaws-endemic area of Papua New Guinea: A prospective cohort study. *Lancet Glob. Health* **2014**, *2*, e235–e241. [CrossRef]
28. Backhouse, J.L.; Hudson, B.J.; Hamilton, P.A.; Nesteroff, S.I. Failure of penicillin treatment of yaws on Karkar Island, Papua New Guinea. *Am. J. Trop. Med. Hyg.* **1998**, *59*, 388–392. [CrossRef] [PubMed]
29. Asiedu, K.; Amouzou, B.; Dhariwal, A.; Karam, M.; Lobo, D.; Patnaik, S.; Meheus, A. Yaws eradication: Past efforts and future perspectives. *Bull. World Health Organ.* **2008**, *86*, 499. [CrossRef] [PubMed]
30. Antal, G.M.; Causse, G. The control of endemic treponematoses. *Rev. Infect. Dis.* **1985**, *7*, S220–S226. [CrossRef] [PubMed]
31. Nurse-Findlay, S.; Taylor, M.M.; Savage, M.; Mello, M.B.; Saliyou, S.; Lavayen, S.; Seghers, F.; Campbell, M.L.; Birgirimana, F.; Ouedraogo, L.; et al. Shortages of benzathine penicillin for prevention of mother-to-child transmission of syphilis: An evaluation from multi-country surveys and stakeholder interviews. *PLoS Med.* **2017**, *14*, e1002473. [CrossRef] [PubMed]
32. Riedner, G.; Rusizoka, M.; Todd, J.; Maboko, L.; Hoelscher, M.; Mmbando, D.; Samky, E.; Lyamuya, E.; Mabey, D.; Grosskurth, H.; et al. Single-dose azithromycin versus penicillin G benzathine for the treatment of early syphilis. *N. Engl. J. Med.* **2005**, *353*, 1236–1244. [CrossRef] [PubMed]
33. Mitjà, O.; Hays, R.; Ipai, A.; Penias, M.; Paru, R.; Fagaho, D.; Lazzari, E.; Bassat, Q. Single-dose azithromycin versus benzathine benzylpenicillin for treatment of yaws in children in Papua New Guinea: An open-label, non-inferiority, randomised trial. *Lancet* **2012**, *379*, 342–347.
34. Kwakye-Maclean, C.; Agana, N.; Gyapong, J.; Nortey, P.; Adu-Sarkodie, Y.; Aryee, E.; Asiedu, K.; Ballard, R.; Binka, F. A single dose oral azithromycin versus intramuscular benzathine penicillin for the treatment of yaws—A randomized non-inferiority trial in Ghana. *PLoS Negl. Trop. Dis.* **2017**, *11*, e0005154. [CrossRef] [PubMed]
35. Mitjà, O.; González-Beiras, C.; Godornes, C.; Kolmau, R.; Houinei, W.; Abel, H.; Kapa, A.; Paru, A.; Bieb, S.V.; Wangi, J.; et al. Effectiveness of single-dose azithromycin to treat latent yaws: A longitudinal comparative cohort study. *Lancet Glob. Health* **2017**, *5*, e1268–e1274.
36. Marks, M.; Mitjà, O.; Bottomley, C.; Kwakye, C.; Houinei, W.; Bauri, M.; Adwere, P.; Abdulai, A.A.; Dua, F.; Boateng, L.; et al. Comparative efficacy of low-dose versus standard-dose azithromycin for patients with yaws: A randomised non-inferiority trial in Ghana and Papua New Guinea. *Lancet Glob. Health* **2018**, *6*, e401–e410. [CrossRef]
37. Grimes, M.; Sahi, S.K.; Godornes, B.C.; Tantalo, L.C.; Roberts, N.; Bostick, D.; Marra, C.M.; Lukehart, S.A. Two mutations associated with macrolide resistance in *Treponema pallidum*: Increasing prevalence and correlation with molecular strain type in Seattle, Washington. *Sex Transm. Dis.* **2012**, *39*, 954–958. [CrossRef] [PubMed]

38. Lukehart, S.A.; Godornes, C.; Molini, B.J.; Sonnett, P.; Hopkins, S.; Mulcahy, F.; Engelman, J.; Mitchell, S.J.; Rompalo, A.M.; Marra, C.M.; et al. Macrolide resistance in *Treponema pallidum* in the United States and Ireland. *N. Engl. J. Med.* **2004**, *351*, 154–158. [CrossRef] [PubMed]
39. Chen, C.Y.; Chi, K.H.; Pillay, A.; Nachamkin, E.; Su, J.R.; Ballard, R.C. Detection of the A2058G and A2059G 23S rRNA gene point mutations associated with azithromycin resistance in *Treponema pallidum* by use of a TaqMan real-time multiplex PCR assay. *J. Clin. Microbiol.* **2013**, *51*, 908–913. [CrossRef] [PubMed]
40. Šmajs, D.; Paštěková, L.; Grillová, L. Macrolide resistance in the syphilis spirochete, *Treponema pallidum* ssp. *pallidum*: Can we also expect macrolide-resistant yaws strains? *Am. J. Trop. Med. Hyg.* **2015**, *93*, 678–683.
41. Šmajs, D.; Pospíšilová, P. Macrolide resistance in yaws. *Lancet* **2018**, *391*, 1555–1556. [CrossRef]
42. Mitjà, O.; Godornes, C.; Houinei, W.; Kapa, A.; Paru, R.; Abel, H.; González-Beiras, C.; Bieb, S.V.; Wangi, J.; Barry, A.E.; et al. Re-emergence of yaws after single mass azithromycin treatment followed by targeted treatment: A longitudinal study. *Lancet Lond. Engl.* **2018**, *391*, 1599–1607. [CrossRef]
43. Solomon, A.W.; Holland, M.J.; Alexander, N.D.E.; Massae, P.A.; Aguirre, A.; Natividad-Sancho, A.; Molina, S.; Safari, S.; Shao, J.F.; Courtright, P.; et al. Mass treatment with single-dose azithromycin for trachoma. *N. Engl. J. Med.* **2004**, *351*, 1962–1971. [CrossRef] [PubMed]
44. Emerson, P.M.; Burton, M.J.; Solomon, A.W.; Bailey, R.; Mabey, D.C. The SAFE strategy for trachoma control: Using operational research for policy, and implementation. *Bull. World Health Organ.* **2006**, *84*, 613–619. [CrossRef] [PubMed]
45. Keenan, J.D.; Bailey, R.L.; West, S.K.; Arzika, A.M.; Hart, J.; Weaver, J.; Kalua, K.; Mrango, Z.; Ray, K.J.; Cook, C.; et al. Azithromycin to reduce childhood mortality in sub-Saharan Africa. *N. Engl. J. Med.* **2018**, *378*, 1583–1592. [CrossRef] [PubMed]
46. The World Health Organization. Eradication of yaws—The Morges Strategy. *Wkly. Epidemiol. Rec.* **2012**, *87*, 189–194.
47. Marks, M.; Mitjà, O.; Fitzpatrick, C.; Asiedu, K.; Solomon, A.W.; Mabey, D.C.; Funk, S. Mathematical modeling of programmatic requirements for yaws eradication. *Emerg. Infect. Dis.* **2017**, *23*, 22–28. [CrossRef] [PubMed]
48. Dyson, L.; Marks, M.; Crook, O.M.; Sokana, O.; Solomon, A.W.; Bishop, A.; Mabey, D.C.W.; Hollingsworth, T.D. Targeted treatment of yaws with household contact tracing: How much do we miss? *Am. J. Epidemiol.* **2018**, *187*, 837–844. [CrossRef] [PubMed]
49. Marks, M.; Vahi, V.; Sokana, O.; Puiahi, E.; Pavluck, A.; Zhang, Z.; Dalipanda, T.; Bottomley, C.; Mabey, D.C.; Solomon, A.W. Mapping the epidemiology of yaws in the Solomon Islands: A cluster randomized survey. *Am. J. Trop. Med. Hyg.* **2015**, *92*, 129–133. [CrossRef] [PubMed]
50. Marks, M.; Vahi, V.; Sokana, O.; Chi, K.H.; Puiahi, E.; Kilua, G.; Pillay, A.; Dalipanda, T.; Bottomley, C.; Solomon, A.W.; et al. Impact of community mass treatment with azithromycin for trachoma elimination on the prevalence of yaws. *PLoS Negl. Trop. Dis.* **2015**, *9*, e0003988. [CrossRef] [PubMed]
51. Marks, M.; Sokanam, O.; Nachamkin, E.; Puiahi, E.; Kilua, G.; Pillay, A.; Bottomley, C.; Solomon, A.W.; Mabey, D.C. Prevalence of active and latent yaws in the Solomon Islands 18 months after azithromycin mass drug administration for trachoma. *PLoS Negl. Trop. Dis.* **2016**, *10*, e0004927. [CrossRef] [PubMed]
52. Abdulai, A.A.; Agana-Nsiire, P.; Biney, F.; Kwakye-Maclea, C.; Kyei-Faried, S.; Amponsa-Achiano, K.; Simpson, S.V.; Bonsu, G.; Ohene, S.A.; Ampofo, W.K.; et al. Community-based mass treatment with azithromycin for the elimination of yaws in Ghana—Results of a pilot study. *PLoS Negl. Trop. Dis.* **2018**, *12*, e0006303. [CrossRef] [PubMed]
53. Mitjà, O.; Houinei, W.; Moses, P.; Kapa, A.; Paru, R.; Hays, R.; Lukehart, S.; Godornes, C.; Bieb, S.V.; Grice, T.; Siba, P.; et al. Mass treatment with single-dose azithromycin for yaws. *N. Engl. J. Med.* **2015**, *372*, 703–710. [CrossRef] [PubMed]

9

Insights into the Control and Management of Human and Bovine African Trypanosomiasis in Zambia between 2009 and 2019

Gloria M. Mulenga [1,2,3,*], Lars Henning [3], Kalinga Chilongo [2], Chrisborn Mubamba [2], Boniface Namangala [4] and Bruce Gummow [3,5]

1 Department of Veterinary Services, Kakumbi Tsetse and Trypanosomiasis Research Station, P.O Box 70, Mfuwe 10101, Zambia
2 Ministry of Fisheries and Livestock, Department of Veterinary Services, Lusaka 10101, Zambia; kchilongo@yahoo.co.uk (K.C.); chrisbornmw@yahoo.com (C.M.)
3 College of Public Health Medical and Veterinary Services, James Cook University, Townsville, Queensland 4814, Australia; lars.hening@jcu.edu.au (L.H.); bruce.gummow@jcu.edu.au (B.G.)
4 Institute of distance learning, The University of Zambia, Lusaka 10101, Zambia; b.namangala@unza.zm
5 Faculty of Veterinary Science, University of Pretoria, 0028 Pretoria, South Africa
* Correspondence: mmukuka2000@yahoo.com;

Abstract: Tsetse transmitted trypanosomiasis is a fatal disease commonly known as *Nagana* in cattle and sleeping sickness in humans. The disease threatens food security and has severe economic impact in Africa including most parts of Zambia. The level of effectiveness of commonly used African trypanosomiasis control methods has been reported in several studies. However, there have been no review studies on African trypanosomiasis control and management conducted in the context of One Health. This paper therefore seeks to fill this knowledge gap. A review of studies that have been conducted on African trypanosomiasis in Zambia between 2009 and 2019, with a focus on the control and management of trypanosomiasis was conducted. A total of 2238 articles were screened, with application of the search engines PubMed, PubMed Central and One Search. Out of these articles, 18 matched the required criteria and constituted the basis for the paper. An in-depth analysis of the 18 articles was conducted to identify knowledge gaps and evidence for best practices. Findings from this review provide stakeholders and health workers with a basis for prioritisation of African trypanosomiasis as an important neglected disease in Zambia and for formulation of One Health strategies for better control and/or management of the disease.

Keywords: trypanosomiasis; control; management; One Health; Zambia

---

1. Introduction

African trypanosomiasis is endemic to Sub-Saharan Africa and continues to threaten human health and food security. African trypanosomiasis has been a major draw-back to agriculture and economic development in affected countries, with annual losses in agricultural gross domestic product estimated at USD 4.7 billion [1,2]. The current strategy of the Zambian government to preserve natural resources and create state protected National Parks (NPs) and Game Management Areas (GMAs) has led to an expansion of wildlife populations that serve as long term reservoirs for African trypanosomiasis, and also to an increase in the population of tsetse flies that transmit the disease [3]. At the same time, increase in human population density and the changing climate, particularly rainfall patterns, have forced people (and their livestock) to migrate into these GMAs in search of fertile land for farming. Such uncontrolled migration of people into protected areas has brought about changes in land use patterns that threaten to alter tsetse habitat quality and patterns of African trypanosomiasis transmission due to increased tsetse–human and tsetse–livestock contacts [4–6].

Tourists visiting NPs and GMAs have not been spared from risks of Human African Trypanosomiasis (HAT) infections occurring through transmission from wildlife reservoir hosts [6]. Despite cases of HAT reported from tourists after their visit to Zambia's NPs, [7,8] there are gaps in protecting tourists and international travellers from tsetse and HAT. Some tour operators have taken it upon themselves to undertake some interventions, particularly in the form of tsetse control, aimed at reducing the risk of HAT infection among tourists visiting their facilities. Such limited interventions produce very limited levels of effectiveness or success, considering that such interventions need to cover considerable large proportions of the affected areas and as such require the collective input of many key stakeholders [9].

Tsetse flies are found in about 37% of Zambia's land area, and it is estimated that the prevalence of African animal trypanosomiasis (AAT) in cattle ranges from 1% to 90% depending on the area [8]. Most of the affected areas are located in rural remote parts of the country and as such the direct negative impacts of the trypanosomiasis problem occur in communities that live in these areas. These impacts include serious economic consequences such as reduced livestock productivity and mortality and the high cost of treating affected livestock [10,11].

In Zambia, AAT has been managed through constant use of trypanocides by individual livestock farmers, while treatment and/or management of the disease in humans has been negatively affected by several factors that include late case detection that tends to result in tragic consequences (death) associated with adverse effects of the administered drugs in the late stage [12,13]. The Zambian government has generally made some notable strides in the control of African trypanosomiasis particularly through tsetse control. However, the government's inability to put in place active surveillance systems, and the lack of adequate resources to effectively sustain control efforts, have contributed to the limitation of success associated with tsetse re-invasion and resurgence of African trypanosomiasis in areas where the disease had earlier been brought under control. In the case of HAT, lack of active surveillance systems has historically hindered progress towards the goal of eliminating African trypanosomiasis as a public health problem in Zambia [14,15].

The period between 2009 and 2019 has seen a significant number of undertakings focused largely on the parasite, transmission and epidemiology of African trypanosomiasis. However, no systematic review of the literature has been conducted on the control and management of African trypanosomiasis in Zambia particularly from a One Health perspective. This review seeks to address this knowledge gap.

2. Materials and Methods

With a focus on studies conducted on HAT and AAT control in Zambia, a systematic review (Figure A1 in Appendix A) of published data was undertaken. Using three searches with three categories of key words, a cumulative total of 2238 peer reviewed articles were identified in December 2019 from the following three search engines: PubMed, PubMed Central and One Search. One Search was used because it has a wider research area while PubMed was used because it is more aligned with veterinary sciences. Using the following key words: trypanosomiasis AND control AND management AND One Health AND Zambia, 610 articles were identified. In addition, two independent searches were performed using key words: trypanosomiasis AND control AND Zambia (995 articles identified), trypanosomiasis AND control AND One Health AND Zambia (633 articles identified). Duplicate articles were removed after which remaining articles were screened by title and abstract to assess the relevance of documents. Articles related to biochemical and biological developments in tsetse and African trypanosomiasis diagnostic assays were excluded from the review as most of the articles were focused on the trypanosome agent rather than management and control. Inclusion criteria were as follows: (i) studies conducted on the control and management of African trypanosomiasis in Zambia, (ii) related to One Health, (iii) related to African trypanosomiasis diagnostic methods, (iv) published in English only, and (v) published between January 2009 and December 2019. A final full text screening from the search conducted left 18 articles that met the inclusion criteria for the review (Table A1 in Appendix B). To support and supplement data from articles included in the review, published and unpublished government records and reports related to tsetse and African trypanosomiasis control for the same period were also referenced.

This review was conducted as part of a PhD project with ethical clearances from James Cook University (H7226 and A2498), Zambian Ethics Committee (Ref. No. 2018-Oct-001) and research approval from the Zambia National Health Research Authority.

3. Results

Based on the analysis of publications included in this review (Table A1 in Appendix B), results indicate that various trypanosome species circulate within a wide and diverse host community in Zambia [4]. The presence of the tsetse fly has facilitated the circulation of the parasite in the ecosystem [16]. Movement of people has led to the development of a new wildlife/livestock/human interface [4,17] *T. congolense* and *T. vivax* are the major causes of clinical AAT in cattle with low packed cell volume (PCV) usually an indicator of infection [18–20]. Infections with *T.b.r* in domestic animals remained a significant indicator that domestic animals could be reservoirs of HAT. Findings show that the impact of AAT is highest in cattle with dogs becoming a potential reservoir host for the human disease [16,21].

Current diagnostic methods used in Zambia do not conform to what is now thought to be the best practice [18,22,23]. Diagnosis of African trypanosomiasis remains a challenge in endemic areas of Zambia due to low staffing levels and non-functional laboratories [24,25].

Food security for communities living in tsetse-infested areas has continued to be negatively impacted [26]. The impact of AAT can be reduced through use of trypanocides and application of insecticide to control tsetse flies. Cattle farmers living in African trypanosomiasis-endemic areas and GMAs have resorted to drastic use of trypanocides to combat the disease [11]. African trypanosomiasis control in Zambia has been focused on cattle and not humans [26], with nothing published on the control and management of the disease in other domestic animals. Wildlife trypanosomiasis hosts pose a risk to communities and tourists living near or in national parks and game reserves [2,7,8].

Despite Zambia having had three major African trypanosomiasis control programmes (aerial spraying, insecticide treated targets and trypanocide drug use), the country has recorded several disease re-occurrences in areas where control was once undertaken. New cases are being reported in new areas while some old foci are disappearing [27,28]. Despite the evidence of the occurrence of African trypanosomiasis in both humans and livestock and the challenges faced by communities living in tsetse-infested areas, there is no One Health approach to control the disease [2,16,26].

A weak health system is in place for the management of HAT. Knowledge of HAT management among health workers is unsatisfactory [24]. A wide diversity of control programmes are available but lack government support [15,24,25,28]. Stakeholders in Zambia have competing views and beliefs regarding tsetse and African trypanosomiasis control, which is critical in developing a One Health approach for the control in both HAT and AAT. Environmentalists believe tsetse flies help keep environments wild and natural by stopping farmers encroaching protected areas. Agriculturalists feel that such moves have contributed to increased poverty as farmers are kept away from protected areas that are tsetse-infested [26].

4. Discussion

The Luangwa and Zambezi river basins support high densities of tsetse flies and wildlife reservoirs of African trypanosomiasis [4]. This review of tsetse and African trypanosomiasis studies undertaken in Zambia clearly indicates that most of these studies have been undertaken from or along the peripherals of the two river basins. With an estimated 37% of Zambia's land area tsetse-infested, the risk of African trypanosomiasis infection for people and livestock living in the tsetse-infested areas in the country cannot therefore be overemphasised [11].

An assessment by the World Health Organization (WHO) indicated that HAT usually affected people whose occupations took them into tsetse-infested areas. Categories of people so affected include among others: small scale farmers, workers under wildlife services, tsetse control workers, poachers, honey gatherers and fishermen [13]. Increased human populations and thus increased demand for land for agriculture continues to force people and their livestock into tsetse-infested areas in search for fertile land. Migration of people with their livestock into tsetse-infested areas, as highlighted in this review, has resulted in changes in the epidemiology of African trypanosomiasis. Livestock rearing in these tsetse-infested areas has thus eroded the diverse ecosystems and led to the development of a new kind of wildlife/livestock/human interface with domestic animals acting as potential link for trypanosome exchange [4,14,29].

The risk of HAT infection in travellers to national parks and game reserves has however not received much attention. Despite reported cases of HAT from tourists after visiting tsetse-infested areas [7,8], there are currently no deliberate interventions in place to protect international travellers from tsetse flies and HAT. In Zambia, most tsetse interventions have been focused in areas with potential for livestock production, with little synchronisation with human intervention programmes [30,31]

Currently, African trypanosomiasis control in humans relies on early diagnosis and treatment. However, challenges in HAT diagnosis in rural settings of Zambia has hindered progress to the control of the disease. Most diagnostic health centres in rural Zambia depend on microscopy for diagnosis. Despite the low sensitivity associated with microscopy, the test remains the gold standard for both HAT and AAT diagnosis because it is affordable. However, the low sensitivity exhibited by microscopy makes it difficult to determine disease incidences, especially in cases where parasitaemia is low, thus stressing the need to improve field diagnosis of African trypanosomiasis [16,19,22,30].

Recent developments of molecular tools such as polymerase chain reaction (PCR) and loop-mediated isothermal amplification (LAMP) for detecting trypanosomiasis has provided hope for improving field diagnosis which may lead to eliminating African trypanosomiasis [32–34]. LAMP has been proven to be more sensitive than microscopy in detecting infections of *T. brucei* and *T. vivax* as compared to *T. congolense*. Such findings indicate the importance of LAMP in epidemiological studies related to HAT rather than AAT. The simplicity and sensitivity of LAMP makes it an ideal diagnostic tool for HAT [16,23,30]. On the other hand, multispecies PCR can identify several species of trypanosomes in a single PCR reaction, thus reducing the cost of molecular diagnosis. The main advantage of molecular tools over microscopy is for epidemiological studies and to identify different trypanosome species [35–37] other than point of care diagnostic tools. Limited support from relevant authorities has negatively impacted on the use of molecular methods in Zambia. Most molecular laboratory consumables cannot be sourced locally, therefore, procurement of consumables has remained a challenge even for institutions that have implemented the use of molecular tools.

For continued efforts to control African trypanosomiasis infections, there is a need to establish strong active and passive surveillance systems in African trypanosomiasis focal point areas. In the absence of diagnostic centres as seen in most rural settings of Zambia, departments of Health and Veterinary services can share resources, diagnostic capacities and personnel for improved case detection, treatment and control of African trypanosomiasis and other zoonotic diseases. Future control efforts for HAT may also consider simultaneous control of the disease in livestock and wildlife reservoirs as a One Health approach [25,26].

Meanwhile, lack of political commitment to sustain tsetse and African trypanosomiasis control programmes [38] has pushed livestock farmers to constant use of trypanocides. The study conducted by Mbewe et al. [12] confirms that livestock farmers living in GMAs or near NPs where tsetse challenge is high have resorted to constant trypanocide use to protect their livestock, which may have serious consequences related to trypanosome resistance to trypanocides [39]. Treatment of infected animals may seem to be the best option for most livestock farmers, but it may tend to be unsustainable and costly in the long run as AAT is largely a herd health problem (Tsetse and Trypanosomiasis section strategic plan 2020, Zambia-unpublished government record). Unfortunately, most farmers living in tsetse-infested areas treat their animals based on clinical signs and symptoms due to lack of access to laboratories and regular surveys from local veterinarians. In this case, most infections remain in their livestock populations and may be responsible for sustaining sporadic African trypanosomiasis incidences within their communities [40].

Earlier studies by Simukoko et al. [18], indicate that livestock treatment with trypanocides is dependent on seasonal variations of tsetse populations and the risk of AAT infection. Such findings indicate the need for tsetse and AAT control programmes to be focused on seasonal differences in the risk of AAT infection when tsetse challenge is highest. Key stakeholders can therefore use such findings to link to biological characteristics of the tsetse vector in developing cost effective and sustainable control programmes during periods of highest challenge [18,41]. From a travel medicine perspective, such findings also highlight risk periods for travellers.

Increased focus on communicable and non-communicable disease management has pushed African trypanosomiasis off the government's priority list. There is a need to holistically quantify the impact and cost of African trypanosomiasis again in the context of disease prioritisation within Zambia and similarly affected countries. Lack of sustainable control programmes and the absence of a national surveillance and control programme for African trypanosomiasis among others, have impacted negatively on control efforts [24–26,38]. Breaking down barriers between social and natural scientists will help in developing a more holistic One Health approach to control tsetse flies and African trypanosomiasis in Zambia. Lessons learnt from past tsetse and African trypanosomiasis control operations can be useful in developing future cost effective and sustainable control programmes as well as informing health practitioners as to the risks travellers face in visiting these travel destinations and the in-country health support system available to them.

5. Recommendations

It is recommended that:

- Work is done to evaluate and identify African trypanosomiasis control programmes that are cost effective and sustainable in the regions where they are applied.
- Data on biological characteristics of tsetse and seasonal differences in African trypanosomiasis infection risk be considered when developing tsetse and trypanosomiasis control programmes in Zambia.
- More robust field diagnostic procedures for African trypanosomiasis be developed that consider the environmental, capacity and infrastructure constraints of working in countries like Zambia.
- Line Ministries consider sharing resources in order to improve diagnosis and treatment of African trypanosomiasis and other zoonotic diseases.
- A One Health approach be considered for the control of African trypanosomiasis in humans, livestock, wildlife and tsetse flies.

Author Contributions: G.M.M. developed, conceptualised and drafted the manuscript. B.G. contributed in the development of the manuscript. B.G., B.N. and L.H. were involved in supervision and project administration. K.C. and C.M. edited the draft manuscript. All authors reviewed, read, edited the draft and final manuscript. All authors have read and agreed to the published version of the manuscript.

Abbreviations

PCV	Packed Cell Volume
HAT	Human African Trypanosomiasis
PCR	Polymerase Chain Reaction;
LAMP	Loop Mediated Isothermal Amplification;
WBC	White Blood Cell;
CSF	Cerebrospinal Fluid;
GMA	Game Management Area;
CAT	Canine Animal Trypanosomiasis;
SRA	human Serum Resistance Associated;
RIME	Repetitive Insertion Mobile Element;
CON2-LAMP	specific primer targeting the 18Rrna gene of *T. congolense*; RHC, Rural Health Centre;
DNA	Deoxyribonucleic acid;
FAO	Food and Agriculture Organization RTTCP, Regional Tsetse and Trypanosomiasis Control Programme;
SAS/SAT	Sequential Aerial Spraying;
ITT	Insecticide Treated Targets and Traps;
TRY	trypanocidal drugs;
PATTEC	Pan African Tsetse and Trypanosomiasis Eradication Campaign;
AAT	Animal African Trypanosomiasis;
ITC	Insecticide Treated Cattle

Appendix A

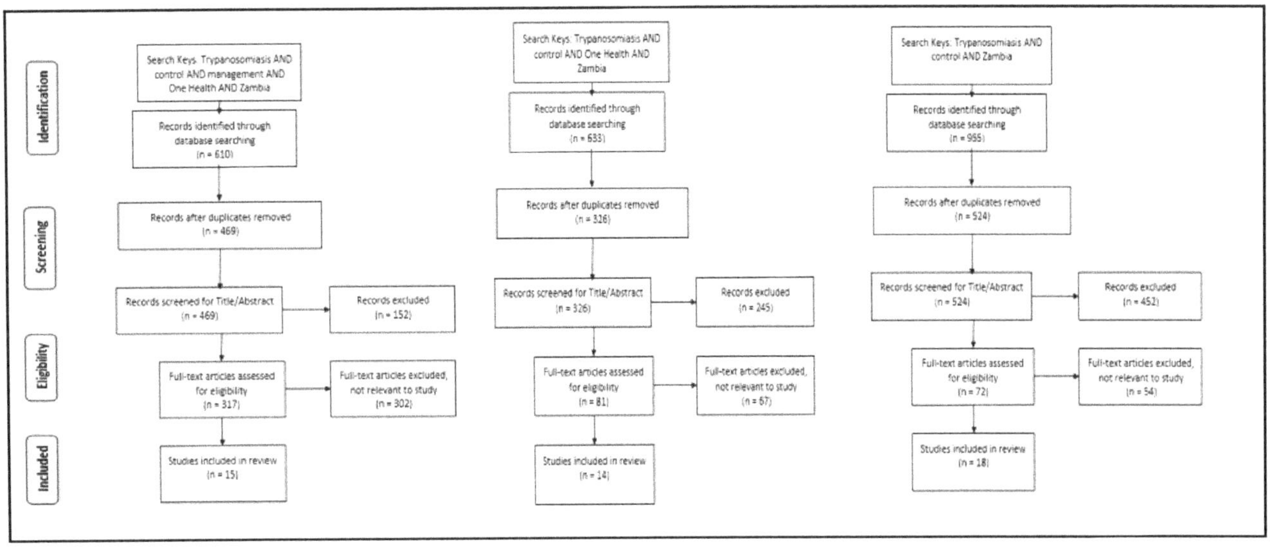

Figure A1. PRISMA diagrams showing three categories of searches conducted and selection criteria of literature included in the review.

Appendix B

Table A1. Articles meeting selection criteria on trypanosomiasis control in Zambia between January 2009 and December 2019 and a summary of key findings.

Author Year	Study Aim	Study Design	Sample and Participation	Study Findings	Needs Domain
(Simukoko et al., 2011 [16]	To assess the monthly risk of bovine trypanosomiasis in cattle kept in tsetse-infested eastern plateau of Zambia.	Longitudinal study of bovine trypanosomiasis incidence in cattle	Eighty-five herds of cattle that grazed together were selected for a 19-month follow-up study	-The risk of trypanosome infection varied significantly between months with the higher risk recorded between December and February. -PCVs of infected and un-infected cattle did not differ significantly -*Trypanosoma congolense* and *T. vivax* were detected in 92.3% and 4.5% of the infected cattle, respectively. Mixed infections were detected in 3.2% of positive samples. -Overall, 155 infections were detected using PCR while microscopy detected 85 infections.	1. More effort in optimizing Animal African Trypanosomiasis (AAT) control during periods of highest challenges. 2. Accuracy of AAT incidence using parasitological diagnosis stresses need for more sensitive diagnostic tools to improve field diagnosis.
(Mwanakasale and Songolo, 2011) [28]	-To identify districts in Zambia that were still reporting cases of Human African Trypanosomiasis (HAT). -To compare the occurrence of HAT cases before and after year 2000.	-Cross sectional survey of districts located close to national parks. -Literature review of occurrence of HAT in Zambia in the 1960s to 1990s.	-Conducted in nine provinces of Zambia except for Lusaka district. -Used google search, PubMed and world health organisation HINARI access to obtain data on HAT occurrence. Only articles with data on HAT distribution, epidemics, treatments and control of HAT before 2000 were reviewed.	-Chama, Mpika and Chipata districts were still reporting HAT cases. Seven districts that used to report HAT no longer had cases after January 2000. -All surveyed districts had no existing tsetse control programs. -In all surveyed health institutions, giemsa stain thick smear microscopy was the routine diagnostic method to detect HAT. Only Chilonga mission hospital used microhaematocrit centrifuge method to detect HAT. -Six of the surveyed hospitals had stocks of suramin but none had melarsoprol. -Findings from literature survey show a significant difference in HAT reporting foci from 1960s to 1990s and 2000 to 2007 with some old foci disappearing whilst new ones emerged or re-emerged	1. Districts reporting HAT 2008 to date 2. Data on Agriculture practices between 2000 to 2007 and compared with 1960s to 1990s to confirm if agriculture practices may have contributed to reduced tsetse flies in previously tsetse-infested areas and thus the drastic reduction of HAT cases. 3. Current data on human activities occurring in game management areas (GMAs) as they may be responsible for persistent HAT transmission and tsetse-human contacts. 4. Human animal contacts as animals may carry trypanosomes with them. 5. Poaching as game destruction was once used to eliminate wildlife reservoirs. 6. Under diagnosing of HAT due to increased focus on management of HIV/AIDS and malaria.

Table A1. *Cont.*

Author Year	Study Aim	Study Design	Sample and Participation	Study Findings	Needs Domain
(Anderson et al., 2011) [4]	To characterise the nature of the reservoir community for trypanosomiasis in the absence of influence from domesticated hosts	A cross-sectional survey of trypanosome prevalence in wildlife hosts. Conducted in the Luangwa valley from 2005 to 2007	A total of 418 wild animals were examined for the presence of trypanosomes	-Overall prevalence in all species was 13.9% with infection likely to be detected in waterbuck, lion, kudu and bushbuck, respectively. -Bushbuck indicated to be important hosts for *T. brucei s.l* with bushbuck, greater Kudu, and Lion to be important hosts for *T. congolense* while *T. vivax* was frequently detected in waterbuck. -*T. b. rhodesiense* were first identified in African buffalo and *T. brucei s.l* in leopard -First use multispecies PCR for the diagnosis of samples collected from free ranging wildlife which offers improved diagnostic specificity and sensitivity compared to traditional techniques. -Results indicated the ability of trypanosomes to survive in a wide variety of wildlife hosts.	1. Tsetse blood meal preference was identified as a risk factor for trypanosome infection. 2. Difficulties in sampling wildlife and method used to sample in this study limited ability to investigate age as a risk factor in trypanosome infection 3. Infection of *T. b. rhodesiense* in buffalo raises concern on possibility of infection been established in cattle populations not far from sampling area i.e., Mambwe district of the eastern province of Zambia. This is because buffalos move over large distances with potential to disseminate infection to other species. 4. Trypanosome reservoir in wildlife hosts maybe wider that estimated in this study 5. Influx of people with their livestock and land use may have an impact on the epidemiology of African trypanosomiasis.
(Namangala et al., 2012) [21]	To evaluate the performance of repetitive insertion mobile element (RIME)–loop mediated isothermal amplification (LAMP) and human serum resistance associated (SRA)–LAMP against microscopy in HAT diagnosis	Case study	Four male patients from Luangwa and Zambezi river basins	-Both RIME-LAMP and SRA-LAMP were able to detect *T. b. rhodesiense* in patients' blood and in cerebrospinal fluid (CSF). -LAMP results correlated with microscopy results but they do not confirm the standard staging criteria using microscopy and white blood cell (WBC) in CSF.	1. Need for a detailed study with larger sample size to evaluate potential of LAMP to be used as a bedside diagnostic test for HAT and for making therapeutic decisions. 2. Need for both active and passive surveillance of HAT and community sensitisation in HAT old foci.

Table A1. *Cont.*

Author Year	Study Aim	Study Design	Sample and Participation	Study Findings	Needs Domain
(Namangala et al., 2013) [41]	To evaluate the performance of LAMP against microscopy to detect CAT in exotic dogs	Cross sectional survey of trypanosomiasis in exotic dogs	Six exotic dogs naturally infected with trypanosomes from Zambia's South Luangwa National Park and Chiawa GMA.	-Results indicated first report of canine animal trypanosomiasis (CAT) in Zambia -All cases initially diagnosed by microscopy and later confirmed by LAMP, showing good correlation between the two methods. -Three dogs reported infection with *T. congolense* according to CON2-LAMP -All SRA-LAMP positive cases were also RIME-LAMP positive indicating similar sensitivity.	1. Further investigation on SRA gene isolated from two dogs in this communication. 2. Scanty parasitaemia sometimes pose challenges caused by weak fluorescence signal thus need to quantify the fluorescence intensity and consider samples to be positive after subtracting the background fluorescence of the negative control. 3. Dogs as potential source of HAT infections 4. Need to investigate performance of LAMP in CAT diagnosis among locally bred dogs in tsetse-infested GMAs and National parks.
(Mwanakasale et al., 2013) [23]	To assess current health delivery system in the management of HAT.	Cross sectional survey of health institutions using structured questionnaires	Nine health institutions from Mpika district of Zambia were involved in the study	-The general knowledge on HAT of health staff from surveyed health institutions was unsatisfactory for proper management of the disease -Study revealed gross understaffing of essential staff to clinically diagnose and manage HAT-No staff from the surveyed institutions had received specific training on HAT diagnosis and treatment. -There was only one treatment centre (Chilonga mission hospital) from the surveyed health institutions -Erratic supply of trypanocides at the only treatment centre in the district -Only 2 of the surveyed institutions has functional laboratories with qualified personnel. Both institutions used less-sensitive methods to diagnose HAT -Distances between rural health centres (RHCs) and treatment centres and non-availability of transport to ferry suspected HAT patients.	1. Need for refresher courses to be conducted every two years for health personnel in districts at risk of HAT transmission in Zambia. 2. Need for awareness on HAT for health policy makers so that they understand the need for refresher courses and trainings on disease management. 3. Need to motivate in kind health staff at the frontline of identifying suspected cases and encourage them to refer such cases to diagnostic and treatment centres 4. Need to establish Mpika district hospital as an additional treatment centre to decongest Chilonga mission hospital and improve health service delivery at both hospitals.Ministry of health to ensure that drugs for both stages of HAT are always in stock. 5. Need for Ministry of health to equip and capacitate health institutions with laboratories and personnel as well as more sensitive diagnostic tools. 6. Need for a proper referral system for HAT suspected cases to diagnostic treatment to ensure they reach their designated centres.

Table A1. *Cont.*

Author Year	Study Aim	Study Design	Sample and Participation	Study Findings	Needs Domain
(Lisulo et al., 2014) [19]	To evaluate the performance of LAMP in determining trypanosome prevalence in indigenous dogs.	Cross sectional survey of Canine African Trypanosomiasis	A total of 237 indigenous dogs from 47 villages within five chiefdoms of Mambwe district of Zambia	-Fourteen cases of trypanosomes were detected using microscopy. -LAMP detected an additional 6 cases indicating higher sensitivity and specificity than microscopy. -Adult dogs were more likely to acquire CAT as they are involved in hunting. -CAT was significantly related to corneal opacity -Dogs are potential links for trypanosome exchange between livestock and humans.	1. Diagnostic accuracy of LAMP against microscopy suggested that its use in CAT diagnosis could improve disease management in African trypanosomiasis in endemic areas. 2. Results from study can trigger a One Health approach towards control of HAT through disease intervention in livestock. 3. Need for continuous surveillance of African trypanosomiasis in tsetse-infested regions using more user friendly and sensitive tests such as LAMP. 4. Need to sensitise locals in GMAs potential dangers of keeping dogs that are left to scavenge without receiving veterinary services. 5. Dogs may harbour other zoonoses apart from *T. b. rhodesiense* with potential serious implications to human health.
(Nyimba et al., 2015) [30]	To determine the prevalence and species distribution of caprine trypanosomiasis	Cross-sectional cluster survey of AAT in goats	Overall, 422 goats from Kalomo and Sinazongwe districts of Southern province of Zambia	-One goat was found infected on microscopy while 100 goats reported positive for AAT on LAMP. -Infection rate for Sinazongwe district was 22.4% while that for Kalomo district was 24.7% -*Trypanosoma brucei*, *T. vivax* and *T. congolense* were detected in 82.0%, 31.0% and 23.0% of the infected goats, respectively. Mixed infections were detected in 33.0% of positive samples. -Study results indicate the re-emergence of AAT in study areas were aerial spraying was once conducted by the government.	1. Need for improved staffing to enhance disease prevention and containment. 2. Need for refresher courses for frontline Veterinary staff in order to improve service delivery. 3. Need for sustainable control operations to avoid tsetse re-invasions and re-occurrence of disease in areas where control was once a success story.

Table A1. *Cont.*

Author Year	Study Aim	Study Design	Sample and Participation	Study Findings	Needs Domain
(Laohasinnarong et al., 2015) [14]	To examine the presence of different trypanosome species in cattle, goats and tsetse using a combination of microscopy, PCR and LAMP	Cross sectional survey of trypanosomes in cattle, goats and tsetse flies.	In total, 243 cattle, 36 goats and 546 tsetse flies were examined for the presence of trypanosomes. Study conducted from Petauke, Chama and Isoka districts of Zambia.	-Microscopy exhibited relatively low sensitivity than PCR and LAMP -There was poor agreement among test methods. For instance, failure of PCR and LAMP to detect microscopically positive samples. -KIN PCR was found to be sensitive for detecting *T. congolense* -TviCatL-PCR and PFL-LAMP were better for detecting *T. Vivax* and *T. b. rhodesiense*, respectively. -The presence of *T. b. rhodesiense* in tsetse samples indicates its ability to take blood meal from multiple hosts (wildlife, humans and domestic animals), facilitating the circulation of the parasite in the ecosystem. -Infection in cattle and goats was highest with *T. congolense* and least with *T. vivax*	1. Need to establish if trypanosome DNA detected from cattle, goats and tsetse were active infections or residual DNA from dead trypanosomes picked from blood meals or treated animals. 2. Need for a One Health approach towards the control of HAT through disease intervention in livestock, wildlife and tsetse.
(Mulenga et al., 2015) [22]	To investigate health personnel's and health centre's capacity to diagnose Human African trypanosomiasis	Cross sectional survey using structured questionnaires.	A sample of 101 health personnel drawn from 12 and nine health centres from Chama and Mambwe districts, respectively	-Staffing levels from both districts were extremely low with most health centres manned by one trained staff -Staff had basic knowledge to identify HAT with staff from Chama districts more likely to identify a case compared to their Mambwe counterparts. -Only Chama district had functional laboratories. Most health centres surveyed reported frequent use of rapid test kits for diagnosing mainly malaria parasites thus reducing diagnosis of other blood parasites that can be detected by microscopy including HAT.	1. Need for authorities to train and post more health staff in rural areas and to come up with deliberate policies that provide incentives to attract and motivate health workers in rural areas 2. Need for capacity building and refresher trainings for health staff with regards to HAT diagnosis. 3. Need for health centres located in HAT foci to be equipped with at least microscopes to enable them more easily identify cases when they occur. Further, referral or district hospitals can also be equipped with more sensitive laboratory tools like PCR and LAMP. 4. Need for HAT national surveillance and control programmes to be enhanced.

Table A1. *Cont.*

Author Year	Study Aim	Study Design	Sample and Participation	Study Findings	Needs Domain
(Mbewe et al., 2015b) [10]	To examine how socio-economic and environmental factors are associated with adherence to the recommended guidelines on trypanocide use	Cross sectional survey using a structured questionnaire.	Farmers interviewed from five veterinary camps from Itezhi tezhi district of central province of Zambia	-Of the interviewed farmers, 25.6% adhered to FAO guidelines on trypanocide use; (i) reducing the number of treatments on whole herd up to a maximum of four times in a year by integrating drug usage with other control measures and (ii) avoiding exposure of the whole parasite population to the drug by limiting treatments to individual sick animals. -None of the socio-economic factors (age, education, cattle herd size, competence in trypanocide use and access to extension on trypanocide use) were associated with a farmer's adherence to FAO guidelines. -Low adherence to recommended FAO guidelines on trypanocide use was associated with the location of crush pen, whether in GMA or not, as an environmental factor. Farmers in GMAs were less likely to adhere to FAO guidelines than those in non-GMA.	1. Need for an integrated approach of measure to control AAT in the GMA of Itezhi tezhi to lessen overuse of trypanocides by farmers. 2. Need to investigate if household income may influence farmer's adherence to FAO guidelines of trypanocide use as defined in this study. 3. Need to investigate if household income may influence control of vector borne diseases.
(Mbewe et al., 2015a) [20]	-To investigate the prevalence of animal trypanosomiasis in anaemic cattle	Cross sectional survey of AAT in cattle	A total of 564 Anaemic cattle from Itezhi tezhi district of Zambia	-Out of 564 cattle screened, 58 (10.3 %) had anaemia. PCR-RFLP results showed that 17 (29.3 %) anaemic cattle were positive for pathogenic trypanosomes compared to 1 (1.7 %) on parasitological examination using thick smears. -Infections were caused by *Trypanosoma congolense* and *Trypanosoma vivax*.	1. Need to investigate other anaemia causing factors in animal trypanosomiasis endemic areas of Itezhi tezhi district of Zambia.
(Grant et al., 2015) [24]	-To examine the narratives on African trypanosomiasis in Zambian policy. -To explore relationships between human, animal and environmental sectors	Case study of key informant interviews	Twenty participants from international organisations, research organisations and local activists.	-Environmentalists believed tsetse stop farmers encroaching protected areas thus keeping areas natural and wild. -Increased poverty because tsetse keeps farmers away from productive areas. -The Zambian government has other diseases of priority other than African trypanosomiasis and does not have funds to keep areas tsetse free. -Major focus of African trypanosomiasis control is emphasised on cattle and not humans. -The need to undertake tsetse control using the best methods have been identified but with no financial resources to support the plan. -Tsetse-infested forests that have been cleared for cotton growing have disrupted tsetse habitats due to chemicals used. -Current conservation strategies have sustained the preservation of tsetse flies and African trypanosomiasis.	1. Need for cross-sector, interdisciplinary decision making to stop rival narratives leading to competing actions. 2. Need for a One Health approach to break down the barriers between social scientists, natural scientists and the expertise of the community.

Table A1. *Cont.*

Author Year	Study Aim	Study Design	Sample and Participation	Study Findings	Needs Domain
(Mweempwa et al., 2015) [41]	To establish the impact of habitat fragmentation on the physiological and demographic parameters of tsetse flies in order to enhance the understanding of the relationship between fragmentation and AAT risk	Longitudinal study of tsetse age, abundance and trypanosome infection in areas of varying degrees of habitat fragmentation in eastern Zambia.	-A set of 3200 *Glossina morsitans morsitans* were caught using black screen fly rounds. -Overall, 577 female tsetse flies were dissected for ovarian age estimation. -A sentinel herd of 40 cattle was established at each of the four sites of Katete and Mambwe districts.	-Results indicated a significant increase in tsetse age as fragmentation increased. -Tsetse density was lower in most fragmented areas whilst the proportion of female flies increased significantly as fragmentation reduced. -AAT incidence in cattle was determined using buffy coat method. Infection rate in both cattle and tsetse flies was higher in highly fragmented areas.	1. Need to develop models that link biological characteristics of tsetse flies with habitat conditions. Such models maybe helpful in planning tsetse control interventions.
(Meyer et al., 2016) [25]	A literature review of past and on-going tsetse and African trypanosomiasis programmes	Systematic literature review of tsetse and African trypanosomiasis programmes between 1980 and 2015	Five African countries including Zambia. 68 documents plus 12 structured questionnaires reviewed.	-Twenty-three major Tsetse and Trypanosomiasis control programmes recorded from the five countries. Three control programmes conducted in Zambia during the stated period include the following: - Insecticide treated targets and traps (ITT) + trypanocidal drugs (TRY) in western province under government services for tsetse elimination (1987–1989). - Sequential aerial spraying (SAS) + ITT in eastern province under Regional Tsetse and Trypanosomiasis Control Programme (RTTCP) for tsetse control (1989–1994) -SAS + ITT in Kwando Zambezi belt under Pan African Tsetse and Trypanosomiasis Eradication Campaign (PATTEC) for tsetse elimination (2008 onwards)	1. Need for evaluation of the control programmes recorded. 2. Need for standardised protocols to conduct such evaluations of control programmes
(Alderton et al., 2016) [15]	To develop an agent-based model (ABM) for investigating *Trypanosoma brucei rhodesiense*	-Mixed methods	-ABM comprised of human/animal trypanosomiasis and tsetse ecological survey data obtained along the 75km transect in the Luangwa valley of Zambia. -Ethnicity, age and gender data were also incorporated.	-ABM produced output that could not be readily generated by other techniques. On average there were 1.99 (S.E. 0.245) human infections and 1.83 (S.E. 0.183) cattle infections per 6-month period. -The model output identified that the approximate incidence rate (per 1000 person-years) was lower amongst cattle owning households (0.079, S.E. 0.017), than those without cattle (0.134, S.E. 0.017). - Immigrant tribes (e.g., Bemba I.R. = 0.353, S.E.0.155) and school-age children (e.g., 5–10-year-old I.R. = 0.239, S.E. 0.041) were the most at-risk for acquiring infection.	1. The ABM can be used as a tool for scenario testing at an appropriate spatial scale to allow the design of logistically feasible mitigation strategies suggested by model output. This is of importance where resources are limited, and management strategies are often pushed to the local scale.

Table A1. *Cont.*

Author Year	Study Aim	Study Design	Sample and Participation	Study Findings	Needs Domain
(Holt et al., 2016) [2]	To assess AAT vulnerability in cattle owing communities	Cross sectional survey of cattle owners using questionnaire interviews.	210 households from Lundazi and Mambwe districts of Zambia	-AAT was constant with seasonal pattern, some trypano-tolerant breeds and communal grazing, small/moderate herd size with crops and mixing farming as primary income source, losses to draft reported, slightly higher mortalities and moderate costs diagnosing and treating, less likely to report treatment failure, low/good knowledge of control and tsetse traps/targets reported. -moderate AAT challenge, some concerns with resistance reported and most likely to keep pigs while some keep sheep and goats.	1. Need to integrate novel treatments with new and existing diagnostic and control programmes with findings of the study to develop tailored recommendations for AAT control and the reduce its impact in vulnerable communities.
(Meyer et al., 2018) [27]	To propose a framework for conducting a cost benefit analysis of possible AAT control analysis	A literature review of AAT of cattle production, herd management, impact of AAT on productivity, incidence and mortality	Two districts from Cameroon and Zambia (Mambwe district)	-For Zambia, the 10-year impact of tsetse elimination on the net value of cattle production was calculated as benefit–cost ratios using a discount rate of 5% and indicated the following:-2.3 (1.8–2.7) Targets, insecticide treated cattle (ITC) barrier -2.0 (1.6–2.4) Targets, barrier traps -2.8 (2.3–3.3) Aerial spraying, ITC barrier -2.5 (2.0–2.9) Aerial spraying, barrier trap -The use of SAT as elimination method for Mambwe district yielded a higher benefit–cost ratio than the use of targets. -The model estimated the total discounted control costs at 3.8 million USD and benefits at 10.5 million USD for Mambwe district if SAT was used as tsetse elimination method	1. Need for barriers to be maintained and monitoring activities conducted continuously unless sequential elimination of the entire tsetse belt is achieved. 2. Cost–benefit studies should be supported by recent estimates of key parameters such as frequency of trypanosome infection and impact, livestock and tsetse demographics. 3. Model generated in study combined data from different locations and from studies conducted years ago, there is need to validate the model using current data from same locations. 4. Need to use existing control programmes for designing future control programmes.

References

1. Swallow, B.M. *Impacts of Trypanosomiasis on African Agriculture*; Food and Agriculture Organization of the United Nations: Rome, Italy, 2000.
2. Holt, H.R.; Selby, R.; Mumba, C.; Napier, G.B.; Guitian, J. Assessment of Animal African Trypanosomiasis (AAT) Vulnerability in Cattle-Owning Communities of Sub-Saharan Africa. *Parasites Vectors* **2016**, *9*, 53. [CrossRef] [PubMed]
3. Munang'andu, H.M.; Siamudaala, V.; Munyeme, M.; Nalubamba, K.S. A review of ecological factors associated with the epidemiology of wildlife trypanosomiasis in the luangwa and zambezi valley ecosystems of zambia. *Interdiscip Perspect Infect. Dis.* **2012**, *2012*, 372523. [CrossRef] [PubMed]
4. Anderson, N.E.; Mubanga, J.; Fevre, E.M.; Picozzi, K.; Eisler, M.C.; Thomas, R.; Welburn, S.C. Characterisation of the wildlife reservoir community for human and animal trypanosomiasis in the Luangwa Valley, Zambia. *PLoS Negl. Trop. Dis.* **2011**, *5*, e1211. [CrossRef] [PubMed]
5. Anderson, N.E.; Mubanga, J.; Machila, N.; Atkinson, P.M.; Dzingirai, V.; Welburn, S.C. Sleeping sickness and its relationship with development and biodiversity conservation in the Luangwa Valley, Zambia. *Parasites Vectors* **2015**, *8*, 224. [CrossRef] [PubMed]
6. Muriuki, G.W.; Njoka, T.J.; Reid, R.S.; Nyariki, D.M. Tsetse control and land-use change in Lambwe valley, south-western Kenya. *Agric. Ecosyst. Environ.* **2005**, *106*, 99–107. [CrossRef]
7. Frean, J.; Sieling, W.; Pahad, H.; Shoul, E.; Blumberg, L. Clinical management of East. *African trypanosomiasis in South. Africa: Lessons learned. Int. J. Infect. Dis.* **2018**, *75*, 101–108.
8. Richter, J.; Göbels, S.; Göbel, T.; Westenfeld, R.; Müller-Stöver, I.; Häussinger, D. A returning traveller with fever, facial swelling, and skin lesions. *BMJ* **2012**, *344*, e2092. [CrossRef]
9. Kakumbi. *Annual Report*; Ministry of Fisheries and Livestock: Mambwe, Zambia, 2017.
10. Mwiinde, A.M.; Simuunza, M.; Namangala, B.; Chama-Chiliba, C.M.; Machila, N.; Anderson, N.; Welburn, S.C. Estimating the economic and social consequences for patients diagnosed with human African trypanosomiasis in Muchinga, Lusaka and Eastern Provinces of Zambia (2004–2014). *Infect. Dis. Poverty* **2017**, *6*, 150. [CrossRef]
11. Livestock and Fisheries. *Ministry Annual Report*; The Republic of Zambia: Lusaka, Zambia, 2016.
12. Mbewe, N.J.; Sitali, L.; Namangala, B.; Michelo, C. Adherence to the Food and Agricultural Organization guidelines on trypanocide usage among cattle farmers in Itezhi tezhi, Central Zambia. *Vet. Parasitol.* **2015**, *209*, 43–49. [CrossRef]
13. WHO. WHO Fact Sheet-Human African Trypanosomiais. Available online: https://www.who.int/news-room/fact-sheets/detail/trypanosomiasis-human-african-(sleeping-sickness) (accessed on 30 May 2020).
14. Franco, J.R.; Cecchi, G.; Priotto, G.; Paone, M.; Diarra, A.; Grout, L.; Argaw, D. Monitoring the elimination of human African trypanosomiasis at continental and country level: Update to 2018. *PLoS Negl. Trop. Dis.* **2020**, *14*, e0008261. [CrossRef]
15. Mwanakasale, V.; Songolo, P. Disapperance of some Human African Trypanosomiasis transmission foci in Zambia in the absence of tsetse fly and trypanosomiasis control program over a period of forty years. *Trans. R. Soc. Trop. Med. Hyg.* **2011**, *105*, 167–172. [CrossRef] [PubMed]
16. Laohasinnarong, D.; Goto, Y.; Asada, M.; Nakao, R.; Hayashida, K.; Kajino, K.; Namangala, B. Studies of trypanosomiasis in the Luangwa valley, north-eastern Zambia. *Parasit Vectors* **2015**, *8*, 555. [CrossRef]
17. Alderton, S.; Macleod, E.T.; Anderson, N.E.; Schaten, K.; Kuleszo, J.; Simuunza, M.; Atkinson, P.M. A Multi-Host Agent-Based Model. *for a Zoonotic, Vector-Borne Disease. A Case Study on Trypanosomiasis in Eastern Province, Zambia. PLoS Negl. Trop. Dis.* **2016**, *10*, e0005252.
18. Simukoko, H.; Marcotty, T.; Vercruysse, J.; Van den Bossche, P. Bovine trypanosomiasis risk in an endemic area on the eastern plateau of Zambia. *Res. Vet. Sci.* **2011**, *90*, 51–54. [CrossRef] [PubMed]
19. Marcotty, T.; Simukoko, H.; Berkvens, D.; Vercruysse, J.; Praet, N.; Van den Bossche, P. Evaluating the use of packed cell volume as an indicator of trypanosomal infections in cattle in eastern Zambia. *Prev. Vet. Med.* **2008**, *87*, 288–300. [CrossRef]
20. Mweempwa, C.; Marcotty, T.; De Pus, C.; Penzhorn, B.L.; Dicko, A.H.; Bouyer, J.; De Deken, R. Impact of habitat fragmentation on tsetse populations and trypanosomiasis risk in eastern Zambia. *Parasites Vectors* **2015**, *8*, 1–10. [CrossRef]

21. Lisulo, M.; Sugimoto, C.; Kajino, K.; Hayashida, K.; Mudenda, M.; Moonga, L.; Namangala, B. Determination of the prevalence of African trypanosome species in indigenous dogs of Mambwe district, eastern Zambia, by loop-mediated isothermal amplification. *Parasit Vectors* **2014**, *7*, 19. [CrossRef]
22. Mbewe, N.J.; Namangala, B.; Sitali, L.; Vorster, I.; Michelo, C. Prevalence of pathogenic trypanosomes in anaemic cattle from trypanosomosis challenged areas of Itezhi-tezhi district in central Zambia. *Parasit Vectors* **2015**, *8*, 638. [CrossRef]
23. Namangala, B.; Hachaambwa, L.; Kajino, K.; Mweene, A.S.; Hayashida, K.; Simuunza, M.; Moonga, L. The use of Loop-mediated Isothermal Amplification (LAMP) to detect the re-emerging Human African Trypanosomiasis (HAT) in the Luangwa and Zambezi valleys. *Parasit Vectors* **2012**, *5*, 282. [CrossRef]
24. Mulenga, G.M.; Likwa, R.N.; Namangala, B. Assessing the capacity to diagnose human African trypanosomiasis among health care personnel from Chama and Mambwe districts of eastern Zambia. *BMC Res. Notes* **2015**, *8*, 433. [CrossRef]
25. Mwanakasale, V.; Songolo, P.; Daka, V. Challenges in the control of human African trypanosomiasis in the Mpika district of Zambia. *BMC Res. Notes* **2013**, *6*, 180. [CrossRef] [PubMed]
26. Grant, C.; Anderson, N.; Machila, N. Stakeholder Narratives on Trypanosomiasis, Their Effect on Policy and the Scope for One Health. *PLoS Negl. Trop. Dis.* **2015**, *9*, e0004241. [CrossRef] [PubMed]
27. Meyer, A.; Holt, H.R.; Selby, R.; Guitian, J. Past and Ongoing Tsetse and Animal Trypanosomiasis Control. *Operations in Five African Countries: A Systematic Review. PLoS Negl. Trop. Dis.* **2016**, *10*, e0005247.
28. Meyer, A.; Holt, H.R.; Oumarou, F.; Chilongo, K.; Gilbert, W.; Fauron, A.; Guitian, J. Integrated cost-benefit analysis of tsetse control and herd productivity to inform control programs for animal African trypanosomiasis. *Parasit Vectors* **2018**, *11*, 154. [CrossRef]
29. Squarre, D.; Kabongo, I.; Munyeme, M.; Mumba, C.; Mwasinga, W.; Hachaambwa, L.; Namangala, B. Human African Trypanosomiasis in the Kafue National Park, Zambia. *PLoS Negl. Trop. Dis.* **2016**, *10*, e0004567. [CrossRef]
30. Nyimba, P.H.; Komba EV, G.; Sugimoto, C.; Namangala, B. Prevalence and species distribution of caprine trypanosomosis in Sinazongwe and Kalomo districts of Zambia. *Vet. Parasitol.* **2015**, *210*, 125–130. [CrossRef]
31. Alderton, S.; Macleod, E.T.; Anderson, N.E.; Machila, N.; Simuunza, M.; Welburn, S.C.; Atkinson, P.M. Exploring the effect of human and animal population growth on vector-borne disease transmission with an agent-based model of Rhodesian human African trypanosomiasis in eastern province, Zambia. *PLoS Negl. Trop. Dis.* **2018**, *12*, e0006905. [CrossRef]
32. Delespaux, V.; Dinka, H.; Masumu, J.; Van den Bossche, P.; Geerts, S. Five-fold increase in Trypanosoma congolense isolates resistant to diminazene aceturate over a seven-year period in Eastern Zambia. *Drug Resist. Updates* **2008**, *11*, 205–209. [CrossRef]
33. Njiru, Z.K.; Mikosza, A.S.J.; Matovu, E.; Enyaru, J.C.K.; Ouma, J.O.; Kibona, S.N.; Ndung'u, J.M. African trypanosomiasis: Sensitive and rapid detection of the sub-genus Trypanozoon by loop-mediated isothermal amplification (LAMP) of parasite DNA. *Int. J. Parasitol.* **2008**, *38*, 589–599. [CrossRef]
34. Njiru, Z. Loop-Mediated Isothermal Amplification Technology: Towards Point of Care Diagnostics. *PLos Negl. Trop. Dis.* **2012**, *6*, 1572. [CrossRef]
35. Njiru, Z.K.; Constantine, C.C.; Guya, S.; Crowther, J.; Kiragu, J.M.; Thompson, R.C.A.; Dávila, A.M.R. The use of ITS1 rDNA PCR in detecting pathogenic African trypanosomes. *Parasitol. Res.* **2005**, *95*, 186–192. [CrossRef] [PubMed]
36. Ahmed, H.A.; Picozzi, K.; Welburn, S.C.; MacLeod, E.T. A comparative evaluation of PCR- based methods for species- specific determination of African animal trypanosomes in Ugandan cattle. *Parasit Vectors* **2013**, *6*, 316. [CrossRef] [PubMed]
37. Picozzi, K.; Carrington, M.; Welburn, S.C. A multiplex PCR that discriminates between Trypanosoma brucei brucei and zoonotic T. *b. rhodesiense. Exp. Parasitol.* **2008**, *118*, 41–46. [CrossRef] [PubMed]
38. Mulenga, G.M.; Namangala, B.; Likwa, R.N. Capacity and Policy Change in Managing Trypanosomiasis in Endemic Rural Health Centres of Eastern Zambia. *ARC J. Public Health Community Med.* **2016**, *1*, 12–19.
39. Van den Bossche, P.; Doran, M.; Connor, R.J. An analysis of trypanocidal drug use in the Eastern province of Zambia. *Acta Trop.* **2000**, *75*, 247–258. [CrossRef]

40. Von Wissmann, B.; Machila, N.; Picozzi, K.; Fèvre, E.M.; Barend, M.; Handel, I.G.; Welburn, S.C. Factors associated with acquisition of human infective and animal infective trypanosome infections in domestic livestock in Western Kenya. *PLoS Negl. Trop. Dis.* **2011**, *5*, e941. [CrossRef]
41. Namangala, B.; Oparaocha, E.; Kajino, K.; Hayashida, K.; Moonga, L.; Inoue, N.; Sugimoto, C. Preliminary investigation of trypanosomosis in exotic dog breeds from Zambia's Luangwa and Zambezi valleys using LAM. *Am. J. Trop. Med. Hyg.* **2013**, *89*, 116–118. [CrossRef]

10

In Situ Diagnosis of Scabies Using a Handheld Digital Microscope in Resource-Poor Settings—A Proof-of-Principle Study in the Amazon Lowland of Colombia

Hollman Miller [1], Julian Trujillo-Trujillo [2] and Hermann Feldmeier [3,*]

1 Public Health Service, Vaupes Department, Mitú 97001, Colombia; hollmanmiller@gmail.com
2 Department of Neglected Tropical Diseases, Ministry of Health and Social Protection, Bogotá 110311, Colombia; trujillotrujillojulian@gmail.com
3 Institute of Microbiology and Infection Immunology, Campus Benjamin Franklin, Charité—University Medicine Berlin, corporate member of Freie Universität Berlin, Humboldt-Universität zu Berlin and Berlin Institute of Health, 12203 Berlin, Germany
* Correspondence: hermann.feldmeier@charite.de

Abstract: Scabies is a neglected tropical disease associated with important morbidity. The disease occurs worldwide and is particularly common in resource-poor communities in the Global South. A validated technique for the diagnosis of scabies in resource-poor settings does not exist. The objective of the study was to determine the practicability and accuracy of handheld digital microscopy in three indigenous communities in the Amazon lowland of Colombia, where scabies is the most common parasitic skin disease. One-hundred-and-eleven children and adults from three indigenous communities with a presumptive diagnosis of scabies were examined clinically by using a handheld digital microscope placed directly on the skin. The microscopical identification of a mite was verified by an "experienced mother", a woman who had acquired the skills to diagnose scabies as part of traditional Amerindian medicine. The "experienced mother" removed the parasite with a fine needle and placed it on a flat surface in order to enable its direct examination with the digital microscope. Using digital microscopy, scabies was diagnosed in 24 out of 111 participants and confirmed by the extraction of a *Sarcoptes* mites from the acarine eminence. A characteristic tunnel (burrow) with or without mite could be clearly identified irrespective of the degree of pigmentation of the skin. Besides, digital microscopy revealed pathological characteristics of scabies hitherto unknown and impossible to be seen in dermoscopy, such as partially or totally obliterated tunnels, tunnels with multiple entry or exit points, circumscribed hyperpigmentation around obliterated tunnels and mites secluded in a nodule. This proof-of-principle study demonstrated the accurate diagnosis of scabies by handheld digital microscopy in patients with pigmented skin and the feasibility of this technique in resource-poor settings.

Keywords: scabies; diagnosis; digital handheld microscope; resource-poor setting; Amerindian communities; Amazon lowland

---

1. Introduction

Scabies, a parasitic skin disease caused by the mite *Sarcoptes scabiei* var. *hominis*, causes considerable morbidity through both direct effects and secondary bacterial infection [1–4]. Scabies provokes intense itch, severely affecting sleep and quality of life [5,6]. The disease occurs worldwide and is particularly common in resource-poor communities in the countries of the Global South [7,8]. In developing countries, children bear the highest disease burden, with an average prevalence of

5–10% [3,5]. In countries with a tropical climate, prevalences are up to 25% in the general population with >40% in some communities in the South Pacific and northern Australia [8–11].

As scabies can mimic a spectrum of skin diseases of infectious and non-infectious etiology, its clinical diagnosis requires experience. Clinical manifestations may differ between babies, children and adults [12,13], but also may vary between settings [14,15] and in the tropics, bacterial superinfection can further complicate the diagnosis [4,8,16]. How to diagnose scabies best in resource-poor settings in endemic areas is still a matter of debate [17]. Usually, the diagnosis is based on a case definition with unknown specificity and sensitivity [3,18]. To enable effective case management in the countries of the Global South, a diagnostic method is needed which is accurate and appropriate in people with moderately to intensely pigmented skin.

Sarcoptes mites can only be identified with certainty using a substantial magnification. We, therefore, decided to use a handheld digital video microscope allowing a magnification of up to 200-fold which, e.g., enables to reliably detect movements of the intestine and contractions of the heart of another skin parasite, *Tunga penetrans* [19]. This parasite is embedded in the lower strata of the epidermis and is difficult to identify even in unpigmented skin. The same technique was also used to diagnose myiasis caused by *Dermatobia hominis*, and trombiculid chigger mites (Hollman Miller, unpublished observation 2017). Here we show that (i) *Sarcoptes* mites can be reliably detected inside the tunnel they have created; (ii) tunnels vary considerably in shape, length and structure; and (iii) if a mite is present, it is almost always located in the acarine eminence at the end of the tunnel (burrow).

2. Material and Methods

2.1. Study Area and Population

The study was performed in Vaupes Department in the Amazon lowland of Colombia. The department has a surface of about 54,000 km^2. The population mainly consists of indigenous people of various ethnicities. They live in small communities along the Vaupes, Apaporis and Isana River and its affluents. Vaupes is covered with dense rain forest and most communities are only accessible by boat. Mitú, the capital of Vaupes Department, is situated at Latitude: 1°15′28″ North and Longitude: 70°14′04″ West with an altitude of 158 m above sea level. The climate is tropical the whole year round.

Scabies is the most common skin disease in the Amazon lowland of Colombia. Prevalence is in the order of 2% in the general population and 80% of the cases are children (Hollman Miller, unpublished observation 2017). Other important parasitic skin diseases are tungiasis, myiasis and cutaneous leishmaniasis. Prior to the present study, no control measures for scabies were undertaken in the area.

2.2. Study Design and Data Collection

The study was performed in the indigenous communities Cariya (N 0°22′22″, W 70°07′46.6″) and Santa Catalina (N 0°21′51.55″, W 70° 5′52.80″), situated along the Tiquié river, as well as in Barrio 12 de octubre, at the periphery of Mitú (N 01°14′00.4″, W 70°14′01.9″) between January and May 2017. Communities were selected on the basis of information from local health personnel that scabies seemed to be frequent and that they were accessible from Mitú by boat or car. In each community, individuals with a presumptive diagnosis of scabies were eligible, independent of their age.

In indigenous communities in the Amazon lowland of Colombia, scabies is traditionally diagnosed and treated by an experienced mother ("mujer experimentada"). These are women without medical training who have learned to diagnose scabies with the naked eye as a part of traditional Amerindian medicine, usually from their mothers. The experienced mother carefully inspects the patient's skin and looks for the presence of a pearly vesicle (*vesicula perlada*) which reflects the entry point of a mite into the skin [20] (Figure 1). Pearly vesicles are whitish and translucent, have a diameter of 0.5 to 3 mm and have a soft resistance against pressure (Figure 2A,B). They are frequently decapitated by scratching and then look like an excoriation. Once the experienced mother has identified a pearly vesicle or its remains, she looks for the acarine eminence (*eminencia acarina*), an oval elevation of the skin with a pearlescent appearance at the limit of visibility (0.3 × 0.4 mm) [20]. By experience, the experienced mother knows that the mite is located in the acarine eminence, usually at short distance to a pearly vesicle (Figure 3). When an experienced mother has identified an acarine eminence, she removes the mite from the corneal layer with the help of a sharp thorn or a sharpened piece of hard wood—a method performed in the Americas for hundreds of years [21] {We had very severe itching in the knuckles and on the back of our hands. The missionary told us, these were *Aradores* (farmers) that dig into the skin. (...) They sent for a mulatto woman who prided herself to be able to [diagnose and heal] all the little beasts that dig into man's skin, the Nigua, the Nuche, the Coya and the Arador; (*Sarcoptes* mite) She heated the tip of a small splinter of very hard wood by the lamp and pierced it in the furrows visible on the skin. After a long search she announced (...) that there was already an *Arador*. I saw a small round sack at the top of the splinter, (...). Because I had the skin full of *Aradores* on both hands, I ran out of patience with the operation, which had lasted well into the night. (...). (Von Humboldt, Südamerikanische Reise, Ullstein Publisher, Berlin, reprint of original, 1979, p. 348)} Hence, in traditional Amerindian medicine, the identification of the acarine eminence is the prerequisite for treatment of scabies.

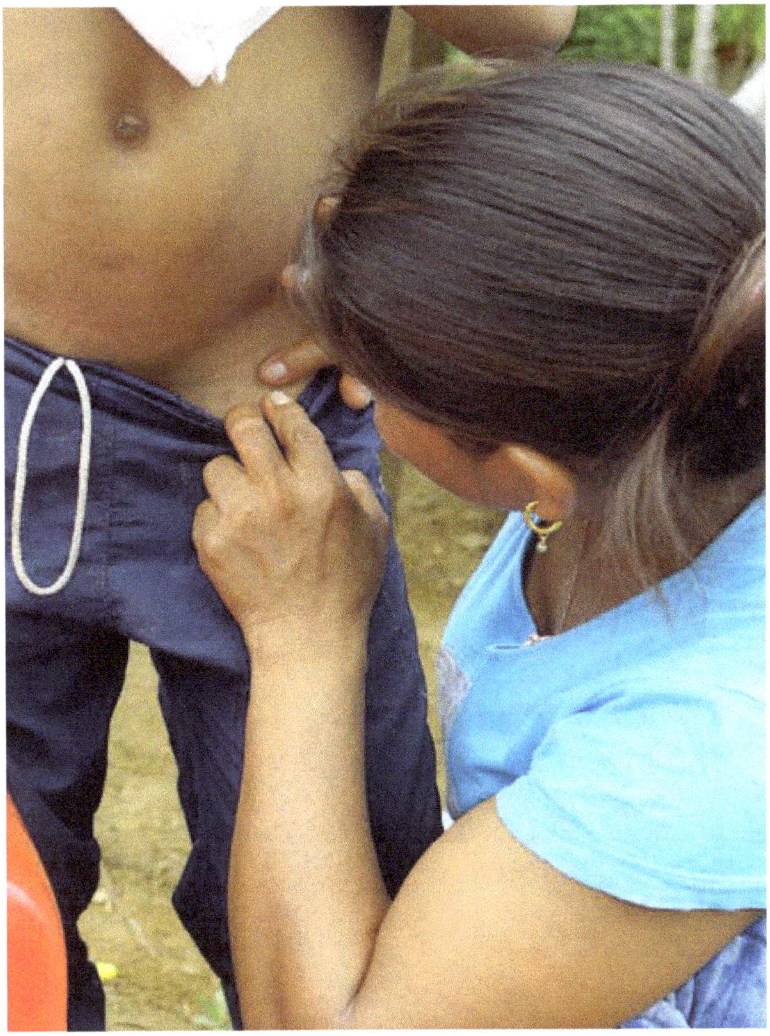

Figure 1. Experienced mother examining the skin of a child for the presence of a pearly vesicle.

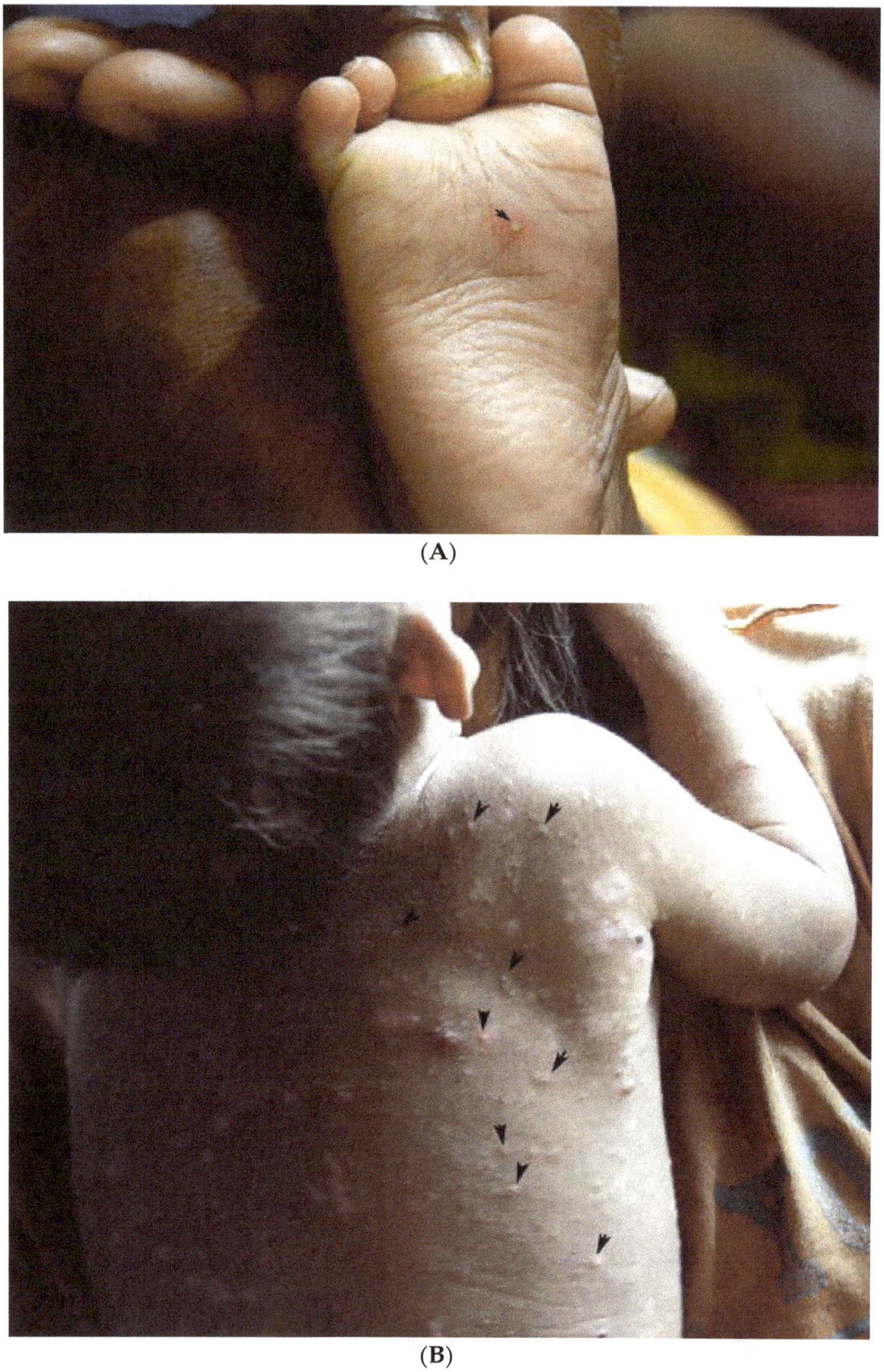

(**A**)

(**B**)

Figure 2. (**A**) A pearly vesicle at the sole of the foot (arrow). (**B**). Multiple pearly vesicles on the back of a child with severe scabies (arrows).

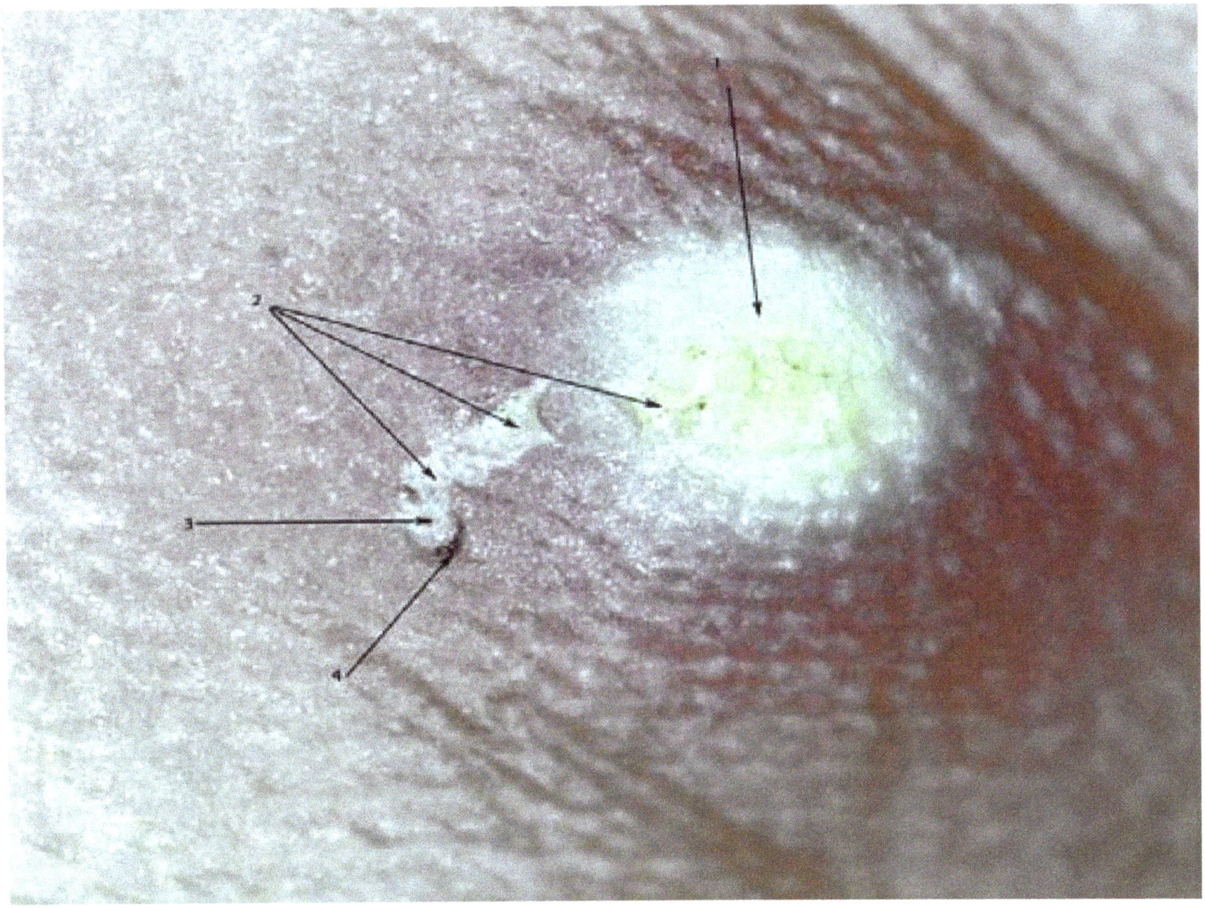

Figure 3. Pearly vesicle (1) and acarine eminence linked by a tunnel (2). The mite is situated at the end of the tunnel with its dorsal part turned towards the surface of the skin (3). The delta-wing sign is clearly visible (4). Photo by digital microscopy; magnification 30-fold.

Community health workers were informed about the arrival of the health team a couple of days in advance. Individuals with itchy lesions of the skin were asked to present themselves at a designated place in the morning and in the afternoon. No active search for cases was performed. After the medical history had been taken, the skin was examined macroscopically. Thereafter, the digital handheld microscope (dnt DigiMicro Mobile 5 Megapixel handheld microscope; Drahtlose Nachrichtentechnik GmbH, Dietzenbach, Germany) was placed directly on the skin and suspicious lesions were examined one by one, first using a 10-fold magnification followed by 30-fold magnification to identify the morphological characteristics of *Sarcoptes* mites (Figure 4A,B). Each lesion was scrutinized for the presence of a tunnel (intact, in the process of obliteration or totally obliterated), the presence of a mite inside a tunnel as well as the presence of faecal pellets or eggs. Other characteristics systematically looked for were the acarine eminence and the pearly vesicle [22,23], the presence of coagulated blood inside or around a tunnel (as an indicator of micro-haemorrhage induced by scratching); exfoliation or desquamation of the corneal layer (as an indicator of repeated scratching); and circumscript hyper-pigmented areas, visible only microscopically.

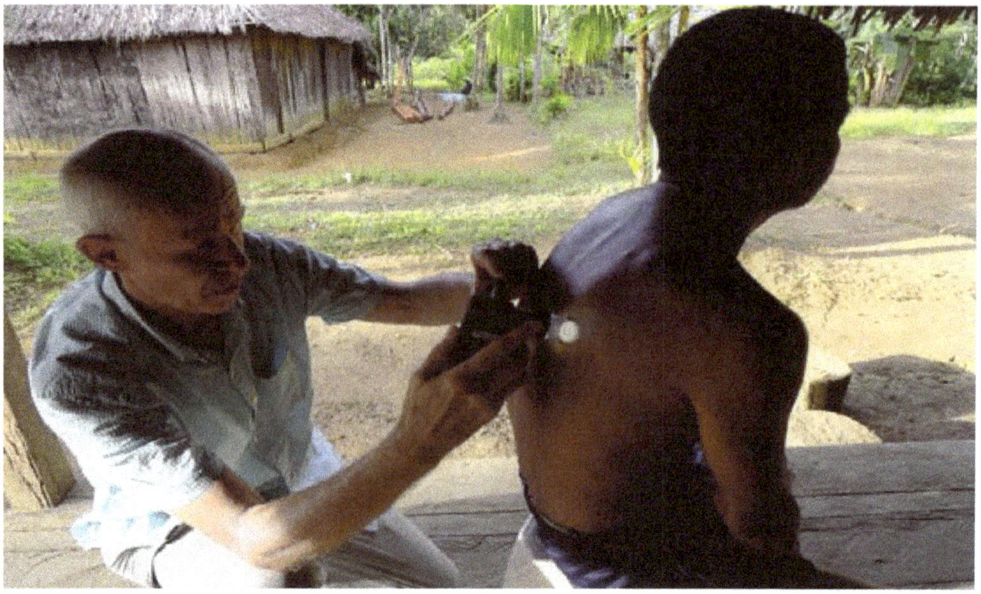

(A)

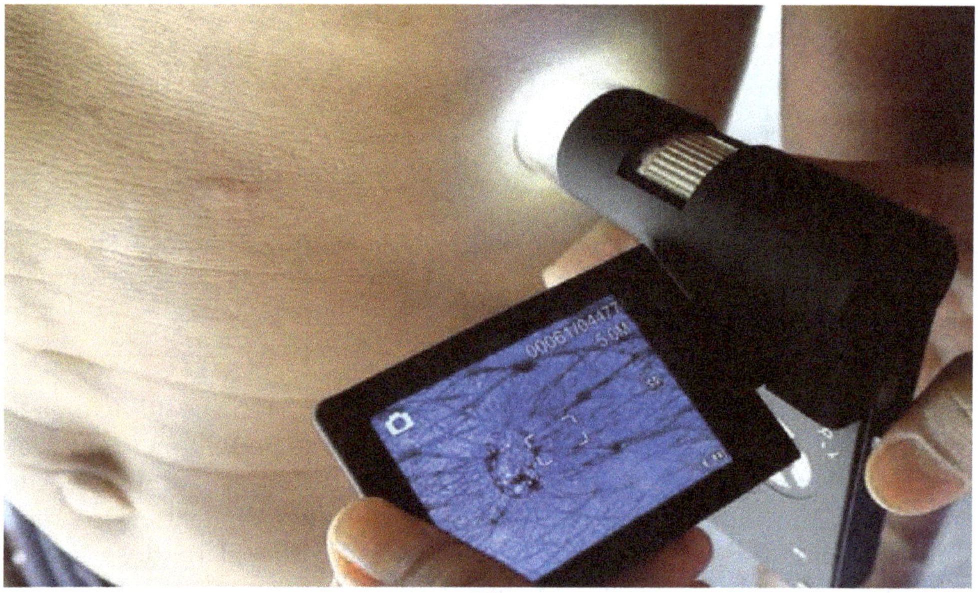

(B)

Figure 4. (**A**) Examination of the skin with the digital handheld microscope. (**B**) Examination of the skin with the digital handheld microscope, close-up.

Pathological findings were photographed, stored on an SD-card inside the microscope and transferred to a computer at the end of the day.

When a mite was detected in an acarine eminence by digital microscopy, the "experienced mother" was asked to remove it with a sterile entomological spin of #3 size and to place it on flat surface, such as a finger nail (Figure 5A,B) to confirm microscopy results. Using the video function of the microscope it was attempted to identify mites moving inside a tunnel or on the surface of the skin.

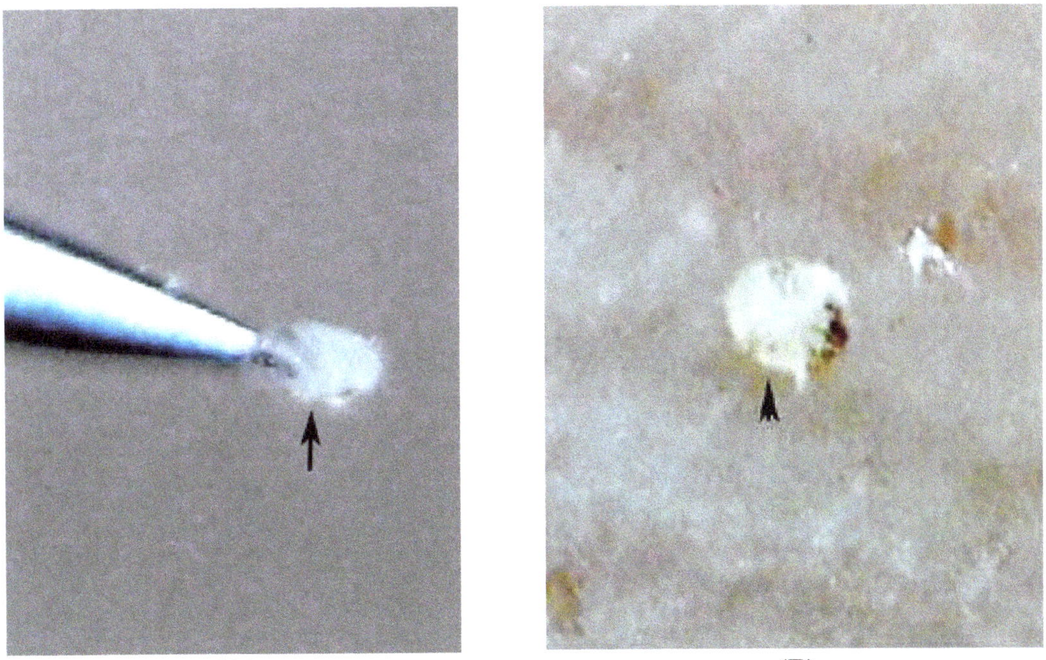

Figure 5. (**A**) *Sarcoptes* mite being extracted with a sterile needle by an experienced mother; magnification 70-fold. (**B**) Dorsal view of a mite extracted by the experienced mother from an acarine eminence; the hyperpigmented area of the anterior part of the mite corresponds to the delta-wing sign as seen in the dermatoscope; magnification 90-fold.

2.3. Diagnosis

Scabies was suspected if a patient showed a suspicious skin alteration accompanied by itching for at least 2 weeks. The following skin alterations were considered suspicious: presence of characteristic primary lesions (papules, crusted papules, vesicles, nodules) with or without the presence of secondary lesions (excoriation of the skin, secondary bacterial infection) that were obviously not associated with other dermatological conditions. Bacterial superinfection was diagnosed when pustules, suppuration or an abscess were present.

Diagnosis of scabies was defined as detection of the morphological characteristics of a mite in an acarine eminence by digital microscopy and subsequent confirmation by the extraction of the parasite; or if faecal pellets were identified inside a tunnel by digital microscopy.

2.4. Treatment

After diagnosis, the patient was treated with 200 μg/kg ivermectin orally, followed by a second dose after 1 week. Children <5 years and pregnant and lactating women were treated topically with sulfur in petrolatum 8%, once a day for 3 days [23]. Ivermectin and sulfur in petrolatum are standard treatments of scabies recommended by the Colombian Ministry of Health.

3. Results

The demographic characteristics of the study participants are summarized in Table 1. All participants had pigmented skin. Scabies was diagnosed in 24 out of 111 participants (21.6%). The frequency of cases was highest in Cariya (54.5%), and considerably lower in Santa Catalina and Barrio 12 de Octubre (15.6 and 20.4% of study participants, respectively). Sixteen of the 24 patients (66%) were children younger than 10 years of age. The clinical characteristics of the patients are depicted in Table 2.

Table 1. Demographic characteristics of participants.

Community	Number of Participants	Age in Years Median (Range)	Males/Females	Scabies Diagnosed [a] (%)
Cariyá	11	29 (3–88)	4/7	6 (54.5)
Santa Catalina	51	19 (2–71)	28/23	8 (15.7)
Barrio 12 de Octubre	49	12 (3 months–77)	21/28	10 (20.4)
Total	111	15 (3 months–88)	53/58	24 (21.6)

[a] see Material and Methods.

Table 2. Clinical characteristics of 24 patients with scabies.

Characteristics	Frequency (n/%)
Number of topographic areas affected	
1–5	10/(41.6%)
6–10	13/(54.1%)
>10	1/(4.31%)
Appearance of lesions (weeks ago)	
<4 weeks	6/(25.0%)
4–12 weeks	14/(58.3%)
>12 weeks	4/(16.6%)
Type of lesion [a]	
Papule	23/(95.8%)
Vesicle	16/(66.6%)
Nodule	2/(8.3%)
Crusted lesion [b]	15/(62.5%)
Excoriation/desquamation	19/(79.1%)
Bacterial superinfection [c]	15/(62.5%)

[a] Multiple classifications possible. [b] Crust developed on top of vesicle or papule. [c] Pustule, suppuration.

In 23 cases, a mite was identified in an acarine eminence. In one case, a mite was detected in the middle of a tunnel without an acarine eminence (Table 3). Pearly vesicles were observed in 17 cases, usually in a short distance of a few mm to an acarine eminence (Figure 6A,B). Frequently, only the residues of a pearly vesicle were visible (Figure 6C).

Table 3. Findings by digital microscopy in 24 scabies patients [a].

Characteristics [b]	Frequency (n/%)
Tunnel without mite	8/(33.7%)
Tunnel with mite	24/(100%)
Tunnel with mite present in the acarine eminence	23/(95.8%)
Tunnel with mite in the middle of the tunnel	1
Tunnel with faecal pellets	8/(33.3%)
Partially or totally obliterated tunnel	16/(66.7%)
Extraction of mite by experienced mother	24/(100%) [c]
Pearly vesicle surrounded by erythema	17/(70.8%)
Circumscribed hyperpigmentation	22/(91.6%)
Micro-haemorrhagia	4/(16.6%)
Excoriation/desquamation of the corneal layer	19/(79.1%) [d]
Nodule containing mite	1/(4.1%)

[a] For case definition see Materials and Methods [b] Multiple classifications possible. [c] In four cases, the mite was lost directly following the extraction. [d] not visible macroscopically.

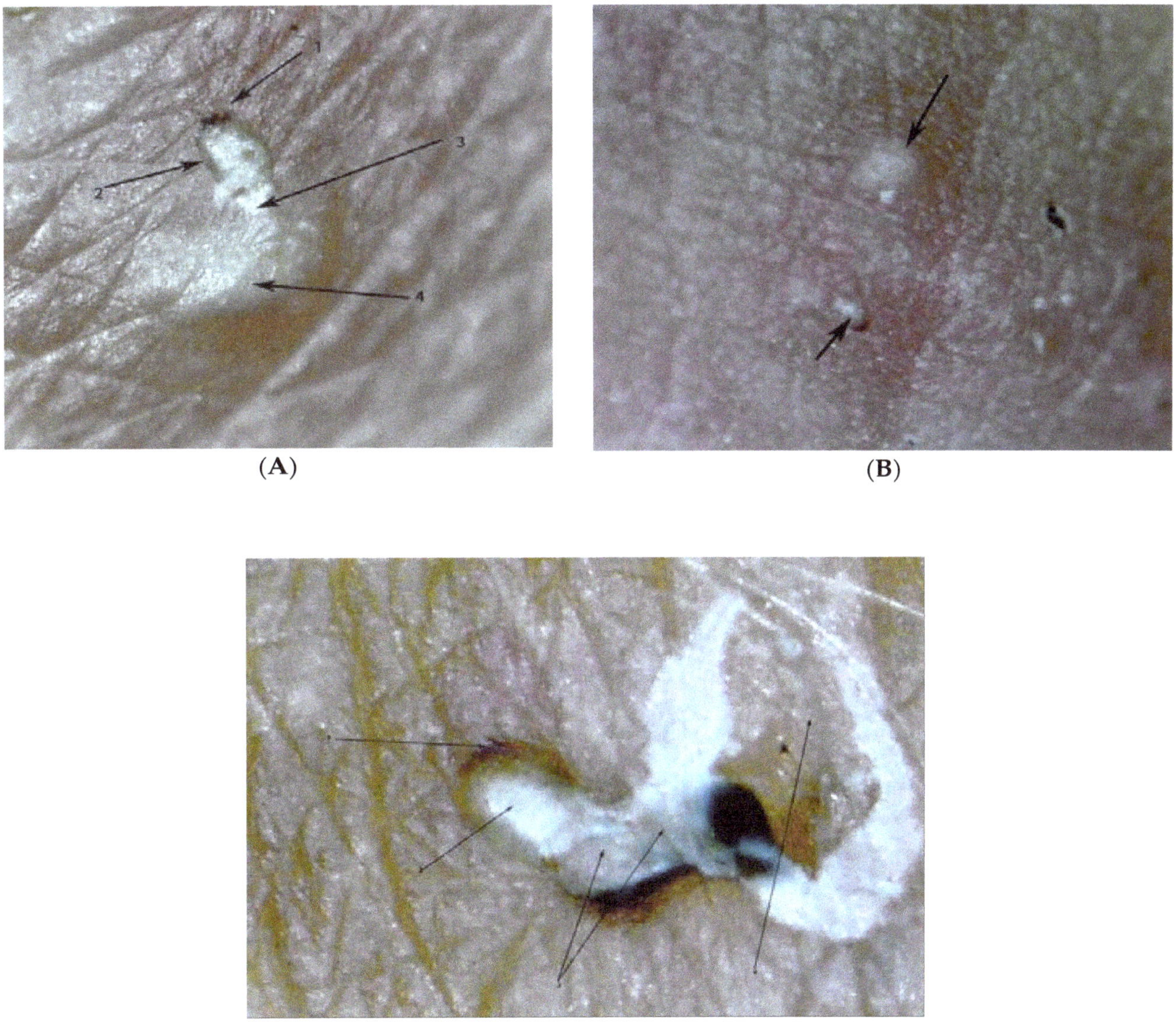

(C)

Figure 6. (**A**) Oval-shaped acarine eminence at the end of the tunnel (2) with the delta-wing sign (1); partially obliterated tunnel (3) connecting the acarine eminence with the pearly vesicle (4); magnification 50-fold. (**B**) Pearly vesicle (top) and acarine eminence (bottom) located at a distance from each other; no tunnel visible; the delta-wing sign is clearly visible (arrow bottom); magnification 15-fold. (**C**) Acarine eminence (3) at the end of an S-shaped tunnel containing a mite (2) with delta-wing sign visible (1); pearly vesicle destroyed by scratching (4); magnification 80-fold.

The microscopic aspect of a mite differed according whether its ventral or dorsal part was turned towards the surface of the skin (Figure 7A,B). Partially or completely obliterated tunnels were observed in 16 patients (Figure 8A,B). Those tunnels did not contain a mite. Tunnels in the process of obliteration showed a circumscript hyperpigmentation, not visible macroscopically (Figure 9). The length of a tunnel varied from less than 1 mm to about 10 mm. In some cases, tunnels showed multiple entry and exit points (Figure 10). In a single case, a mite was detected outside a tunnel moving on the skin. One nodule was identified which contained 2 mites (Figure 11).

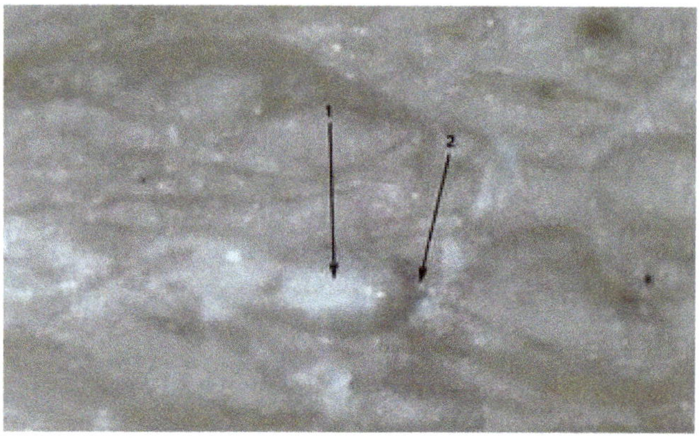

(A)

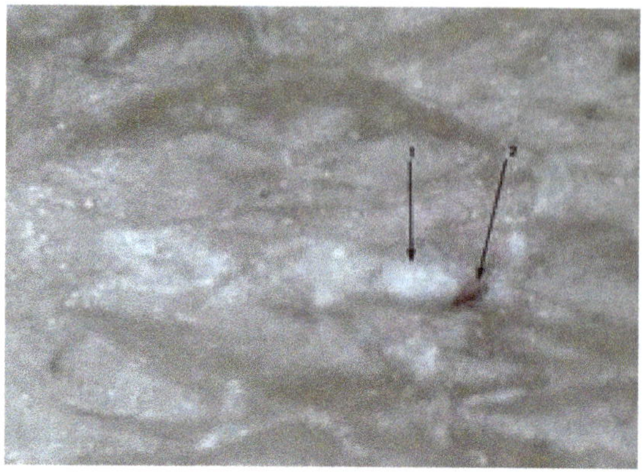

(B)

Figure 7. (**A**) Sarcoptes mite inside an acarine eminence with its dorsal part turned towards the surface of the skin (1); delta-wing sign visible (2); magnification 65-fold. (**B**) The same mite after having changed its position (1); now the ventral part is turned towards the surface of the skin (2); delta-wing sign not clearly visible.

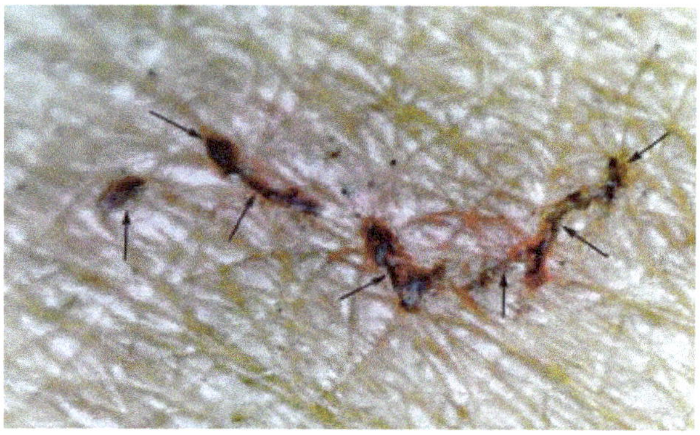

(A)

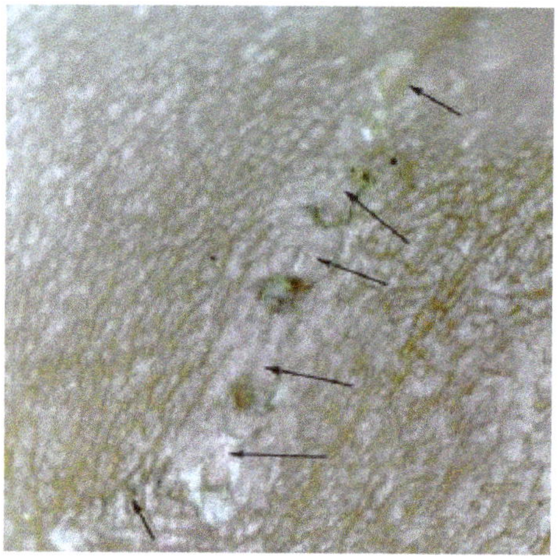

(B)

Figure 8. (**A**) Partially obliterated tunnel, obliterated parts show micro-haemorrhages (arrows); magnification 15-fold. (**B**) Totally obliterated tunnel; only residues of micro-haemorrhages visible; magnification 15-fold.

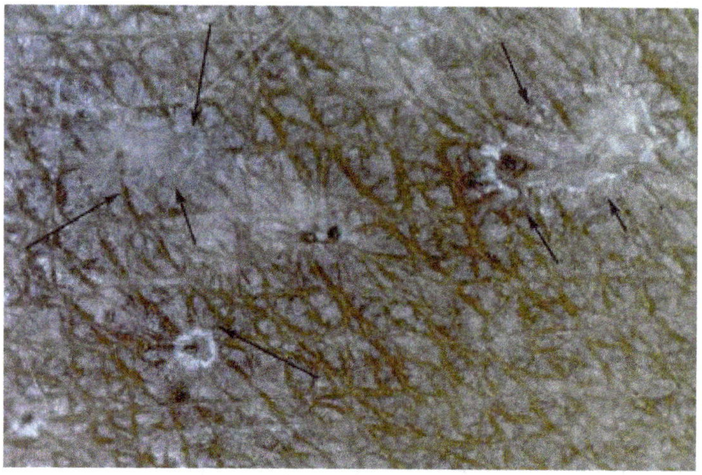

Figure 9. Microscopic circumscribed hyperpigmented areas (arrows) around a sinusoidal tunnel; magnification 30-fold.

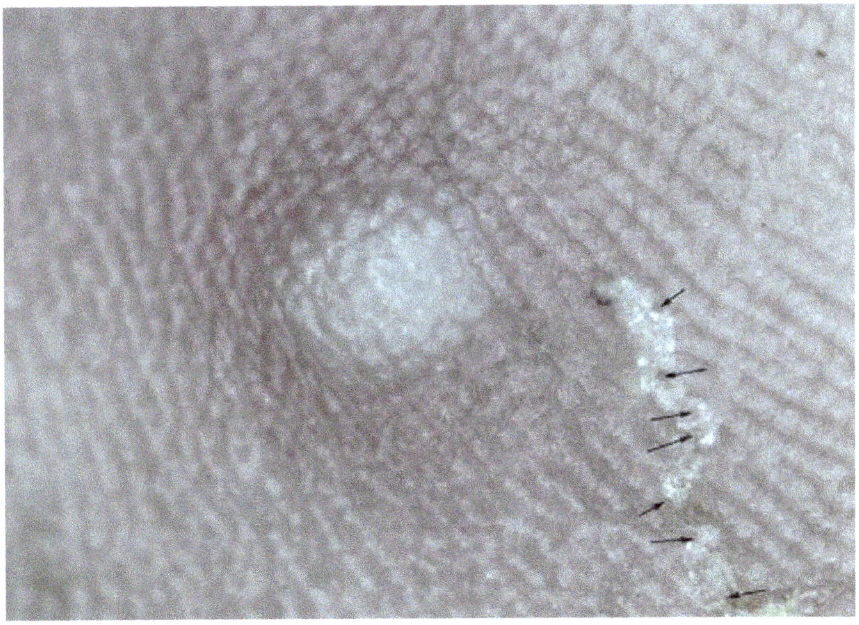

Figure 10. Serpiginous tunnel with multiple entry and exit points (arrows); magnification 15-fold.

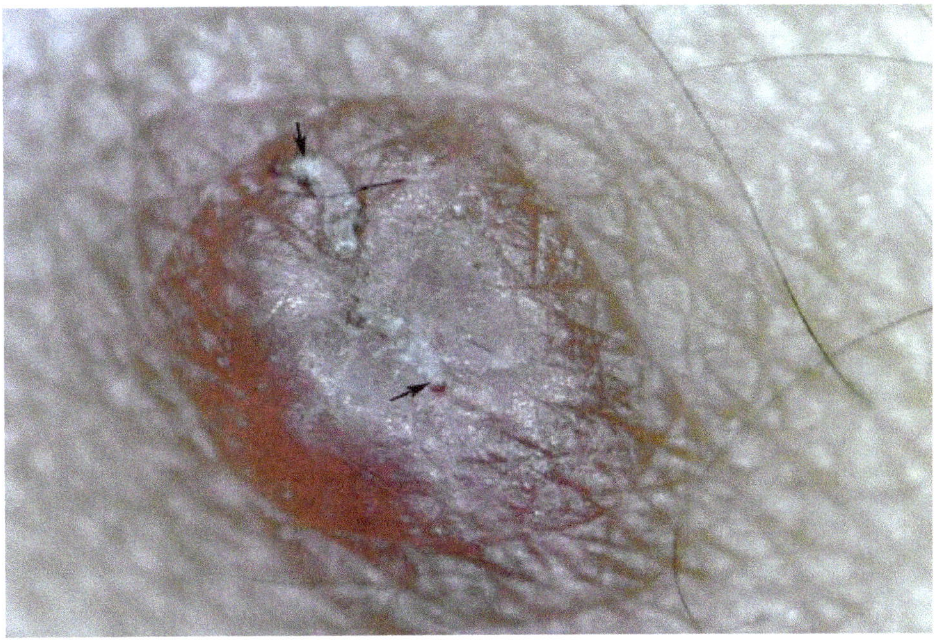

Figure 11. Nodule containing two mites (arrows); magnification 25-fold.

Usually, when excoriations were present macroscopically, micro-hemorrhages were visible microscopically (Figure 8A). Besides, the handheld digital microscope demonstrated the presence of tiny excoriations which were not visible macroscopically (Figure 12).

Lesions caused by *Trombicula alfreddugesi*, a mite endemic in the tropical rain forest of the Amazon and the Orinoco Basin, were ancillary findings by digital microscopy. The morphological characteristics of *T. alfreddugesi* are easily differentiated from those of a *Sarcoptes* (Figure 13).

All participants of the study were at ease with the examination of the skin by digital microscopy. Elder patients found it informative to spot the parasite that caused their disease.

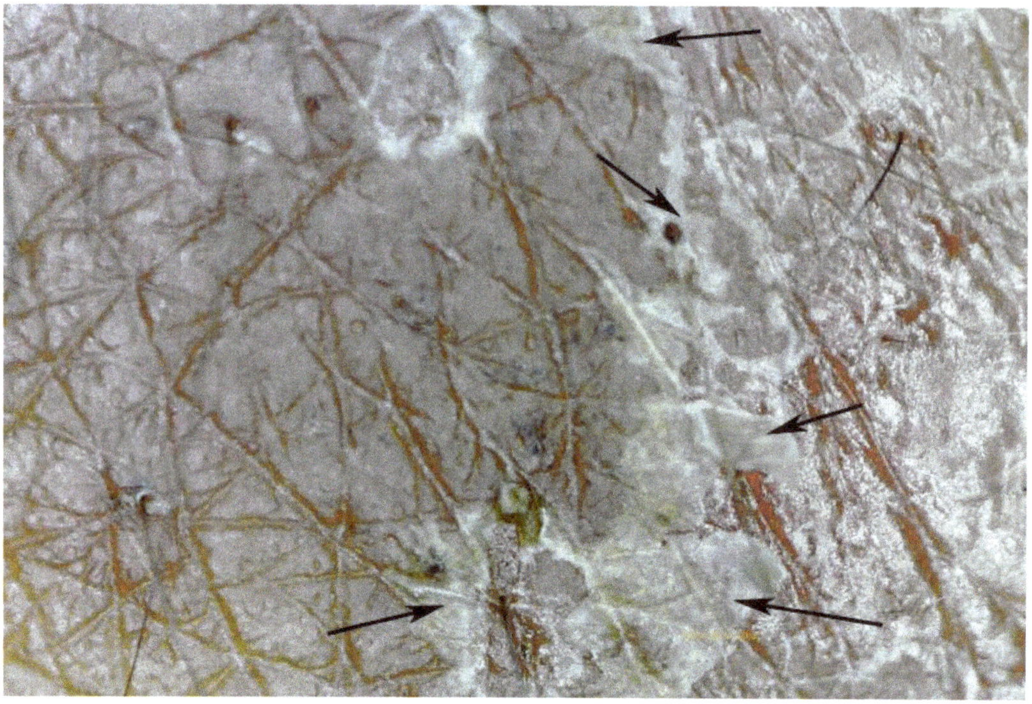

Figure 12. Microscopic excoriations of the stratum corneum not visible microscopically (arrows); magnification 100-fold.

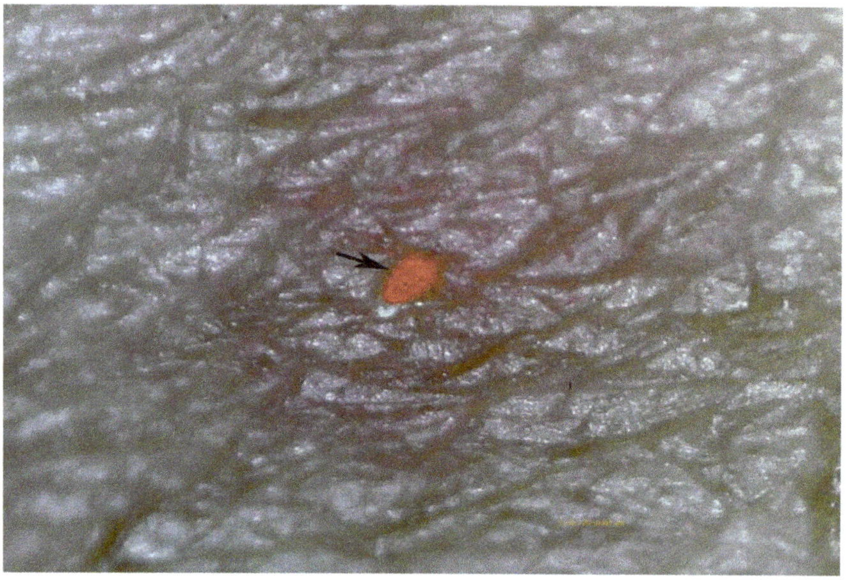

Figure 13. *Trombicula alfreddugesi* identified by the digital handheld microscope (arrow); magnification 10-fold.

4. Discussion

Scabies can mimic a broad range of infectious and non-infectious diseases [12] and the clinical picture is frequently masked by superinfection [13]. Hence, the specificity of clinical diagnosis is low, and its sensitivity depends on the experience of the observer. Since simple and accurate diagnostic techniques do not exist, in resource-poor settings, the diagnosis of scabies is based on the presence of suspicious clinical findings such as itchy papules or on a case definition of which neither sensitivity nor specificity is known [18,24].

Our findings also explain why a diagnosis based solely on the identification of a tunnel, such as by means of a burrow ink test, has a notoriously low sensitivity and specificity [25,26].

Based on our findings in tungiasis, a skin disease where the parasite is embedded in the lower strata of the epidermis and is difficult to identify macroscopically [19], we decided to use a digital handheld microscope for the detection of *Sarcoptes* mites in situ. The application of the digital handheld microscope is totally inoffensive and well tolerated even by small children [19]. The digital microscope is directly placed on the skin and illuminates a circumscript area of the skin of a diameter of 30 mm with 8 LED. The area examined is displayed on a color monitor with a resolution of 5 megapixels. Resolution of pictures can be further enhanced by connecting the microscope with a laptop or a tablet computer and enlarging the picture on the computer in real time. Photos and videos are stored on a Micro-SD card inside the microscope. The price of the handheld digital microscope is in the order of 120 US$. Previously described optical methods for the in vivo detection of mites used highly sophisticated stationary and expensive equipment such as reflectance-mode confocal microscopy or epiluminescence microscopy which are not suitable for resource-poor settings [27–29].

The digital handheld microscope allowed the identification of 24 cases of scabies out of 111 participants who fulfilled the admission criteria. Except for one case, mites were seen in the acarine eminence at the end of the tunnel. We presume that the acarine eminence is caused by a mite feeding on corneal cells and thereby exerting pressure on the surrounding layers of corneal cells. It reflects a dilatation of the upper corneal layer by a biologically active foreign body moving forward in the skin. The pearly vesicle was described first by the French dermatologist Pierre-Antoine-Ernest Bazin in 1862 [22]. We suppose that the pearly vesicle reflects an acute local inflammation at the point where a female mite has penetrated into the stratum corneum. Due to scratching, a pearly vesicle is frequently decapitated and only a residue remains. Ideally, the pearly vesicle and the acarine eminence should be linked by a tunnel. In practice though, pearly vesicles and tunnels are destroyed by scratching or become invisible due to bacterial superinfection [20,23]. The appearances of the pearly vesicle may vary under different environmental conditions and in colder climates and older persons, for instance, the mite entry point is often drier and scaly. This emphasizes the importance of adapting training to suit local conditions and using descriptive words that are easily understandable by local health workers.

An intriguing observation was the finding that the ventral and the dorsal part of an embedded *Sarcoptes* mite showed a different pigmentation pattern: The triangular pigmentation at the anterior part of the mite (the delta-wing sign visible in dermoscopy) being pronounced, when its dorsal part was turned towards the skin. Since the other body areas of a mite are almost translucent and a mite may change its position with regard to the skin's surface, this explains why in dermoscopy the delta-wing sign is not consistently present [24,30–32]. Obviously, even in non-pigmented skin, the delta-wing sign cannot be seen in the dermatoscope when the ventral end of the mite is positioned towards the surface of the skin or when the mite has changed its direction and its rear end is situated towards the end of the tunnel.

Faecal pellets were only inconsistently detectable in the handheld digital microscope and eggs were only seen in a single occasion. Neither faecal pellets nor eggs are reliable indicators of active scabies in digital microscopy and dermoscopy. Actually, it has been previously shown that eggs and faecal pellets need to be stained to become clearly visible [33,34].

The digital microscope also showed that tunnels considerably vary in size and shape and degree of obliteration. Surprisingly, we observed that tunnels may have various entry and exit points and that there are intact tunnels not inhabited by a mite. This confirms previous observations [29]. The presence of a tunnel as such, therefore, cannot be considered pathognomonic for the presence of active scabies and does not allow for a conclusion on the necessity of treatment [28]. Our findings also explain why a diagnosis based solely on the identification of a tunnel, such as by means of a burrow ink test, have a notoriously low sensitivity and specificity [25,26].

Our study corroborates previous findings that dermoscopy is an inappropriate means to diagnose scabies in a resource-poor setting [24]. Although the sensitivity of the technique is rather high (0.85; 95% CI 0.70–0.94), its specificity is low (0.46; 95% CI, 0.34–0.58) [24]. This can be explained by the finding that dermoscopy only yields optimal results when examiners are trained in the diagnosis of scabies [30] and that artefacts induced by scratching, such as crusts, or punctuate bleeding or small particles of dirt can be confounded with a mite [35,36].

Our study has several limitations. First, due to the lack of privacy, we excluded the genital area in both sexes and the peri-mamillary area in women. Since the morphological characteristics of lesions at these topographic areas may differ from those of other parts of the skin, e.g., noduli are very common on the penis, but rare at the abdomen, we cannot exclude that the distribution patterns of acarine eminence and/or the pearly vesicle are the same at all topographic areas of the skin. Second, we used the extraction of a mite from the acarine eminence by the experienced mother as a proof that the morphological characteristics seen in the digital handheld microscope were actually that of a *Sarcoptes* mite. We therefore can only conclude on the specificity of the method, but not on its sensitivity. A study to compare the sensitivity of the digital handheld microscopy with other diagnostic techniques used in resource-poor settings is currently being performed. Third, since all patients presented themselves voluntarily, we cannot rule out that a selection bias towards patients with a severe form of scabies might have occurred.

In conclusion, the proof-of-principle study showed that the digital handheld microscope is an accurate diagnostic instrument to diagnose scabies in resource-poor settings in people with pigmented skin. In addition, the technique allows the detection of micro-pathological alterations of the skin presumably caused by scratching or due to an immune response of the host. If applied in a systematic way, handheld digital microscopy will provide new insights into the biological host-parasite-relationships of *Sarcoptes* mites and eventually lead to the understanding of pathogenesis and pathophysiology of skin alterations caused by *S. scabiei*.

Author Contributions: Study concept and design: H.F. and H.M.; Acquisition of data: H.M. and H.F.; Analysis and interpretation of data: H.M., H.F. and J.T.-T.; Drafting of the manuscript: H.F.; Critical revision of the manuscript for important intellectual content: All authors.

Acknowledgments: We are very grateful that the experienced mothers Belkis Bernal Rodriguez, Martha Lucia Sanchez Perez, Maria Sanchez Perez and Denia Valenzuela Lima shared their knowledge with us. We are also very grateful for the support by the community health workers, particularly Cesar de Jesus Tamayo Londoño.

Ethical Considerations: The study was performed as part of a routine health care provided by public health personnel of Vaupés Health Department. When the medical team arrived in a community, the procedure was explained to community leaders, community health assistants and study participants. The examination of the skin for the diagnosis of scabies and other dermatological conditions is part of the routine health care and was carried out with the aim to identify and treat patients with scabies. The examination of minors was made with the authorization and in the presence of at least one of their parents. As illiteracy is frequent in indigenous populations, participants—and in the case of minors the respective care-giver—were asked to provide oral informed consent. There was a written authorization from the traditional indigenous authorities. In accordance with Resolution 008430 of 1993 of the Ministry of Health and Social Protection of Colombia which regulates research in humans, the study was classified as risk-free, because the examination with digital microscopy is totally inoffensive. The study was approved by the Ethical Committee of the Universidad del Cauca, certificate 6.1-1.25/021.

References

1. Engelman, D.; Kiang, K.; Chosidow, O.; McCarthy, J.; Fuller, C.; Lammie, P.; Hay, R.; Steer, A. Toward the global control of human scabies: Introducing the international alliance for the control of scabies. *PLoS Negl. Trop. Dis.* **2013**, *7*, e2167. [CrossRef] [PubMed]
2. Feldmeier, H.; Heukelbach, J. Epidermal parasitic skin diseases: A neglected category of poverty-associated plagues. *Bull. World Health Organ.* **2009**, *87*, 152–159. [CrossRef] [PubMed]
3. Heukelbach, J.; Feldmeier, H. Scabies. *Lancet* **2006**, *367*, 1767–1774. [CrossRef]
4. Berrios, X.; Lagomarsino, E.; Solar, E.; Sandoval, G.; Guzman, B.; Riedel, I. Post-streptococcal acute glomerulonephritis in chile—20 years of experience. *Pediatr. Nephrol.* **2004**, *19*, 306–312. [CrossRef] [PubMed]

5. Hay, R.J.; Steer, A.C.; Engelman, D.; Walton, S. Scabies in the developing world—Its prevalence, complications, and management. *Clin. Microbiol. Infect.* **2012**, *18*, 313–323. [CrossRef] [PubMed]
6. Worth, C.; Heukelbach, J.; Fengler, G.; Walter, B.; Liesenfeld, O.; Feldmeier, H. Impaired quality of life in adults and children with scabies from an impoverished community in Brazil. *Int. J. Dermatol.* **2012**, *51*, 275–282. [CrossRef] [PubMed]
7. Feldmeier, H.; Jackson, A.; Ariza, L.; Calheiros, C.M.L.; de Lima Soares, V.; Hengge, U.R.; Heukelbach, J. The epidemiology of scabies in an impoverished community in rural brazil: Presence and severity of disease are associated with poor living conditions and illiteracy. *J. Am. Acad. Dermatol.* **2009**, *60*, 436–443. [CrossRef] [PubMed]
8. Carapetis, J.R.; Connors, C.; Yarmirr, D.; Krause, V.; Currie, B.J. Success of a scabies control program in an australian aboriginal community. *Pediatr. Infect. Dis. J.* **1997**, *16*, 494–499. [CrossRef] [PubMed]
9. Heukelbach, J.; Wilcke, T.; Winter, B.; Feldmeier, H. Epidemioloy and morbidity of scabies and pediculosis capitis in resource-poor communities in Brazil. *Br. J. Dermatol.* **2007**, *153*, 150–156. [CrossRef] [PubMed]
10. Jackson, A.; Heukelbach, J.; Feldmeier, H. Transmission of scabies in an endemic area. *Br. J. Infect. Dis.* **2007**, *11*, 307–308.
11. Currie, B.J.; Connors, C.M.; Krause, V.L. Scabies programs in aboriginal communities. *Med. J. Aust.* **1994**, *161*, 636–637. [PubMed]
12. Feldmeier, H.; Wilcke, T. Scabies in childhood. In *Recent Advances in Pediatrics*; David, T.J., Ed.; The Royal Society of Medicine Press: London, UK, 2007; pp. 25–38.
13. Jackson, A.; Heukelbach, J.; Ferreira da Silva Filho, A.; Barros Campelo Junior, E.; Feldmeier, H. Clinical features and associated morbidity of scabies in a rural community in alagoas, Brazil. *Trop. Med. Int. Health* **2007**, *12*, 493–502. [CrossRef] [PubMed]
14. Cestari, T.F.; Martignago, B.F. Scabies, pediculosis, bedbugs, and stinkbugs: Uncommon presentations. *Clin. Dermatol.* **2005**, *23*, 545–554. [CrossRef] [PubMed]
15. Schmeller, W.; Bendick, C.; Stingl, P. *Dermatosen aus drei Kontinenten—Bildatlas der Vergleichenden Dermatologie*, 1st ed.; Schattauer: Stuttgart, Germany, 2005; p. 238.
16. Feldmeier, H. Diagnosis of parasitic skin diseases. In *Evidence Based Dermatology*, 2nd ed.; Maibach, H., Farzam, G., Eds.; PMPH-USA: Raleigh, NC, USA, 2010; pp. 73–86.
17. Walton, S.F.; Currie, B.J. Problems in diagnosing scabies, a global disease in human and animal populations. *Clin. Microbiol. Rev.* **2007**, *20*, 268–279. [CrossRef] [PubMed]
18. Mahe, A.; Faye, O.; N'Diaye, H.T.; Ly, F.; Konare, H.; Keita, S.; Traore, A.K.; Hay, R. Definition of an algorithm for the management of common skin diseases at primary health care level in sub-saharan africa. *Trans. R. Soc. Trop. Med. Hyg.* **2005**, *99*, 39–47. [CrossRef] [PubMed]
19. Thielecke, M.; Nordin, P.; Ngomi, N.; Feldmeier, H. Treatment of tungiasis with dimeticone: A proof-of-principle study in rural kenya. *PLoS Negl. Trop. Dis.* **2014**, *8*, e3058. [CrossRef] [PubMed]
20. Aguado Taberné, C.; del Pozo Guzmán, R.; García Aranda, J.M. Tratamiento de las infestaciones cutáneas. In *Manual de Terapéutica en Atención Primaria*; Central Publications Service of the Basque Government: Vitoria-Gasteiz, Spain, 2006.
21. Von Humboldt, A. *Südamerikanische Reise*; Ullstein GmbH: Berlin, Germany, 1981.
22. Bazin, E. *Leçons Théoriques et Cliniques sur les Affections Génériques de la Peau*; Adrien Delahaye: Pairs, France, 1862; p. 454.
23. Dorado, J.G.; Fraile, P.A. Sarna, pediculosis y picaduras de insectos. *Pediatríaintegral* **2012**, *16*, 301–320.
24. Walter, B.; Heukelbach, J.; Fengler, G.; Worth, C.; Hengge, U.; Feldmeier, H. Comparison of dermoscopy, skin scraping, and the adhesive tape test for the diagnosis of scabies in a resource-poor setting. *Arch. Dermatol.* **2011**, *147*, 468–473. [CrossRef] [PubMed]
25. Palicka, P.; Mali, L.; Samsinak, K.; Zitek, K.; Vobrazkov, E. Laboratory diagnosis of scabies. *J. Hyg. Epidemiol. Microbiol. Immunol.* **1980**, *24*, 63–70. [PubMed]
26. Woodley, D.; Saurat, J.H. The burrow ink test and the scabies mite. *J. Am. Acad. Dermatol.* **1981**, *6*, 715–722. [CrossRef]
27. Argenziano, G.; Fabbrocini, G.; Delfino, M. Epiluminescence microscopy: A new approach to in vivo detection of sarcoptes scabiei. *Arch. Dermatol.* **1997**, *133*, 751–753. [CrossRef] [PubMed]

28. Lacarrubba, F.; Musumeci, M.L.; Caltabiano, R.; Impallomeni, R.; West, D.P.; Micali, G. High-magnification videodermatoscopy: A new noninvasive diagnostic tool for scabies in children. *Pediatr. Dermatol.* **2001**, *18*, 439–441. [CrossRef] [PubMed]
29. Longo, C.; Bassoli, S.; Monari, P.; Seidenari, S.; Pellacani, G. Reflectance-mode confocal microscopy for the in vivo detection of sarcoptes scabiei. *Arch. Dermatol.* **2005**, *141*, 1336–1337. [CrossRef] [PubMed]
30. Dupuy, A.; Dehen, L.; Bourrat, E.; Lacroix, C.; Benderdouche, M.; Dubertret, L.; Morel, P.; Feuilhade de Chauvin, M.; Petit, A. Accuracy of standard dermoscopy for diagnosing scabies. *J. Am. Acad. Dermatol.* **2007**, *56*, 53–62. [CrossRef] [PubMed]
31. Yoshizumi, J.; Harada, T. "Wake sign": An important clue for the diagnosis of scabies. *Clin. Exp. Dermatol.* **2008**, *34*, 711–714. [CrossRef] [PubMed]
32. S1-Leitlinie zu Diagnostik und Therapie der Skabies. Available online: http://www.awmf.org/leitlinien/detail/ll/013-052.html (accessed on 31 January 2006).
33. Bhutto, A.M.; Honda, M.; Kubo, Y.; Nonaka, S.; Yoshida, H. Introduction of a fluorescense-microscopic technique for the detection of eggs, egg shells, and mites in scabies. *J. Dermatol.* **1993**, *20*, 122–124. [CrossRef] [PubMed]
34. Uenotsuchi, T.; Moroi, Y.; Urabe, K.; Tsuji, G.; Takahara, M.; Furue, M. The scybala (fecal pellets) of *Sacroptes scabiei* var. *Hominis* are obviously stained with chlorazol black E. *J. Dermatol.* **2004**, *31*, 511–512. [PubMed]
35. Neynaber, S.; Wolff, H. Diagnosis of scabies with dermoscopy. *Can. Med. Assoc. J.* **2008**, *178*, 1540–1541. [CrossRef] [PubMed]
36. Prins, C.; Stucki, L.; French, L.; Saurat, J.H.; Braun, R.P. Dermoscopy for the in vivo detection of sarcoptes scabiei. *Dermatology* **2004**, *208*, 241–243. [CrossRef] [PubMed]

11

Community Involvement in the Care of Persons Affected by Podoconiosis—A Lesson for other Skin NTDs

Abebayehu Tora [1], Asrat Mengiste [2], Gail Davey [3] and Maya Semrau [3,*]

1 Department of Sociology, Wolaita Sodo University, Sodo, Ethiopia; abezed@yahoo.com
2 National Podoconiosis Action Network, Addis Ababa, Ethiopia; asrat_m@napanEthiopia.org
3 Department of Global Health and Infection, Brighton and Sussex Medical School, Falmer Campus, University of Sussex, Brighton BN1 9PX, UK; G.Davey@bsms.ac.uk
* Correspondence: M.Semrau@bsms.ac.uk;

Abstract: Podoconiosis is a neglected tropical disease (NTD) characterized by lower-leg swelling (lymphedema), which is caused by long-term exposure to irritant red-clay soils found within tropical volcanic high-altitude environments with heavy rainfall. The condition places a substantial burden on affected people, their families and communities, including disability, economic consequences, social exclusion, and stigma; mental disorders and distress are also common. This paper focuses on community-based care of podoconiosis, and, in particular, the role that community involvement can have in the reduction of stigma against people affected by podoconiosis. We first draw on research conducted in Ethiopia for this, which has included community-based provision of care and treatment, education, and awareness-raising, and socioeconomic rehabilitation to reduce stigma. Since people affected by podoconiosis and other skin NTDs often suffer the double burden of mental-health illness, which is similarly stigmatized, we then point to examples from the mental-health field in low-resource community settings to suggest avenues for stigma reduction and increased patient engagement that may be relevant across a range of skin NTDs, though further research is needed on this.

Keywords: podoconiosis; lymphedema; neglected tropical diseases; NTDs; mental health; community engagement; patient involvement; stigma

---

1. Introduction

Podoconiosis is a neglected tropical disease (NTD), characterized by lower-leg swelling (lymphedema), which is found in highland areas of the tropics. It has often been confused with lymphatic filariasis, and is currently dealt with by the World Health Organization (WHO) under the lymphatic filariasis (LF) program (link: http://www.who.int/lymphatic_filariasis/epidemiology/podoconiosis/en/), but differs in that it is associated with long-term exposure to irritant tropical soils [1] rather than any parasite, virus, or bacterium. These red-clay soils are found in highland tropical areas, where ancient volcanic deposits have weathered [2] at high altitude (over 1000 m) under conditions of heavy rainfall (over 1000 mm/year). There is now strong evidence of underlying genetic susceptibility for podoconiosis [3], and endemic communities are usually aware that the condition clusters in families.

Countries with a high burden of podoconiosis include Ethiopia, Uganda, Cameroon, Kenya, and Tanzania [4]. Although rarely a direct cause of mortality, podoconiosis disables those affected through progressive leg swelling and repeated episodes of acute dermatolymphangioadenitis. These acute episodes occur frequently (reports vary from five [5] to 23 [6] episodes per year), and contribute substantially to the disability and social impact associated with podoconiosis [7,8]. Research has explored the enormous economic burden of podoconiosis on affected communities. In a southern Ethiopian zone of 1.5 million inhabitants, where the prevalence of podoconiosis is known to be 5.4%, the overall cost of podoconiosis was estimated to be in excess of US$16 million per year. In this zone, where the average income is less than US$100 per year, the direct costs to a patient were found to be US$143 per year [9]. In addition to its economic consequences, one of the most devastating characteristics of podoconiosis is stigma [10–12].

This article is a nonsystematic narrative review [13]. It focuses on community-based care of podoconiosis, and, in particular, the role that community involvement can have in the reduction of stigma against people affected by podoconiosis, but it also draws on other types of lymphedema, such as leprosy and LF. We start by exploring the sources and consequences of stigma among people with podoconiosis and then describe community-based approaches used to reduce stigma and provide care in Ethiopia. We then draw on examples from the field of mental health in low-resource community settings to suggest avenues for stigma reduction and increased patient engagement relevant across a range of skin NTDs. To our knowledge, this is the first review on community involvement in the care of people affected by podoconiosis, which also looks beyond NTDs to learn lessons from the mental-health field.

2. Sources and Consequences of Stigma in Podoconiosis

Stigma has commonly been defined as an undesirable or discrediting attribute that reduces an individual's status in the eyes of society [14,15]. The major sources of stigma among people affected with podoconiosis include the progressive physical disability that prevents affected individuals from making a living [9,16]; the misconceptions among community members about the causes of the disease and treatment options [7,17–19]; fear of public identification of a disease that is known to be familial [18]; and the physical disfigurement caused as the disease advances [20].

People affected by podoconiosis, as is the case for people affected by other lower-limb lymphedemas such as leprosy and LF, are stigmatized in all areas of their daily life. Overt discrimination is common during social functions, around mate selection and marriage, when seeking employment, and in relation to leadership roles. Due to deep-seated stigmatizing attitudes within the community, affected individuals also experience self-stigma, manifested in the form of low self-esteem, suicidal ideation, and avoidance of interactions with nonaffected community members [11]. The prejudice, discrimination, and self-stigma related to podoconiosis and other lymphedemas not only compromise the psychological and social wellbeing of patients and their families, but also limit their access to healthcare and adherence with treatment. This causes a vicious circle, creating further disability, illness, and reduced economic productivity. Breaking the vicious cycle of stigma related to podoconiosis has been a top priority for community organizations and researchers to improve the quality of life of patients and their families.

3. Community Interventions

Several community-based podoconiosis interventions have been implemented within Ethiopia, including provision of care and treatment, education, and socioeconomic rehabilitation. Though podoconiosis is an age-old disease, appropriate and effective means of treatment have not been understood or available until recently. Personal efforts to treat the disease using traditional knowledge have usually been counterproductive [21]. Most people affected by the disease therefore live with disfigurement and disability without receiving standardized services through the formal health system [22]. This has led to misconceptions around the possibility of cure, which, in turn, has increased the stigmatization of affected people [21].

3.1. Community-Based Care and Treatment

Over the last two decades, NGOs and faith-based organizations have played a pioneering role in providing care and treatment for people affected by the disease in vertically established outreach clinics [22,23]. In southern Ethiopia, Mossy Foot International has transformed patients who have successfully treated themselves into Community Podoconiosis Agents. Patients who have been educated to high-school completion are given full-time clinical training over a period of one week, and then become responsible for identifying patients in their own community and supporting self-care [22]. Training expert patients to provide simple, close-to-patient services is a potentially powerful solution to lack of care in countries with low formal health-services coverage. Harnessing the power of the local community to advocate for patients is likely to improve social support and diminish stigma in relation to a range of dermatologic conditions [24].

By halting the progress of disability and reducing the chances of illness related to acute attacks, the care that patients receive increases participation in community affairs and enhances their economic productivity, thereby improving their acceptance in society. Similar benefits have been documented for people affected by leprosy and LF, for example a leprosy self-care program in the 1990s and other leprosy and LF programs since then. Although the main function of the leprosy self-care groups was to encourage members to take responsibility for their own wound management, the group members reported a number of qualitative benefits, in particular improved self-respect and dignity and increased participation in society [25]. However, while these disease-specific examples are important, other studies suggest that integration of care and treatment into existing health systems may provide better opportunities to counter stigma than stand-alone vertical programs [26]. A systematic review conducted in 2016 suggested that joint approaches to reduce stigmatization across NTDs may be feasible given the similarities in causes, manifestations, and interventions against it [12]. Recent efforts to integrate podoconiosis care and treatment into government health structures alongside other types of lymphedema such as leprosy and LF are likely to play an important role in this regard [27].

3.2. Community-Based Education and Awareness

In addition to patient care and treatment, both Mossy Foot International and the International Orthodox Christian Charities (IOCC) program (in northern Ethiopia) have utilized Community Conversations or their equivalents to raise the awareness of the general population about podoconiosis causes, treatment, and prevention. These programs seek to encourage people to reflect on their place in the wider community, and to identify training, employment, and personal-development opportunities within the community sector.

The effectiveness of community-based health education run by lay people in reducing stigma has been confirmed in Ethiopia [28]. This study demonstrated that a health-education intervention that included community awareness campaigns and household skill-building activities run by lay health advisors decreased both felt and enacted stigma related to podoconiosis. In addition, awareness-raising and education amongst healthcare staff may be equally important to counter the stigmatizing attitudes and prejudices commonly held by them.

3.3. Community-Based Socioeconomic Rehabilitation

The final form of stigma reduction implemented in the context of podoconiosis is socioeconomic rehabilitation. This involves skills training (e.g., carpentry, masonry, hairdressing, shoemaking, etc.), enhancing entrepreneurship through revolving funds and loans, and providing educational opportunities [22]. Though the impact of socioeconomic rehabilitation in the context of podoconiosis has not been formally assessed, anecdotal evidences suggests that access to these services reduces stigma by increasing self-reliance, self-esteem, and financial independence, and acquiring new skills that widen opportunities for self-employment and access to public institutions. Participation in socioeconomic rehabilitation also influences the process of social integration and social acceptance through contributing to attitudinal change towards affected people [29].

4. Lessons from Community Engagement for Mental Health

Mental illness shares similar characteristics to skin NTDs in that affected persons are also heavily stigmatized and discriminated against, and are often excluded from social and economic activities [30–32]. Furthermore, rates of mental disorder (such as depression) and distress have been shown to be elevated amongst people with podoconiosis, LF, and other skin NTDs (which may both be an additional cause of stigma, as well as a consequence of the NTD-related stigma) [8,33,34]. Community engagement has been shown to be effective in addressing stigma, and thereby increasing uptake of and adherence to services, not only for NTDs such as podoconiosis and LF (as described above) but also for mental illness. It may therefore be helpful to look beyond NTDs, to learn lessons about community engagement from interventions used within the mental-health field, and how these might shape holistic interventions for stigmatized skin NTDs, particularly—but not only—for those who suffer the added burden of mental illness. However, further research on this is greatly needed.

The few studies published from low- and middle-income countries (LMICs) that have aimed to increase uptake of mental-health services by reducing stigma in the local community have included awareness-raising to change community knowledge and attitudes towards people with mental illness as their core component [35–37]. A program implemented in several states in Nigeria [35,36], for example, led to a significant increase in the use of community-based primary-care mental-health services by training voluntary lay community health workers (CHWs) to deliver positive health messages and challenge misconceptions around mental health, alongside a media campaign of radio announcements, jingles, and newspaper coverage. The program highlighted the importance of regular 'booster' training (e.g., every six months) and supervision, plus possibly other initiatives (such as incentives or paid work), to sustain CHWs' enthusiasm and the effectiveness of the program over time. Other key lessons learned from such programs have been the importance of involving and gaining buy-in from community members and leaders and health-system leaders from the start (for example, through forming of a stakeholder committee); linking raising awareness to the available services; and using 'Training of Trainers' approaches to achieve scale-up.

A further important finding from the mental-health field has been that interventions that include a social-contact element seem to be the most effective in reducing mental-health-related stigma and discrimination [38,39]. This can be either through direct contact with a patient, or indirect contact such as video testimonies, or affected persons sharing their experiences in newspapers, radio, TV, or posters. Whilst community-based awareness-raising interventions such as the ones outlined in the sections above may be essential in improving literacy of mental health and/or skin NTDs, it may therefore be valuable to explore further the inclusion of social-contact components within community-engagement interventions for skin NTDs and/or comorbid mental illness in order to increase their effectiveness. Contact interventions have indeed already shown successes in reducing leprosy-related stigma [40].

Service-user (patient) engagement is another area that may be as important for skin NTDs as for mental health, to empower and support affected people, and to facilitate self-care, and there are several good cases from the leprosy and LF field [27,41–45]. Examples of mental-health programs come from the five-year 'Emerging mental health systems in LMICs' (Emerald) program [46] and the seven-year 'PRogramme for Improving Mental health carE' (PRIME) [47], which were both implemented in countries in Africa and Asia (Ethiopia, India, Nepal, South Africa, and Uganda; plus Nigeria for Emerald). Both programs aimed to improve mental health care in these countries; whilst PRIME did so by collecting evidence on the integration and scale-up of mental health services into primary health care [47], Emerald did so by building capacity and generating evidence to enhance health-system strengthening [46]. PRIME, which also used WHO's widely-implemented mhGAP Intervention Guide [48] within primary health care, included a range of community-based interventions within its larger program, such as awareness-raising workshops, mental-health components within Community Conversation groups, information dissemination, case detection by CHWs, community mobilization, and community-based rehabilitation [49].

Both Emerald and PRIME included the engagement of mental-health patients and their families/caregivers as an important component, and acknowledged that patient involvement is essential when developing interventions and when expanding access to integrated care services within primary-care settings in LMICs [50]. A cross-country qualitative study conducted by Emerald identified the main strategies for increasing patient involvement in health-system strengthening to be patient and caregiver mobilization and empowerment; the need for capacity-building (training) of patients/caregivers and service providers; and ensuring human rights for greater involvement [51]. Alongside this, common barriers were identified that need to be tackled and that are reminiscent of skin NTDs, such as stigma, poverty, and power differentials in the health system, including lack of knowledge of services and support in the local community [50–53]. To achieve capacity-building of mental-health patients and their families/caregivers, Emerald took a country-specific multifaceted approach that aimed to include awareness-raising, stigma reduction, information, and mobilization and engagement of patients as its key ingredients; some of the main interventions used were workshops with mental-health patients and their caregivers to raise awareness and mobilize for greater advocacy and involvement, and workshops for primary-care workers and managers to support greater patient involvement [54]. The concepts of appropriateness, reciprocity, sustainability, and equality in partnerships were identified as being important and underpinned all capacity-building activities [54,55]; these may be relevant beyond the mental-health field, including within skin NTD programs.

5. Looking to the Future

While several approaches to community-based delivery of care, of education and awareness, and of socioeconomic rehabilitation have been successfully used by podoconiosis (as well as leprosy and LF) programs in Ethiopia and elsewhere, there is much potential for more. Socioeconomic community-based rehabilitation in particular is an area that warrants further research.

Looking to the experience of community-based mental health services, there are still many interventions that could potentially be applied to podoconiosis and across other stigmatized skin conditions. Holistic approaches are needed that take into account not only the physical care of skin NTDs, but also integrate mental-health components and take into account the complex interplay of physical disability, mental illness, and associated stigma. At the community level, this could include awareness-raising, not only of the implications in regards to the physical health of people affected by skin NTDs, but also the mental-health implications (for example through awareness-raising workshops, the inclusion of mental-health components within Community Conversation groups, or information dissemination). Social-contact elements may be particularly useful in this respect. Similarly, patient engagement, for example through patient groups, is vital in order to empower and support affected people, and to facilitate self-care. Services should be integrated so that patients receive care not only for their physical disabilities but also any mental distress or disorder; this can be achieved by making integrated services readily available in nearby primary healthcare facilities and/or in the community, for instance by training (and then providing regular supervision for) primary healthcare staff and/or community health workers in case detection and/or treatment of mental disorders, as well as physical healthcare. Stigma-reduction activities within this training may be important to counter any negative attitudes or prejudices. Further research is required to adapt and evaluate these programs in a range of disease and country contexts.

Author Contributions: All authors contributed to the writing of the paper, and have seen and approved the final version.

References

1. Molla, Y.; Wardrop, N.; Le Blond, J.; Baxter, P.; Newport, M.; Atkinson, P.; Davey, G. Modelling environmental factors correlated with podoconiosis: A geospatial study of non-filarial elephantiasis. *Int. J. Health Geogr.* **2014**, *13*, 24. [CrossRef] [PubMed]
2. Le Blond, J.; Cuadros, J.; Molla, Y.; Berhanu, T.; Umer, M.; Baxter, P.; Davey, G. Weathering of the Ethiopian volcanic province: A new weathering index to characterize and compare soils. *Am. Mineral.* **2015**, *100*, 2518–2532. [CrossRef]
3. Tekola Ayele, F.; Adeyemo, A.; Finan, C.; Hailu, E.; Sinnott, P.; Diaz Burlinson, N.; Aseffa, A.; Rotimi, C.; Newport, M.; Davey, G. HLA class II locus and susceptibility to podoconiosis. *N. Engl. J. Med.* **2012**, *366*, 1200–1208. [CrossRef] [PubMed]
4. Deribe, K.; Cano, J.; Trueba, M.; Newport, M.; Davey, G. Global epidemiology of podoconiosis: A systematic review. *PLoS Negl. Trop. Dis.* **2018**, *12*, e0006324. [CrossRef] [PubMed]
5. Molla, Y.; Tomczyk, S.; Amberbir, T.; Tamiru, A.; Davey, G. Podoconiosis in East and West Gojam Zones, northern Ethiopia. *PLoS. Negl. Trop. Dis.* **2012**, *6*, e1744. [CrossRef] [PubMed]
6. Bekele, K.; Deribe, K.; Amberbir, T.; Tadele, G.; Davey, G.; Samuel, A. Burden assessment of podoconiosis in Wayu Tuka Woreda, East Wollega Zone, western Ethiopia: A community-based cross-sectional study. *BMJ Open* **2016**, *6*, e012308. [CrossRef] [PubMed]
7. Molla, Y.; Tomczyk, S.; Amberbir, T.; Tamiru, A.; Davey, G. Patients' perceptions of podoconiosis causes, prevention and consequences in East and West Gojam, northern Ethiopia. *BMC Public Health* **2012**, *12*, 828. [CrossRef] [PubMed]
8. Bartlett, J.; Deribe, K.; Tamiru, A.; Amberbir, T.; Medhin, G.; Malik, M.; Hanlon, C.; Davey, G. Depression and disability in people with podoconiosis: A comparative cross-sectional study in rural northern Ethiopia. *Int. Health* **2015**, *8*, 124–131. [CrossRef] [PubMed]
9. Tekola, F.; HaileMariam, D.; Davey, G. Economic costs of endemic non-filarial elephantiasis in Wolaita Zone, Ethiopia. *Trop. Med. Int. Health* **2006**, *11*, 1136–1144. [CrossRef] [PubMed]
10. Deribe, K.; Tomczyk, S.; Mousley, E.; Tamiru, A.; Davey, G. Stigma towards a neglected tropical disease: Felt and enacted stigma scores among podoconiosis patients in northern Ethiopia. *BMC Public Health* **2013**, *13*, 1178. [CrossRef] [PubMed]
11. Tora, A.; Franklin, H.; Deribe, K.; Reda, A.; Davey, G. Extent of podoconiosis-related stigma in Wolaita Zone, southern Ethiopia: A cross-sectional study. *SpringerPlus* **2014**, *3*, 647. [CrossRef] [PubMed]
12. Hofstraat, K.; van Brakel, W. Social stigma towards neglected tropical diseases: A systematic review. *Int. Health* **2016**, *8*, i53–i70. [CrossRef] [PubMed]
13. Grant, M.; Booth, A. A typology of reviews: An analysis of 14 review types and associated methodologies. *Health Inf. Libr. J.* **2009**, *26*, 91–108. [CrossRef] [PubMed]
14. Link, B.; Phelan, J. Conceptualizing stigma. *Annu. Rev. Sociol.* **2001**, *27*, 363–385. [CrossRef]
15. Weiss, M. Stigma and the social burden of neglected tropical diseases. *PLoS Negl. Trop. Dis.* **2008**, *2*, e237. [CrossRef] [PubMed]
16. Desta, K.; Ashine, M.; Davey, G. Prevalence of podoconiosis (endemic non-filarial elephantiasis) in Wolaitta, southern Ethiopia. *Trop. Doctor* **2003**, *32*, 217–220. [CrossRef] [PubMed]
17. Yakob, B.; Deribe, K.; Davey, G. High levels of misconceptions and stigma in a community highly endemic for podoconiosis in southern Ethiopia. *Trans. R. Soc. Trop. Med. Hyg.* **2008**, *102*, 439–444. [CrossRef] [PubMed]
18. Tora, A.; Davey, G.; Tadele, G. A qualitative study on stigma and coping strategies of patients with podoconiosis in Wolaita Zone, southern Ethiopia. *Int. Health* **2011**, *3*, 176–181. [CrossRef] [PubMed]
19. Ayode, D.; McBride, C.; de Heer, D.; Watanabe, E.; Gebreyesus, T.; Tadele, G.; Tora, A.; Davey, G. The association of beliefs about heredity with preventive and interpersonal behaviors in communities affected by podoconiosis in rural Ethiopia. *Am. J. Trop. Med. Hyg.* **2012**, *87*, 623–630. [CrossRef] [PubMed]

20. Tekola, F.; Bull, S.; Farsides, B.; Newport, M.; Adeyemo, A.; Rotimi, C.; Davey, G. Impact of social stigma on the process of obtaining informed consent for genetic research on podoconiosis: A qualitative study. *BMC Med. Ethics* **2009**, *10*, 13. [CrossRef] [PubMed]
21. Tora, A.; Davey, G.; Tadele, G. Factors related to discontinued clinic attendance by patients with podoconiosis in southern Ethiopia: A qualitative study. *BMC Public Health* **2012**, *12*, 902. [CrossRef] [PubMed]
22. Davey, G.; Burridge, E. Community-based control of a neglected tropical disease: The mossy foot treatment and prevention association. *PLoS Negl. Trop. Dis.* **2009**, *3*, e424. [CrossRef] [PubMed]
23. Tomczyk, S.; Tamiru, A.; Davey, G. Addressing the neglected tropical disease podoconiosis in northern Ethiopia: Lessons learned from a new community podoconiosis program. *PLoS Negl. Trop. Dis.* **2012**, *6*, e1560. [CrossRef] [PubMed]
24. Molla, Y.; Davey, G. Podoconiosis control in rural Ethiopia: The roles of expert patients, appropriate treatment and community mobilization. *Commun. Dermatol.* **2012**, *10*, 3.
25. Benbow, C.; Temiru, T. The experience of self-care groups with people affected by leprosy: Alert, Ethiopia. *Lepr. Rev.* **2001**, *72*, 311–321. [CrossRef] [PubMed]
26. Arole, S.; Premkumar, R.; Arole, R.; Maury, M.; Saunderson, P. Social stigma: A comparative qualitative study of integrated and vertical care approaches to leprosy. *Lepr. Rev.* **2002**, *73*, 186–196. [PubMed]
27. Pryce, J.; Mableson, H.; Choudhary, R.; Pandey, B.; Aley, D.; Betts, H.; Mackenzie, C.; Kelly-Hope, L.; Cross, H. Assessing the feasibility of integration of self-care for filarial lymphoedema into existing community leprosy self-help groups in Nepal. *BMC Public Health* **2018**, *18*, 201. [CrossRef] [PubMed]
28. McBride, C.; Price, C.; Ayode, D.; Tora, A.; Farrell, D.; Davey, G. A cluster randomized intervention trial to promote shoe use by children at high risk for podoconiosis. *Int. J. Health Sci. Res.* **2015**, *5*, 518–528.
29. Ebenso, B.; Fashona, A.; Ayuba, M.; Idah, M. Impact of socio-economic rehabilitation on leprosy stigma in northern Nigeria: Findings of a retrospective study. *Asian Pac. Disabil. Rehabilit. J.* **2007**, *18*, 98–119.
30. Thornicroft, G.; Brohan, E.; Rose, D.; Sartorius, N.; Leese, M. INDIGO Study Group. Global pattern of experienced and anticipated discrimination against people with schizophrenia: A cross-sectional survey. *Lancet* **2009**, *373*, 408–415. [CrossRef]
31. Thornicroft, G.; Bakolis, I.; Evans-Lacko, S.; Gronholm, P.; Henderson, C.; Kohrt, B.; Koschorke, M.; Milenova, M.; Semrau, M.; Votruba, N.; et al. Key lessons learned from the indigo global network on mental health related stigma and discrimination. *World Psychiatry*, in press.
32. Semrau, M.; Evans-Lacko, S.; Koschorke, M.; Ashenafi, L.; Thornicroft, G. Stigma and discrimination related to mental illness in low and middle income countries. *Epidemiol. Psychiatr. Sci.* **2015**, *24*, 382–394. [CrossRef] [PubMed]
33. Mousley, E.; Deribe, K.; Tamiru, A.; Tomczyk, S.; Hanlon, C.; Davey, G. Mental distress and podoconiosis in northern Ethiopia: A comparative cross-sectional study. *Int. Health* **2015**, *7*, 16–25. [CrossRef] [PubMed]
34. Obindo, J.; Abdulmalik, J.; Nwefoh, E.; Agbir, M.; Nwoga, C.; Armiya'u, A.; Davou, F.; Maigida, K.; Otache, E.; Ebiloma, A.; et al. Prevalence of depression and associated clinical and socio-demographic factors in people living with lymphatic filariasis in Plateau State, Nigeria. *PLoS Negl. Trop. Dis.* **2017**, *6*, e0005567. [CrossRef] [PubMed]
35. Eaton, J.; Agomoh, A. Developing mental health services in Nigeria. *Soc. Psychiatry Psychiatr. Epidemiol.* **2008**, *43*, 552–558. [CrossRef] [PubMed]
36. Eaton, J.; Nwefoh, E.; Okafor, G.; Onyeonoro, U.; Nwaubani, K.; Henderson, C. Interventions to increase use of services; mental health awareness in Nigeria. *Int. J. Ment. Health Syst.* **2017**, *11*, 66. [CrossRef] [PubMed]
37. Armstrong, G.; Kermode, M.; Raja, S.; Suja, S.; Chandra, P.; Jorm, A. A mental health training program for community health workers in India: Impact on knowledge and attitudes. *Int. J. Ment. Health Syst.* **2011**, *5*, 17. [CrossRef] [PubMed]
38. Thornicroft, G.; Mehta, N.; Clement, S.; Evans-Lacko, S.; Doherty, M.; Rose, D.; Koschorke, M.; Shidhaye, R.; O'Reilly, C.; Henderson, C. Evidence for effective interventions to reduce mental-health-related stigma and discrimination. *Lancet* **2016**, *387*, 1123–1132. [CrossRef]
39. Mehta, N.; Clement, S.; Marcus, E.; Stona, A.-C.; Bezborodovs, N.; Evans-Lacko, S.; Palacios, J.; Docherty, M.; Barley, E.; Rose, D.; et al. Evidence for effective interventions to reduce mental health-related stigma and discrimination in the medium and long term: Systematic review. *Br. J. Psychiatry* **2015**, *207*, 377–384. [CrossRef] [PubMed]

40. Peters, R.; Dadun, D.; Zweekhorst, M.; Bunders, J.; Irwanto, I.; van Brakel, W. A cluster-randomized controlled intervention study to assess the effect of a contact intervention in reducing leprosy-related stigma in Indonesia. *PLoS Negl. Trop. Dis.* **2015**, *9*, e0004003. [CrossRef] [PubMed]
41. Cross, H.; Chowdhary, R. Step: An intervention to address the issue of stigma related to leprosy in southern Nepal. *Lepr. Rev.* **2005**, *76*, 316–324. [PubMed]
42. Sermrittirong, S.; van Brakel, W.; Bunbers-Aelen, J. How to reduce stigma in leprosy—A systematic literature review. *Lepr. Rev.* **2014**, *85*, 149–157. [PubMed]
43. Peters, R.; Zweekhorst, M.; van Brakel, W.; Bunders, J.; Irwanto, I. 'People like me don't make things like that': Participatory video as a method for reducing leprosy-related stigma. *Glob. Public Health* **2016**, *11*, 5–6. [CrossRef] [PubMed]
44. Lusli, M.; Peters, R.; van Brakel, W.; Zweekhorst, M.; Iancu, S.; Bunders, J.; Irwanto; Regeer, B. The impact of a rights-based counselling intervention to reduce stigma in people affected by leprosy in Indonesia. *PLoS Negl. Trop. Dis.* **2016**, *10*, e0005088. [CrossRef] [PubMed]
45. Lusli, M.; Zweekhorst, M.; Miranda-Galarza, B.; Peters, R.; Cummings, S.; Seda, F.; Bunders, J.; Irwanto. Dealing with stigma: Experiences of persons affected by disabilities and leprosy. *Biomed. Res. Int.* **2015**, *2015*, 261329. [CrossRef] [PubMed]
46. Semrau, M.; Evans-Lacko, S.; Alem, A.; Ayuso-Mateos, J.; Chisholm, D.; Gureje, O.; Hanlon, C.; Jordans, M.; Kigozi, F.; Lempp, H.; et al. Strengthening mental health systems in low and middle-income countries: The Emerald programme. *BMC Med.* **2015**, *13*, 79. [CrossRef] [PubMed]
47. Lund, C.; Tomlinson, M.; de Silva, M.; Fekadu, A.; Shidhaye, R.; Jordans, M.; Petersen, I.; Bhana, A.; Kigozi, F.; Prince, M.; et al. PRIME: A programme to reduce the treatment gap for mental disorders in five low- and middle-income countries. *PLOS Med.* **2012**, *9*, e1001359. [CrossRef] [PubMed]
48. World Health Organization (WHO). *Mhgap Intervention Guide*; WHO: Geneva, Switzerland, 2016.
49. Lund, C.; Tomlinson, M.; Patel, V. Integration of mental health into primary care in low- and middle-income countries: The PRIME mental healthcare plans. *Br. J. Psychiatry* **2016**, *208*, s1–s3. [CrossRef] [PubMed]
50. Abayneh, S.; Lempp, H.; Alem, A.; Alemayehu, D.; Eshetu, T.; Lund, C.; Semrau, M.; Thornicroft, G.; Hanlon, C. Service user involvement in mental health system strengthening in a rural african setting: Qualitative study. *BMC Psychiatry* **2017**, *17*, 187. [CrossRef] [PubMed]
51. Lempp, H.; Abayneh, S.; Gurung, D.; Kola, L.; Abdulmalik, J.; Evans-Lacko, S.; Semrau, M.; Alem, A.; Thornicroft, G.; Hanlon, C. Service user and caregiver involvement in mental health system strengthening in low and middle income countries: A cross-country qualitative study. *Epidemiol. Psychiatr. Sci.* **2018**, *27*, 29–39. [CrossRef] [PubMed]
52. Gurung, D.; Upadhaya, N.; Magar, J.; Giri, N.; Hanlon, C.; Jordans, M. Service user and care giver involvement in mental health system strengthening in Nepal: A qualitative study on barriers and facilitating factors. *Int. J. Ment. Health Syst.* **2017**, *11*, 30. [CrossRef] [PubMed]
53. Samudre, S.; Shidhaye, R.; Ahuja, S.; Nanda, S.; Khan, A.; Evans-Lacko, S.; Hanlon, C. Service user involvement for mental health system strengthening in India: A qualitative study. *BMC Psychiatry* **2016**, *16*, 269. [CrossRef] [PubMed]
54. Semrau, M.; Alem, A.; Abdulmalik, J.; Docrat, S.; Evans-Lacko, S.; Gureje, O.; Kigozi, F.; Lempp, H.; Lund, C.; Petersen, I.; et al. Developing capacity-building activities for mental health system strengthening in low- and middle-income countries for service users and caregivers, service planners and researchers. *Epidemiol. Psychiatr. Sci.* **2017**, *27*, 11–21. [CrossRef] [PubMed]
55. Hanlon, C.; Semrau, M.; Alem, A.; Abayneh, S.; Abdulmalik, J.; Docrat, S.; Evans-Lacko, S.; Gureje, O.; Jordans, M.; Lempp, H.; et al. Evaluating capacity-building for mental health system strengthening in low- and middle-income countries for service users and caregivers, service planners and researchers. *Epidemiol. Psychiatr. Sci.* **2017**, *27*, 3–10. [CrossRef] [PubMed]

12

Intestinal Schistosomiasis and Giardiasis Co-Infection in Sub-Saharan Africa: Can a One Health Approach Improve Control of Each Waterborne Parasite Simultaneously?

John Archer [1,2], Lisa O'Halloran [2], Hajri Al-Shehri [2,3], Shannan Summers [4], Tapan Bhattacharyya [4], Narcis B. Kabaterine [5], Aaron Atuhaire [5], Moses Adriko [5], Moses Arianaitwe [5], Martyn Stewart [2], E. James LaCourse [2], Bonnie L. Webster [1], Amaya L. Bustinduy [4] and J. Russell Stothard [2,*]

1 Wolfson Wellcome Biomedical Laboratories, Department of Zoology, Natural History Museum, Cromwell Road, London SW7 5BD, UK; j.archer@nhm.ac.uk (J.A.); b.webster@nhm.ac.uk (B.L.W.)
2 Department of Tropical Disease Biology, Liverpool School of Tropical Medicine, Pembroke Place, Liverpool L3 5QA, UK; lisa.ohalloran@live.co.uk (L.O.); haj_3933@hotmail.com (H.A.-S.); martyn.stewart@lstmed.ac.uk (M.S.); james.lacourse@lstmed.ac.uk (E.J.L.)
3 Department of Tropical Infectious Diseases, Ministry of Health, Asir District, Abha 61411, Saudi Arabia
4 Department of Clinical Research, London School of Hygiene and Tropical Medicine, Keppel Street, London WC1E 7HT, UK; shannan.summers1@student.lshtm.ac.uk (S.S.); tapan.bhattacharyya@lshtm.ac.uk (T.B.); amaya.bustinduy@lshtm.ac.uk (A.L.B.)
5 Vector Control Division, Ministry of Health, Kampala 759125, Uganda; vcdmoh@gmail.com (N.B.K.); aaronatuhaire@gmail.com (A.A.); adrikomoses@gmail.com (M.A.); vcdmoh@gmail.com (M.A.)
* Correspondence: russell.stothard@lstmed.ac.uk;

Abstract: Both intestinal schistosomiasis and giardiasis are co-endemic throughout many areas of sub-Saharan Africa, significantly impacting the health of millions of children in endemic areas. While giardiasis is not considered a neglected tropical disease (NTD), intestinal schistosomiasis is formally grouped under the NTD umbrella and receives significant advocacy and financial support for large-scale control. Although there are differences in the epidemiology between these two diseases, there are also key similarities that might be exploited within potential integrated control strategies permitting tandem interventions. In this review, we highlight these similarities and discuss opportunities for integrated control of giardiasis in low and middle-income countries where intestinal schistosomiasis is co-endemic. By applying new, advanced methods of disease surveillance, and by improving the provision of water, sanitation and hygiene (WASH) initiatives, (co)infection with intestinal schistosomiasis and/or giardiasis could not only be more effectively controlled but also better understood. In this light, we appraise the suitability of a One Health approach targeting both intestinal schistosomiasis and giardiasis, for if adopted more broadly, transmission of both diseases could be reduced to gain improvements in health and wellbeing.

Keywords: One Health; *Schistosoma mansoni*; *Giardia duodenalis*; water, sanitation and hygiene (WASH); Uganda

---

1. Introduction

Throughout many tropical and sub-tropical low- and middle-income countries (LMICs) where provision of water, sanitation and hygiene (WASH) infrastructure is inadequate, communities of people are often found to be co-infected with multiple parasitic diseases acquired through ingestion of, or contact with, contaminated water and food [1,2]. Notably, intestinal schistosomiasis and giardiasis are both waterborne parasitic diseases highly prevalent and co-endemic in these regions.

Intestinal schistosomiasis is a debilitating neglected tropical disease (NTD) caused by infection with parasitic blood flukes of the species *Schistosoma mansoni, S. japonicum, S. intercalatum, S. mekongi* and *S. guineensis* [3]. This disease is highly prevalent throughout many areas of sub-Saharan Africa and locally endemic in some areas of South America and the Caribbean, where the vast majority of cases are caused by infection with *S. mansoni.* Intestinal schistosomiasis compromises the general integrity of the small bowel via egg-induced perforations with associated local and systemic inflammation [3].

Giardiasis, another debilitating but underreported intestinal parasitic disease, is caused by infection with the single-celled eukaryotic diplomonad *Giardia duodenalis*, a flagellated protist [4]. While cosmopolitan in distribution, giardiasis prevalence is particularly high in low and middle-income countries [5,6]. Like intestinal schistosomiasis, giardiasis also compromises the general integrity of the digestive tract. It does this through a major disruption of the gut microbiota, causing a variety of debilitating pathologies such as dehydration and anemia [7,8]. Unlike intestinal schistosomiasis, however, giardiasis is not considered an NTD, although there have been previous discussions proposing its inclusion [9,10].

Whilst there are differences in the transmission biology and epidemiology between both intestinal schistosomiasis and giardiasis, there are also key similarities that might be exploited within potential integrated control strategies, allowing for control of both diseases in tandem. By highlighting these similarities, and by outlining opportunities for integrated control of giardiasis in areas where intestinal schistosomiasis is co-endemic, we aim to diminish the detrimental effects of (co)infection, thereby improving the health and wellbeing of those, particularly children, in endemic areas. To do this, an integrated 'One Health' approach is needed that requires a detailed knowledge of the transmission biology of each parasite, appropriate use of reliable point-of-care (POC) diagnostics, mitigation of environmental and zoonotic transmission through improved WASH infrastructure and effective use of anti-parasitic chemotherapies. Each of these should be carefully considered and applied simultaneously to improve public health outcomes [11–14].

2. Intestinal Schistosomiasis and Giardiasis: Pathology and Epidemiology

Intestinal schistosomiasis disproportionally afflicts school-aged children between the ages of six and fifteen years old, where pathology can be both acute and chronic [3]. As based on 'classic' age-infection profiles and measured using faecal egg counts, the intensity of infection typically begins to decline in late adolescence while morbidity associated with *S. mansoni,* such as multi-organ fibrosis, accumulates. This decline in egg-patent prevalence is due to a variety of factors such as partial-immunity to infection, notwithstanding extensive fibrosis of the bowel itself which can occlude egg exit sites, giving rise to granulomatous masses known as intestinal 'bilharzomas' [15,16].

Pathologies associated with intestinal schistosomiasis occur primarily as a result of the body's response to the copious number of eggs produced by female adult worms inhabiting the mesenteric veins surrounding the intestines. Rather than being passed in stool (or occasionally in urine) to perpetuate the parasites lifecycle, a large proportion of eggs will instead become sequestered throughout the venous bloodstream of the intestinal and hepatoportal tracts. Many eggs will then enter into general venous circulation and subsequently become lodged in other major organs. Once eggs become trapped, for example in the intestinal wall and/or liver sinuses, a range of clinical systemic and organ-specific morbidity ensues, including acute abdominal pain, stunted growth, environmental enteropathy, presence of faecal occult blood and overt hepato/splenomegaly [17,18].

Human giardiasis is caused by infection with *G. duodenalis* (syn. *Giardia intestinalis, Giardia lamblia*). While *G. duodenalis* is the only human-infecting *Giardia* species, eight distinct evolutionary assemblages based on multi-locus genotyping, named A through H, are known to exist [19]. Of these eight, the vast majority of human infections are caused by assemblages A and B, although human infections with assemblages C, D, E and F do also occur, albeit rarely [19,20].

Unlike the distribution of *S. mansoni*, which is intrinsically linked to its *Biomphalaria* spp. intermediate freshwater snail hosts, the distribution of *G. duodenalis* is truly cosmopolitan. Giardiasis prevalence in humans is particularly high; however, in LMICs lacking access to clean, safe drinking water and associated WASH infrastructures, including many areas of sub-Saharan Africa and South America, where *S. mansoni* is also endemic [5,6]. A notable feature of giardiasis, in humans, can be asymptomatic infections, although acute and/or chronic and debilitating pathologies owing to infection are well described. These include diarrhoea, dehydration, malabsorption, tropical enteropathy, stunted growth, impaired cognitive development, anaemia and chronic fatigue [7,8]. The primary cause of these pathologies is a major disruption to the gut microbiota, a complex community of symbiotic microbes responsible for vitamin production, nutrient absorption and regulation of lipid metabolism, brought about through *G. duodenalis* invading, inhabiting and multiplying within the intestinal tract [21–23]. Importantly, severe morbidity is most often observed in certain high-risk groups including children, the elderly, those with physical disabilities and the immunocompromised [24,25].

2.1. Common Modes of Environmental Contamination

A major factor linking the transmission of both intestinal schistosomiasis and giardiasis is their transfaecal environmental contamination routes via the excretion of schistosome eggs (*S. mansoni*) or cysts (*G. duodenalis*) into a viable body of freshwater. Although waterborne transmission is not required for *G. duodenalis* to complete its life cycle, and while not all *S. mansoni* eggs or *G. duodenalis* cysts will successfully reach a viable freshwater habitat, in a disease-endemic setting, many environmental water bodies will undergo some extent of direct or indirect faecal contamination with both parasites (Figure 1) [3,4,26,27]. Indirect faecal contamination of freshwater can occur, for example, while bathing, through infected stools deposited on the banks of rivers and ponds being washed into these waters by heavy rains or floods, through overflowing pit latrines, and possibly through animals such as cattle walking through sites of defecation and transporting faecal matter to bodies of water on their hooves [28,29]. *S. mansoni* eggs can survive up to approximately eight days in the stool post-defecation and before reaching freshwater, whereas *G. duodenalis* cysts can survive up to eight weeks in the environment [4,30] (Table 1).

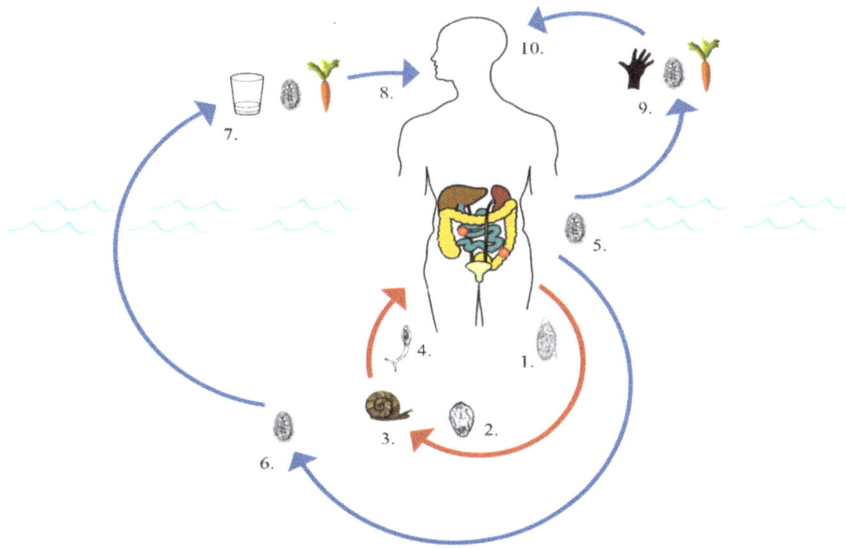

Figure 1. Transmission routes of *S. mansoni* (red, 1–4) and *G. duodenalis* (blue, 5–8 and 9–10). Both parasites are transmitted through faecal contamination of freshwater (*S. mansoni*: 1, *G. duodenalis*: 5). Infection with *S. mansoni* primarily occurs through cercarial penetration of the skin upon contact with contaminated water (4). Waterborne infection with *G. duodenalis* occurs through consumption of contaminated water or foods washed with contaminated water (7–8). Infection with *G. duodenalis* can also occur through consumption of contaminated foods or unwashed hands (9–10). Adapted from [26,27].

Once exposed to freshwater, *S. mansoni* eggs (Figure 1, (1)) will hatch to release free-swimming ciliated miracidia (Figure 1, (2)) that will then employ a range of morphological adaptations and host-seeking behaviours to locate and penetrate the soft tissues of its freshwater snail intermediate host, *Biomphalaria* spp. (Figure 1, (3)) [31–33]. Miracidia are ephemeral, living only a short period of time, typically less than six hours, before dying as their glycogen energy reserves are exhausted (Table 1).

Miracidia that successfully invade a suitable intermediate snail host metamorphose into mother sporocysts, which, in turn, produce daughter sporocysts. These daughter sporocysts then differentiate upon sporogenesis, producing numerous cercariae that are shed from the snail approximately one month after initial invasion by the miracidium (Figure 1, (4)). Once established, cercarial production and shedding from *Biomphalaria* spp. snail hosts occur daily and typically continue over the remainder of the snails' lives. Over the course of an infected snail's life, tens of thousands of cercariae can be liberated [3,34].

Shed cercariae will then go on to infect humans and other mammalian definitive hosts, primarily through cutaneous penetration (Figure 1, (4)), although infection may also occur through penetration of the buccal cavity when consuming contaminated water [30]. Like miracidia, cercariae are ephemeral in freshwater as their glycogen energy reserves are quickly depleted, lasting no longer than three days (Table 1). In addition, survival of both miracidia and cercariae is highly dependent on favourable biotic and abiotic environmental conditions. Freshwater too high in salinity or too polluted, for example, can prevent the hatching of eggs into miracidia and can be lethal to both miracidia and cercariae [32,33,35,36].

G. duodenalis has a direct, faecal–oral life cycle that can be completed either through waterborne transmission when consuming water contaminated with cysts (or foods/utensils washed using contaminated water without sufficient soaps) (Figure 1, (5–8)), or through the consumption of contaminated foods or unwashed hands (Figure 1, (9–10)) [4,37]. Unlike *S. mansoni*, which will asexually reproduce within an intermediate host, and although *Giardia* cysts may survive and even accumulate within certain filter-feeding freshwater invertebrates (for example, oysters), *G. duodenalis* does not require an intermediate host for transmission [38]. Cysts passed in the stool are, however, extremely resilient and can remain viable within the stool or in freshwater for up to eight weeks after excretion (Table 1) [4,37,39].

Table 1. Survival and viability of *S. mansoni* eggs and *G. duodenalis* cysts in the environment post-defecation.

Species	Life-Stage	Survival Post-Defecation in the Stool or in Freshwater	Reference(s)
S. mansoni	Eggs	~8 days in stool prior to reaching freshwater	[30]
	Miracidia	<6 h in freshwater	[31–33]
	Cercariae	~1–3 days in freshwater	[32,33,35,36]
G. duodenalis (Assemblages A and B)	Cysts	Up to eight weeks in stool or in freshwater	[4,37,39]

Maintained transmission of intestinal schistosomiasis is therefore dependent on the continued contamination of freshwater and continued exposure to contaminated/infested water, whereas giardiasis transmission is heavily exacerbated by the continued contamination of freshwater and continued consumption of contaminated water. There are a variety of ways in which an individual can be exposed to and infected with both parasites, for example, when water is used for consumption, sanitation purposes, income generation from fishing or farming and/or recreation [40,41]. As such, transmission of both diseases is particularly high in impoverished areas lacking adequate WASH infrastructures, such as access to functional pit latrines and clean drinking water, as well as behavioural impediments in those unaware of how to avoid contamination and infection [42,43].

2.2. Transmission via Non-Human Hosts

The transmission of both intestinal schistosomiasis and giardiasis is also exacerbated by a range of non-human definitive hosts acting as either major or minor reservoirs of infection, although the precise extent to which these hosts contribute to human transmission is not fully understood (Table 2). Further to the significant health and economic impact of infection with African schistosomes and/or *Giardia* on, for example livestock, animal reservoirs of both parasites also pose challenges in controlling and reducing human transmission as each parasite follows similar routes of infection, contamination and, ultimately, environmental transmission via non-human hosts [5,44,45].

Table 2. Primary reservoir hosts of *S. mansoni* and *G. duodenalis* (assemblages A-H). '+' denotes known primary reservoir host; '-' denotes no known primary reservoir host.

Species	Humans	Non-Human Primates	Ruminants	Rodents	Other Mammals	Fish	References
S. mansoni	+	+	-	+	-	-	[46,47]
G. duodenalis (assemblage A)	+	+	+	+	+	+	[20,48–51]
G. duodenalis (assemblage B)	+	+	+	+	+	+	[20,48–50]
G. duodenalis (assemblage C)	- *	-	+	-	+	-	[19,20]
G. duodenalis (assemblage D)	- *	-	+	-	+	-	[19,20]
G. duodenalis (assemblage E)	- *	-	+	-	+	-	[19,20]
G. duodenalis (assemblage F)	- *	-	-	-	+	-	[19,20]
G. duodenalis (assemblage G)	-	-	-	+	-	-	[19,20]
G. duodenalis (assemblage H)	-	-	-	-	+	-	[19,20]

* Human infection possible but rarely observed [20].

To reduce human transmission effectively, animal reservoirs and the degree to which they contribute to and maintain disease transmission must therefore be carefully considered when developing, implementing and monitoring any disease control strategies. Moreover, particular attention is needed on those animal hosts able to reintroduce parasites into viable bodies of freshwater following prior control or elimination campaigns [52]. Limiting contact of cattle with freshwater, for example, as well as limiting run-off from fields on which cattle manure has been spread and disposing of animal waste away from bodies of freshwater are known to reduce transmission of *Giardia*, as well as non-human infecting *Schistosoma* species [53,54]. Doing so, however, can be extremely challenging to implement and maintain through time.

In light of recent findings, additional consideration should also be given to the potential emergence of schistosome hybrids and their impact on schistosomiasis transmission [55–57]. *Schistosoma mansoni*, for example, can form hybrids with rodent-infecting species *S. rodhani*, which have been observed along the shoreline of Lake Victoria, one of the Great East African lakes. However, *S. rodhaini* appears exclusive to rodents, together with the *S. mansoni-rodhaini* hybrids, but with many gaps in routine surveillance this appraisal may be incomplete [58,59]. Uniquely among trematodes, schistosomes are dioecious, and so adult worms form inter-species copulatory pairs which facilitate permissive introgression(s). In nature, pre- and post-zygotic reproductive isolating barriers, such as host specificity, anatomical site of infection, geographical distribution, mating preference, worm competition and snail incompatibility, are thought to prevent prolific inter-species admixture. Recently, however, and owing to advanced methods of molecular analysis on schistosome larval stages from snail-intermediate and mammalian-definitive hosts, surprising inter-species hybrid forms are now being identified in several endemic African countries [58]. Such hybrids, resulting from interactions between human- and animal-infecting species, not only raise concerns about zoonotic transmission, but also the expanded host ranges and increased transmission potential acquired through heritable traits [59].

Changes to natural landscapes can readily lead to the formation of new freshwater bodies, snail habitats and multi-host transmission sites, breaking down the ecological barriers between species and leading to further inter-species interactions. Although the full impact that these hybridization events may have on human disease epidemiology and disease pathology is currently unknown, hybridization certainly suggests that future schistosomiasis control may warrant an expanded One Health approach with more tailored interventions specific to local settings and schistosome epidemiology [56,58,60].

3. Intestinal Schistosomiasis and Giardiasis: Surveillance and Control

Highlighting these key similarities in disease transmission, biology and epidemiology between *S. mansoni* and *Giardia* presents clear opportunities for integrated surveillance and control of both diseases, particularly with regard to disease diagnosis, surveillance and control.

3.1. Diagnosis: Parasitological, Immunological and Molecular Methods

Owing to its low cost, portability and high specificity, light microscopy for the detection of *S. mansoni* eggs in faecal samples is widely used during disease surveillance programmes to detect infection with *S. mansoni* in sub-Saharan Africa [61]. Using microscopy, routine parasitological surveillance to assess endemicity and prevalence of intestinal schistosomiasis, as well as other intestinal helminth infections, in a community is typically carried out via the Kato-Katz technique using faecal samples provided by school-aged children [62]. While inexpensive and portable, the sensitivity of Kato-Katz is, however, severely reduced in low-intensity infections, hampering its use in areas of low disease endemicity or in areas having undergone successful disease control intervention(s) [63–65].

Giardiasis cannot be reliably detected using the Kato-Katz method, and so alternative methods, such as formalin/ether concentration techniques, flotation techniques or immunofluorescent antibody microscopy, are needed [11,66–68]. Unfortunately, however, none of these techniques are straightforward or inexpensive to carry out under rural field conditions, particularly as it has been reported that formalin/ether concentration techniques have a higher sensitivity in detecting infection with *S. mansoni* than the more field-deployable Kato-Katz technique [69,70]. Moreover, these techniques can also often be insufficiently sensitive to reliably detect giardiasis infection [68].

For these reasons, a variety of immunological and molecular diagnostic assays with improved sensitivity in detecting both *S. mansoni* and *Giardia* infection using non-invasive urine and faecal samples have been developed (Table 3).

Table 3. Overview of primary diagnostic assays to detect infection with *Schistosoma mansoni* and *Giardia duodenalis*.

Species	Direct Diagnosis	Antigen Detection	Molecular Diagnosis
S. mansoni	Identification of ova in concentrated faecal smear via Kato-Katz technique [62,71]	Detection of circulating cathodic antigen (CCA) or circulating anodic antigen (CAA) in urine samples using ELISA or lateral-flow test strips [72,73]	Detection and amplification of species-specific DNA in faecal samples using PCR/qPCR [74], (LAMP and RPA assays have also been developed [71,75–77]).
G. duodenalis	Identification of cysts in concentrated faecal smear via formalin/ether concentration techniques, flotation techniques or immunofluorescent antibody microscopy [68]	Detection of species-specific antigens in faecal samples using ELISA or lateral-flow test strips [11,78–80]	Detection and amplification of species-specific DNA in faecal samples using PCR/qPCR [78], (LAMP and RPA assays have also been developed [81–83]).

Though highly sensitive, immunoassays such as the enzyme-linked immunosorbent assay (ELISA) and molecular assays such as PCR/qPCR require specialist laboratory infrastructure seldom available in disease-endemic areas, preventing their use at POC [84,85]. As such, several rapid and field-deployable RDTs have also been developed to detect trace levels of parasite-derived antigens and parasite-derived DNA in urine and faecal samples. Some examples include straightforward lateral-flow dipsticks to detect *S. mansoni* circulating cathodic antigen (CCA) in urine samples and *G. duodenalis* (with or without *Cryptosporidium* spp.) cyst antigen in faecal samples, as well as loop-mediated isothermal amplification (LAMP) and recombinase polymerase amplification (RPA) assays to detect species-specific *Schistosoma*- and *Giardia*-derived DNA in urine and faecal samples [11,64,85].

While POC-RDTs have many advantages over light-microscopy, microscopy remains less financially expensive to carry out and so it is the favoured method of diagnosis during routine monitoring and control programmes with only limited financial resources available [68,75,78]. In addition, and though promising, assays such as LAMP and RPA to detect species-specific parasite DNA currently require further assessment and validation before their upscaled and routine use in such control programmes [81,85]. Nevertheless, continued development, assessment and validation of POC-RDTs is widely advocated as affordable and sensitive point-of-care diagnostics, capable of detecting low levels of infection within individuals able to maintain disease transmission, are sorely needed [86]. Given these challenges in reliably detecting infection using human samples, particularly in low-endemicity settings, alternative methods of detecting and monitoring disease transmission within endemic foci, such as parasite host surveillance and use of environmental DNA (eDNA), have also been explored.

3.2. *Exploring the One Health InterFace with Increased Host Surveillance*

Intermediate hosts and definitive reservoir hosts, such as *Biomphalaria* freshwater snails (*S. mansoni*) and rodents or cattle (*S. mansoni* and *G. duodenalis*, respectively), offer an alternative means of detecting and monitoring disease transmission in areas where detecting transmission through human diagnosis may be unreliable [87]. Collecting freshwater snails capable of transmitting schistosomes and carrying out shedding analyses to assess cercarial emergence, for example, may help identify active transmission sites [87,88]. This approach, however, can also be unreliable, as very few snails are typically found to be shedding cercariae [89].

For this reason, highly sensitive molecular xenomonitoring approaches to detect *Schistosoma* DNA in snail host tissues have also been developed and assessed [90]. Using PCR to detect *Schistosoma* DNA within snail hosts, for example, can identify prepatent infections and is not affected by diurnal fluctuations in cercarial shedding in the same way that cercarial shedding is; allowing a more reliable assessment of schistosome presence in a given locality than shedding analyses can allow. An added advantage of molecular xenomonitoring by use of PCR is the ability to genotype parasite and snail DNA, providing valuable opportunities to better understand disease transmission and molecular epidemiology, such as more reliable species identification of human-infecting cercariae and snail intermediate hosts than can be achieved using morphological analysis and the detection of *Schistosoma* hybridisation events [55]. In addition, collecting and screening freshwater snail hosts for the presence of parasite DNA can be more straightforward and more lucrative than collecting and screening human faecal samples for parasite DNA [90]. Currently, however, mass collection and molecular screening of freshwater snail hosts using PCR remains logistically, technically and financially demanding, and so development of a high-throughput methodology, possibly incorporating use of rapid and POC DNA amplification technologies such as LAMP or RPA, or pooling of snail samples, should also be further explored and assessed [91,92].

Similarly, molecular detection of *S. mansoni* and *G. duodenalis* DNA in DNA extracted from faeces collected from definitive reservoir hosts capable of perpetuating transmission, such as rodents (*S. mansoni*) and cattle (*Giardia*), has also been used to monitor disease transmission with success [49,58]. An added benefit of collecting and analysing faecal samples in this way is that this method also provides an opportunity to assess and better understand wild-type *Schistosoma* hybridisation events and zoonotic transmission of human-infecting *G. duodenalis* through genotyping [55,93,94]. Again, however, this approach too requires significant financial and technological resources. As such, it is unlikely to be widely integrated into control programmes undertaken in low-resource areas such as rural regions of sub-Saharan Africa without further development and use of field-deployable DNA amplification technologies.

3.3. Detecting Parasitic Contamination through Water Sampling and by Environmental DNA (eDNA) Analysis

Extensive screening of environmental water samples for contamination with *Giardia* cysts using the United States Environmental Protection Agency method 1623 (US-EPA method 1623) has been carried out in many areas of the world, such as the USA [95]. Through collection and filtration of water samples, protozoan cysts can be detected and quantified, allowing viable transmission sites to be identified [96]. Although straightforward to carry out, this method does not differentiate between morphologically identical *Giardia* assemblages A-H and so identification of human-infecting *Giardia* transmission sites, specifically, is not possible. As such, revised methods of detecting and monitoring assemblage-specific *Giardia*-contaminated water sources, such as through detection and genotypic analysis of parasite-derived eDNA, have been developed.

Assessing and monitoring disease transmission within a given focus through the detection of parasite-derived eDNA rather than, or in conjunction with, using human bodily samples, has been explored with respect to a range of waterborne pathogens, including both schistosomiasis and giardiasis [97–99]. Dependence of both parasites on freshwater provides an ideal target for sample collection and assessment using PCR/qPCR, LAMP or RPA assays [83,100,101]. In addition, collection of water samples to detect eDNA derived from *Schistosoma* freshwater snail hosts to identify and monitor the presence of snail species capable of transmitting infection within a given waterbody has also been assessed [102,103].

Again, though promising, the upscaled and routine use of molecular assays to detect parasite- and/or parasite host-derived eDNA remains beyond the financial reach of most LMIC control programmes and too requires further methodological development, assessment and validation. Nevertheless, continued development of this approach to better understand the potential of eDNA as an effective monitoring tool and to reduce associated financial costs has been encouraged [75]. In particular, and like molecular xenomonitoring approaches, the monitoring of eDNA to identify disease transmission may prove extremely useful in areas of low disease endemicity where identifying infection in individual patients may be challenging.

3.4. A Case Example of Co-Infection and Morbidity Surveillance in Uganda

Given these key similarities in disease transmission biology and co-endemicity of both intestinal schistosomiasis and giardiasis throughout much of sub-Saharan Africa, co-infection with both parasites is likely commonplace, yet only little formal attention has been given towards co-surveillance of both diseases. This is despite each parasite potentially influencing reciprocal infection susceptibilities and disease-associated pathologies, before and after anti-parasitic treatment(s). As an example, it is possible that *S. mansoni* egg-induced perforations to the bowel with associated mucosal bleeding, inflammation and bacterial translocation may influence an individual's susceptibility to chronic *Giardia* infection. The extent to which this occurs, however, is currently unknown.

This lack of attention on co-infection and co-surveillance may be, in part, due to an unfortunate division within parasitology that often siloes macro-parasite (helminth) and micro-parasite (protist) research. Though sparse, recent epidemiological studies are now beginning to shed more detailed light on the prevalence of co-infection of intestinal schistosomiasis and giardiasis, with detection of associated morbidities, throughout rural areas of sub-Saharan Africa [11,104,105]. A suitable example arises from two recent studies assessing co-infection in school-aged children along the shoreline of Lake Albert, Uganda, which, despite ongoing preventive chemotherapy for intestinal schistosomiasis, can still be considered hyper-endemic for *S. mansoni* today (Figure 2) [88]. Here, initial infection with *S. mansoni* occurs very soon after birth, with all ages vulnerable to infection and chronic disease [106].

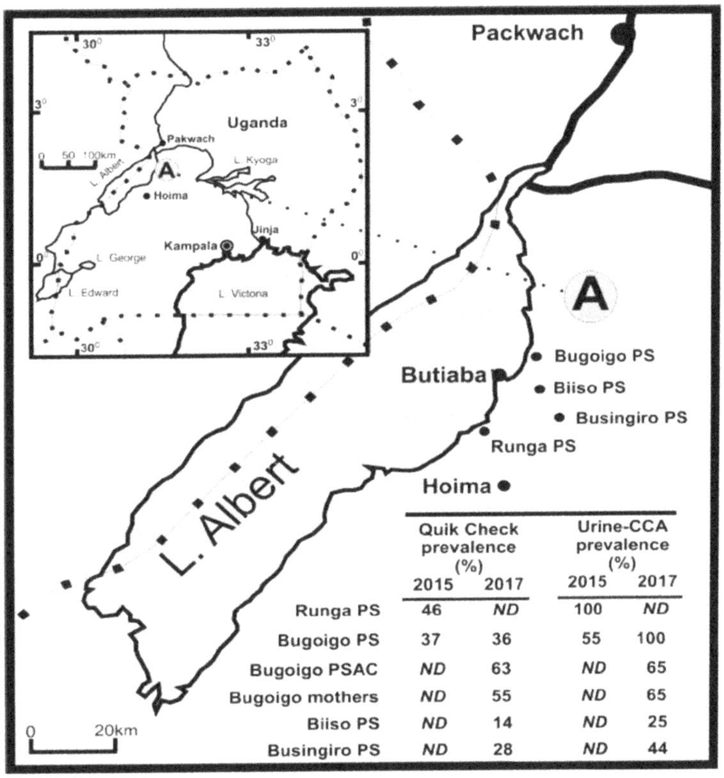

Figure 2. High prevalence of intestinal schistosomiasis (assessed using urine-CCA POC-RDT) and giardiasis co-infection (assessed using Quik Chek POC-RDT (TechLab, USA)) in school-aged children across multiple communities along the shoreline of Lake Albert, Uganda in 2015 and 2017 [8].

Beginning in 2015, Al-Shehri et al. [8] conducted a novel attempt to integrate surveillance for intestinal schistosomiasis, giardiasis and malaria using available POC rapid diagnostic tests (RDTs) combined with later real-time qPCR analysis of stool and finger-prick collected blood with parasite-specific TaqMan DNA® probes. This was the first attempt to quantify giardiasis with the POC Quik Chek RDT (TechLab, USA), finding 42% of children attending Runga and Bugoigo primary schools to be positive (Figure 2). Upon qPCR analysis of ethanol preserved stool using an 18S rDNA *Giardia*-specific TaqMan® probe, up to 87.0% of children were found excreting *Giardia* DNA. Notably, the prevalence of heavy infection by real-time PCR (Ct $\leq$ 19) was 19.5% and strongly associated with Quik-Chek RDTs, as well as postively correlated with increasing intensities of egg-patent schistosomiasis and host anaemia [11].

Giardia species assemblages present were also later identified and characterised with specific triose phosphate isomerase (TPI) Taqman® probes and by sequence characterisation of the β-giardin gene [107]. While less sensitive than the 18S rDNA assay, general prevalence by TPI probes was 52%, with prevalence by taxon assemblage of 8% (assemblage A), 36% (assemblage B) and 8% co-infection (A and B assemblages), and while assemblage B was dominant across the sample, proportions of assemblages A and B, and co-infections thereof, varied by school and by age of child. Mixed infections were particularly common at Runga school and in children aged 6 and under. Most importantly, infection with assemblage B was associated with underweight children. The presence of each assemblage was also confirmed by sequence analysis of the β-giardin gene finding sub-assemblage AII and further genetic diversity within assemblage B; also of note was the absence cryptosporidiosis, another pertinent water-borne disease, concurrently detectable by the same Quik Chek RDT.

To assess any changes through time, a repeat epidemiological survey was undertaken in 2017 which included reinspection of Bugoigo school and expanded point-of-care testing with Quik Chek (Figure 2). The prevalence of giardiasis at Bugoigo primary school was shown to be identical with a third of children examined positive by Quik Chek, with even higher local prevalence in pre-school-age children (63%) and their mothers (55%), good evidence for pervasive nature of giardiasis across all ages. Away from the lake at Biiso and Busingiro, the prevalence of giardiasis and intestinal schistosomiasis declined, suggesting that the risk of infection is perhaps higher on the lake shoreline. This study also attempted to evaluate a new POC-RPA RDT onsite, as well as a pilot assessment of giardiasis in local livestock and companion animals [81]. Ultimately, the RPA assay did not perform as well as expected, being in need for further optimisation of stool DNA extraction protocols.

Further to human-surveillance, screening for *S. mansoni* transmission has also taken place along the same shoreline by collection and cercarial shedding of *Biomphalaria* freshwater snail hosts with success [88,108]. Future surveillance should also be carried out through molecular xenomonitoring of collected snails (and so omitting the need for shedding analyses), collection and screening of non-human definitive hosts to identify *S. mansoni* and *G. duodenalis* DNA and through collection and screening of surface water samples to identify *S. mansoni* and *G. duodenalis* eDNA.

3.5. Access to Treatment and Large-Scale Campaigns

In areas where schistosomiasis transmission is identified, preventive chemotherapy through repeated mass drug administration (MDA) of the donated anthelmintic drug praziquantel (40 mg/kg body weight) is the principal strategy for disease control [109]. Because the highest burden of infection is typically seen in children and young adolescents, MDA is customarily carried out in schools, but aims to limit overall transmission within a community through a reduced human reservoir of infection while also reducing overall disease morbidity [110]. Though praziquantel's mechanism of action is not currently fully understood, significant reductions in disease prevalence and morbidity have been seen globally since MDA programmes began in 2001 [111,112]. Reinfection of schistosomiasis following treatment is, however, commonplace owing to communities' reliance on freshwater, and so MDA must be repeated annually or biannually, depending on disease prevalence, to achieve a sustained impact.

Severe adverse effects are seen only very rarely when distributing praziquantel, making it well suited for mass distribution. Praziquantel, however, typically does not achieve 100% infection clearance primarily because dosing is usually based only on height and so does not account for differences in body mass. As a result, treatment success varies between individuals meaning many are still able to continue maintaining transmission [113]. In addition, and while local school systems provide a viable means of mass-distributing praziquantel, important human reservoirs of infection, including pre-school-aged children and adults, typically remain untreated [106,114].

The need for repeated annual or biannual distribution of MDA in this way has also raised regular concerns about the development of praziquantel resistance in schistosomes; particularly as there is currently no known efficacious alternative treatment to replace praziquantel if *Schistosoma* populations were to become more drug-tolerant or resistant [115,116]. A significant reduction in praziquantel efficacy, identified by a decreased reduction in *Schistosoma* egg output from infected individuals pre- and post-praziquantel treatment, has already been reported in *S. mansoni* populations in many communities across sub-Saharan Africa that have undergone repeated rounds of MDA [113]. This reduced efficacy may be a direct result of selection pressure placed on schistosomes during repeated and prolonged MDA campaigns, highlighting an urgent need to consider alternative methods of disease control outside of MDA.

A variety of drugs can be used to treat giardiasis [117,118]. Of these, metronidazole is the most predominantly used and most thoroughly studied owing to its straightforward oral administration and relatively low price. Like with schistosomiasis, reinfection with giardiasis is also commonplace; however, repeated mass drug administration to alleviate giardiasis transmission is not seen as a feasible strategy because the drug is not currently involved in any donation scheme, severe adverse effects of treatment are often seen, and metronidazole has only limited efficacy in clearing infection [117]. As an example, it has been reported that just one course of treatment has only an approximately 60% clearance rate, and so repeated treatment is needed to significantly clear infection [119]. Repeated treatment, however, not only significantly increases the likelihood of severe adverse events but is difficult to carry out during MDA campaigns [5]. In addition, the potential emergence of giardiasis resistance to treatment with metronidazole has also recently been reported, and while alternative and more efficacious chemotherapies, such as tinidazole exist, these can also cause adverse events [117–119]. Albendazole, a broad-spectrum and efficacious anthelmintic treatment used in MDA campaigns to reduce transmission of soil-transmitted helminth and some filarial nematode infections, can also be used to treat giardiasis [117,120,121]. To significantly reduce *Giardia* infection, however, a minimum dosage of 200–800 mg/day albendazole is needed for at least three concurrent days which, again, is difficult to carry out in the context of MDA campaigns and, by having limited donated stocks, also diminishes albendazole availability for anti-helminth control programmes [117,118,122].

Though treatment of schistosomiasis and giardiasis using praziquantel and metronidazole are important components of disease control, aligning treatment of both diseases in tandem during control campaigns may be challenging, owing to differences in drug type, dosages and treatment courses. In addition, as neither drug can safely and reliably achieve a 100% clearance rate using just one dosage, it is now widely accepted that alternative methods of control to reduce transmission and overall prevalence must be implemented alongside treatment campaigns if disease elimination targets are to be met. One such example is the implementation of WASH initiatives in communities where both diseases are endemic. The extent to which WASH provision, when used in conjunction with MDA, can successfully reduce schistosomiasis transmission is now beginning to be understood, and although only minimal data has been reported on the impact of WASH provision on giardiasis transmission in sub-Saharan Africa, it is widely assumed that improved WASH infrastructure would help significantly reduce giardiasis transmission [1,123,124].

3.6. *Water, Sanitation and Hygeine (WASH)*

WASH provision and infrastructure is extremely inadequate throughout many areas of rural sub-Saharan Africa [125]. In 2012, the World Health Assembly (WHA) formally advocated for the integration of WASH provision and education initiatives into amenable NTD control and elimination programmes; subsequently publishing guidance on ways in which these can be integrated [126,127]. Since, much attention has been given towards how WASH initiatives can be tailored for use, specifically, in schistosomiasis control programmes and the impact such initiatives have had when used in tandem with routine strategies such as preventive chemotherapy [2,30,128,129].

WASH initiatives relevant to schistosomiasis control, such as the adequate provision of safe drinking water, fully functional and properly maintained pit latrines and improved community hygiene education, effectively reduce disease transmission by minimising the direct and indirect contamination of freshwater by infected individuals and animals, by reducing contact with/consumption of infectious waters by human and non-human hosts and by helping communities better understand human and non-human disease transmission [30,130] (Figure 3).

Like intestinal schistosomiasis, giardiasis is widely prevalent throughout many rural and impoverished regions of sub-Saharan Africa and is intrinsically linked to contact with contaminated and unsafe water in areas lacking adequate water, sanitation and hygiene (WASH) infrastructure [4,41]. Giardiasis, however, receives only relatively little attention with regard to disease control, surveillance and elimination throughout sub-Saharan Africa.

As an example, despite numerous clear advantages of implementing WASH initiatives on reducing schistosomiasis transmission and despite these key similarities between schistosomiasis and giardiasis with regard to disease transmission biology, surprisingly little attention has been given to the impact of improved WASH provision and education on giardiasis transmission in sub-Saharan Africa [43]. This oversight presents not only a missed opportunity with regard to better understanding, and reducing, giardiasis transmission and its associated pathological impact on some of the world's most disadvantaged communities, but also presents the question: why is giardiasis ignored in intestinal schistosomiasis monitoring and control programmes?

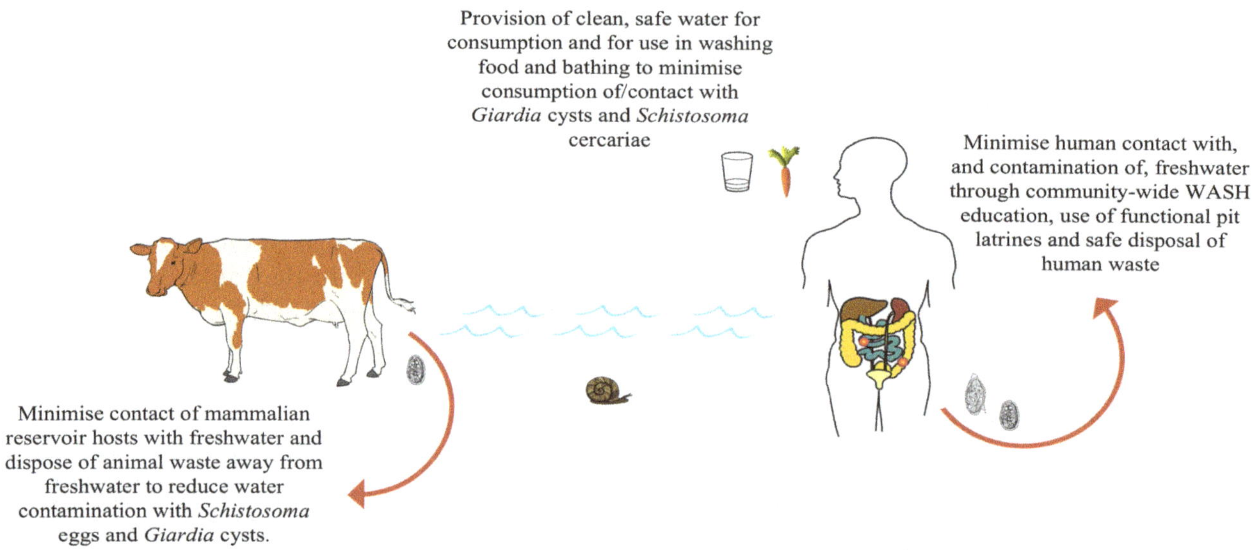

Figure 3. Examples of water, sanitation and hygiene (WASH) initiatives implemented to prevent the contamination of freshwater with *S. mansoni* eggs and *G. duodenalis* cysts, as well as to prevent contact with and consumption of contaminated water. Adapted from [26,27].

4. Intestinal Schistosomiasis and Giardiasis: Towards a One Health Approach

Research funding opportunities for NTDs are limited when compared to those for other diseases such as human immunodeficiency virus (HIV), malaria or tuberculosis [131]. One way in which the impact of NTD control programmes can be significantly increased, however, is by appropriate integration with other disease surveillance, control, research and policy efforts. Successful examples of this integrated One Health approach can be seen when integrating lymphatic filariasis surveillance and elimination efforts into malaria elimination programmes, as well as by integrating soil-transmitted helminth and schistosomiasis control and elimination efforts [128,132–135].

In keeping with this integrated One Health approach, here, we propose a variety of ways in which the transmission of, and pathologies associated with, co-infection of intestinal schistosomiasis and giardiasis can be better understood, monitored and reduced via the integration of giardiasis control efforts into existing schistosomiasis control programmes. These include:

- Integrating screening of giardiasis endemicity and infection prevalence into existing schistosomiasis control programmes by using stool samples used for diagnosing infection with *S. mansoni*, and other intestinal parasites, to also record and report levels of *Giardia* infection in school-aged children. This can be conducted with POC-RDTs such as the Quik Chek immunoassay or using PCR/qPCR. In addition, the continued development, assessment and application of sensitive and straightforward POC-RDTs able to detect low-levels of infection in asymptomatic individuals capable of maintaining transmission of both parasites, such as the RPA, is encouraged.
- Further development and application of sensitive molecular assays to detect trace levels of species/assemblage-specific parasite DNA within freshwater snail intermediate hosts of human-infecting *Schistosoma*, and in faecal samples from non-human animal definitive hosts of both diseases. Further development and application of sensitive molecular assays to detect trace levels of species-/assemblage-specific parasite DNA from human-infecting *Schistosoma* cercariae and *Giardia* cysts in water samples easily collected from viable transmission sites is also encouraged.
- The upscaled provision of water, sanitation and hygiene (WASH) infrastructure and education initiatives to communities afflicted by both schistosomiasis and giardiasis to reduce environmental contamination events and to reduce contact with/consumption of contaminated water, simultaneously reducing transmission of both diseases.

- Monitoring *Giardia* disease prevalence and associated morbidities in tandem with schistosomiasis surveillance in school-aged children following any control programme intervention to better understand how giardiasis transmission and related pathologies can be reduced.
- An increased focus on understanding how the transmission of intestinal schistosomiasis and giardiasis, as well as immune responses and morbidities related to both diseases, interact and are potentially exacerbated by co-infection.

5. Conclusions

Here, we have highlighted various potential opportunities to improve the health and wellbeing of individuals in low- and middle-income countries where intestinal schistosomiasis and giardiasis are co-endemic by exploiting key similarities between both diseases with regard to disease transmission biology, epidemiology, surveillance and control. In addition, future steps needed to develop and implement an integrated, One Health approach for intestinal schistosomiasis and giardiasis co-infection surveillance, control and elimination strategies, are also outlined. In adopting this One Health approach, and by integrating giardiasis surveillance, control and elimination efforts into existing schistosomiasis elimination programmes, not only can the debilitating pathological impacts of intestinal schistosomiasis/giardiasis co-infection be better understood, but a reduction in co-infection and concurrent reduction in disease-related morbidities experienced by the world's most disadvantaged communities can also be achieved.

Author Contributions: Concept of the study (J.A., A.L.B. & J.R.S.), literature searching and review (J.A., L.O., S.S., M.S.), fieldwork (J.A., H.A.-S., N.B.K., A.A., M.A. (Moses Adriko), M.A. (Moses Arianaitwe), E.J.L., A.L.B., J.R.S.), and molecular analyses performed by (H.A.-S., T.B., B.L.W.). All authors have read and agreed to the published version of the manuscript.

Acknowledgments: J.A. would like to thank Michael Fowler of EH Studios for support with figures.

Abbreviations

eDNA	environmental DNA
ELISA	enzyme-linked immunosorbent assay
FGS	female genital schistosomiasis
LAMP	loop-mediated isothermal reaction
LMIC	lower-middle-income countries
MDA	mass drug administration
NTD	neglected tropical disease
PCR	polymerase chain reaction
POC	point-of-care
qPCR	quantitative polymerase chain reaction
RDT	rapid diagnostic test
RPA	recombinase polymerase amplification
Th1	T-helper 1
Th2	T-helper 2
WASH	water, sanitation and hygiene
WHA	world health assembly

References

1. Omarova, A.; Tussupova, K.; Berndtsson, R.; Kalishev, M.; Sharapatova, K. Protozoan parasites in drinking water: A system approach for improved water, sanitation and hygiene in developing countries. *Int. J. Environ. Res. Public Health* **2018**, *15*, 495. [CrossRef] [PubMed]
2. Campbell, S.J.; Biritwum, N.K.; Woods, G.; Velleman, Y.; Fleming, F.; Stothard, J.R. Tailoring water, sanitation, and hygiene (WASH) Targets for toil-transmitted helminthiasis and schistosomiasis control. *Trends Parasitol.* **2018**, *34*, 53–63. [CrossRef] [PubMed]
3. Colley, D.G.; Bustinduy, A.L.; Secor, W.E.; King, C.H. Human schistosomiasis. *Lancet* **2014**, *383*, 2253–2264. [CrossRef]
4. Thompson, R.C.A.; Reynoldson, J.A.; Sciences, B. *Giardia* and giardiasis. *Adv. Parasitol.* **1993**, *32*, 71–160.
5. Squire, S.A.; Ryan, U. *Cryptosporidium* and *Giardia* in Africa: Current and future challenges. *Parasites Vectors* **2017**, *10*, 1–32. [CrossRef]
6. Nkrumah, B.; Nguah, S. *Giardia lamblia*: A major parasitic cause of childhood diarrhoea in patients attending a district hospital in Ghana. *Parasites Vectors* **2011**, *4*, 1–7. [CrossRef]
7. Bartelt, L.A.; Sartor, R.B. Advances in understanding *Giardia*: Determinants and mechanisms of chronic sequelae. *F1000Prime Rep.* **2015**, *7*, 1–14. [CrossRef]
8. Naess, H.; Nyland, M.; Hausken, T.; Follestad, I.; Nyland, H.I. Chronic fatigue syndrome after *Giardia* enteritis: Clinical characteristics, disability and long-term sickness absence. *BMC Gastroenterol.* **2012**, *12*. [CrossRef]
9. Chifunda, K.; Kelly, P. Parasitic infections of the gut in children. *Paediatr. Int. Child Health* **2019**, *39*, 65–72. [CrossRef]
10. Savioli, L.; Smith, H.; Thompson, A. *Giardia* and *Cryptosporidium* join the "Neglected Diseases Initiative". *Trends Parasitol.* **2006**, *22*, 203–208. [CrossRef]
11. Al-Shehri, H.; Stanton, M.C.; LaCourse, J.E.; Atuhaire, A.; Arinaitwe, M.; Wamboko, A.; Adriko, M.; Kabatereine, N.B.; Stothard, J.R. An extensive burden of giardiasis associated with intestinal schistosomiasis and anaemia in school children on the shoreline of Lake Albert, Uganda. *Trans. R. Soc. Trop. Med. Hyg.* **2016**, *110*, 597–603. [CrossRef] [PubMed]
12. La Hoz, R.M.; Morris, M.I. Intestinal parasites including *Cryptosporidium, Cyclospora, Giardia*, and *Microsporidia, Entamoeba histolytica, Strongyloides*, Schistosomiasis, and *Echinococcus*: Guidelines from the American Society of Transplantation Infectious Diseases Community of Pract. *Clin. Transplant.* **2019**, *33*, 1–16. [CrossRef] [PubMed]
13. Zhou, X.N. Prioritizing research for "One health—One world". *Infect. Dis. Poverty* **2012**, *1*, 1–5. [CrossRef] [PubMed]
14. Mackenzie, J.S.; Jeggo, M. *One Health and Zoonoses*; MDPI Books: Basel, Switzeland, 2019; ISBN 9783039212958. [CrossRef]
15. Samuels, A.M.; Matey, E.; Mwinzi, P.N.M.; Wiegand, R.E.; Muchiri, G.; Ireri, E.; Hyde, M.; Montgomery, S.P.; Karanja, D.M.S.; Secor, W.E. *Schistosoma mansoni* morbidity among school-aged children: A SCORE Project in Kenya. *Am. J. Trop. Med. Hyg.* **2012**, *87*, 874–882. [CrossRef] [PubMed]
16. De Moira, A.P.; Fulford, A.J.C.; Kabatereine, N.B.; Ouma, J.H.; Booth, M.; Dunne, D.W. Analysis of complex patterns of human exposure and immunity to *Schistosomiasis mansoni*: The influence of age, sex, ethnicity and IgE. *PLoS Negl. Trop. Dis.* **2010**, *4*, e820. [CrossRef]
17. Costain, A.H.; MacDonald, A.S.; Smits, H.H. Schistosome egg migration: Mechanisms, pathogenesis and host immune responses. *Front. Immunol.* **2018**, *9*, 3042. [CrossRef]
18. Olveda, David Bilharzia: Pathology, diagnosis, management and control. *Trop. Med. Surg.* **2013**, *1*, 1–19. [CrossRef]
19. Heyworth, M.F. *Giardia duodenalis* genetic assemblages and hosts. *Parasite* **2016**, *23*. [CrossRef]
20. Sprong, H.; Cacciò, S.M.; Van Der Giessen, J.W.B. Identification of zoonotic genotypes of *Giardia duodenalis*. *PLoS Negl. Trop. Dis.* **2009**, *3*, 1–12. [CrossRef]
21. Fink, M.Y.; Singer, S.M. The intersection of immune responses, microbiota, and pathogenesis in giardiasis. *Trends Parasitol.* **2017**, *33*, 901–913. [CrossRef]

22. Keselman, A.; Li, E.; Maloney, J.; Singer, S.M. The microbiota contributes to CD8+ T cell activation and nutrient malabsorption following intestinal infection with *Giardia duodenalis*. *Infect. Immun.* **2016**, *84*, 2853–2860. [CrossRef] [PubMed]
23. Allain, T.; Amat, C.B.; Motta, J.P.; Manko, A.; Buret, A.G. Interactions of *Giardia* sp. with the intestinal barrier: Epithelium, mucus, and microbiota. *Tissue Barriers* **2017**, *5*, 1–16. [CrossRef] [PubMed]
24. Mmbaga, B.T.; Houpt, E.R. *Cryptosporidium* and *Giardia* infections in children: A Review. *Pediatr. Clin. N. Am.* **2017**, *64*, 837–850. [CrossRef] [PubMed]
25. Lane, S.; Lloyd, D. Current trends in research into the waterborne parasite *Giardia*. *Crit. Rev. Microbiol.* **2002**, *28*, 123–147. [CrossRef]
26. Centers for Disease Control and Prevention (CDC), USA: Schistosomiasis, About, Life Cycle. Available online: https://www.cdc.gov/parasites/schistosomiasis/biology.html (accessed on 1 July 2020).
27. Centers for Disease Control and Prevention (CDC), USA: Giardiasis, About, Life Cycle. Available online: https://www.cdc.gov/dpdx/giardiasis/index.html#:~{}:text=Thespectrumvariesfromasymptomaticcarriagetosevere, includediarrhea%2Cabdominalpain%2Cbloating%2Cnausea%2Candvomiting. (accessed on 1 July 2020).
28. Sow, S.; Polman, K.; Vereecken, K.; Vercruysse, J.; Gryseels, B.; de Vlas, S.J. The role of hygienic bathing after defecation in the transmission of *Schistosoma mansoni*. *Trans. R. Soc. Trop. Med. Hyg.* **2008**, *102*, 542–547. [CrossRef]
29. Vercruysse, J.; Shaw, D.J.; De Bont, J. Index of potential contamination for schistosomiasis. *Trends Parasitol.* **2001**, *17*, 256–261. [CrossRef]
30. Grimes, J.E.; Croll, D.; Harrison, W.E.; Utzinger, J.; Freeman, M.C.; Templeton, M.R. The roles of water, sanitation and hygiene in reducing schistosomiasis: A review. *Parasites Vectors* **2015**, *8*, 1–16. [CrossRef]
31. Wright, C.A. Chapter 4: Fluke Life-Cycles. In *Flukes and Snails*; George Allen and Unwin LTD: London, UK, 1971.
32. Galaktionov, K.V.; Dobrovolskij, A. *The Biology and Evolution of Trematodes. An Essay on the Biology, Morphology, Life Cycles, Transmission, and Evolution of Digenetic Trematodes. Chapter 2: The Trematode Life Cycle as a System of Adaptations*; Kluwer Academic Publishers: Dordrecht, The Netherlands; Boston, MA, USA, 2003.
33. Fried, B.T.; Graczyk, T. Chapter 7: Host Recognition by Trematode Miracidia and Cercariae. In *Advances in Trematode Biology*; CRC Press: New York, NY, USA, 1997.
34. Lockyer, A.E.; Jones, C.S.; Noble, L.R.; Rollinson, D. Trematodes and snails: An intimate association. *Can. J. Zool.* **2004**, *82*, 251–269. [CrossRef]
35. Théron, A. *Chronobiology of Trematode Cercarial Emergence: From Data Recovery to Epidemiological, Ecological and Evolutionary Implications*; Elsevier Ltd.: Amsterdam, The Netherlands, 2015; Volume 88.
36. Frandsen, F.; Christensen, N. An introductory guide to the identification of cercariae from African freshwater snails with special reference to cercariae of trematode species of medical and veterinary importance. *Acta Trop.* **1984**. [CrossRef]
37. Einarsson, E.; Ma'ayeh, S.; Svärd, S.G. An up-date on *Giardia* and giardiasis. *Curr. Opin. Microbiol.* **2016**, *34*, 47–52. [CrossRef]
38. Mohammed Mahdy, A.K.; Lim, Y.A.L.; Surin, J.; Wan, K.L.; Al-Mekhlafi, M.S.H. Risk factors for endemic giardiasis: Highlighting the possible association of contaminated water and food. *Trans. R. Soc. Trop. Med. Hyg.* **2008**, *102*, 465–470. [CrossRef] [PubMed]
39. Ankarklev, J.; Jerlström-Hultqvist, J.; Ringqvist, E.; Troell, K.; Svärd, S.G. Behind the smile: Cell biology and disease mechanisms of *Giardia* species. *Nat. Rev. Microbiol.* **2010**, *8*, 413–422. [CrossRef] [PubMed]
40. Huang, Y.; Manderson, L. Schistosomiasis and the social patterning of infection. *Acta Trop.* **1992**, *51*, 175–194. [CrossRef]
41. Ahmed, S.A.; Guerrero Flórez, M.; Karanis, P. The impact of water crises and climate changes on the transmission of protozoan parasites in Africa. *Pathog. Glob. Health* **2018**, *112*, 281–293. [CrossRef] [PubMed]
42. Esrey, S.A.; Collett, J.; Miliotis, M.D.; Koornhof, H.J.; Makhale, P. The risk of infection from *Giardia lamblia* due to drinking water supply, use of water, and latrines among preschool children in rural Lesotho. *Int. J. Epidemiol.* **1989**, *18*, 248–253. [CrossRef]
43. Campbell, S.J.; Nery, S.V.; D'Este, C.A.; Gray, D.J.; McCarthy, J.S.; Traub, R.J.; Andrews, R.M.; Llewellyn, S.; Vallely, A.J.; Williams, G.M.; et al. Water, sanitation and hygiene related risk factors for soil-transmitted helminth and *Giardia duodenalis* infections in rural communities in Timor-Leste. *Int. J. Parasitol.* **2016**, *46*, 771–779. [CrossRef]

44. Robinson, M.W.; Dalton, J.P. Zoonotic helminth infections with particular emphasis on fasciolosis and other trematodiases. *Philos. Trans. R. Soc. B Biol. Sci.* **2009**, *364*, 2763–2776. [CrossRef]
45. Chomel, B.B. Control and prevention of emerging parasitic zoonoses. *Int. J. Parasitol.* **2008**, *38*, 1211–1217. [CrossRef]
46. MARTINS, A.V. Non-human vertebrate hosts of Schistosoma haematobium and Schistosoma mansoni. *Bull. World Health Organ.* **1958**, *18*, 931–944.
47. Standley, C.J.; Dobson, A.; Dobson, A.P.; Stothard, J.R. *Out of Animals and Back again: Schistosomiasis as a Zoonosis in Africa. Schistosomiasis*; Rokni, M.B., Ed.; InTech Europe: Rijeka, Croatia, 2012; Available online: http://www.intechopen.com/books/schistosomiasis/out-of-animals-andback-again-schistosomiasis-as-a-zoonosis-in-africa (accessed on 13 January 2012)ISBN ISBN 978-953-307-852-6.
48. Ryan, U.; Cacciò, S.M. Zoonotic potential of *Giardia*. *Int. J. Parasitol.* **2013**, *43*, 943–956. [CrossRef]
49. Yaoyu, F.; Xiao, L. Zoonotic potential and molecular epidemiology of *Giardia* species and giardiasis. *Clin. Microbiol. Rev.* **2011**, *24*, 110–140. [CrossRef]
50. Thompson, R.C.A. The zoonotic significance and molecular epidemiology of *Giardia* and giardiasis. *Vet. Parasitol.* **2004**, *126*, 15–35. [CrossRef]
51. Sak, B.; Petrzelkova, K.J.; Kvetonova, D.; Mynarova, A.; Shutt, K.A.; Pomajbikova, K.; Kalousova, B.; Modry, D.; Benavides, J.; Todd, A.; et al. Long-term monitoring of *Microsporidia, Cryptosporidium* and *Giardia* Infections in western lowland gorillas (*Gorilla gorilla gorilla*) at different stages of habituation in Dzanga Sangha protected areas, Central African Republic. *PLoS ONE* **2013**, *8*, e71840. [CrossRef] [PubMed]
52. Hanelt, B.; Mwangi, I.N.; Kinuthia, J.M.; Maina, G.M.; Agola, L.E.; Mutuku, M.W.; Steinauer, M.L.; Agwanda, B.R.; Kigo, L.; Mungai, B.N.; et al. Schistosomes of small mammals from the Lake Victoria Basin, Kenya: New species, familiar species, and implications for schistosomiasis control. *Parasitology* **2010**, *137*, 1109–1118. [CrossRef]
53. De Bont, J.; Vercruysse, J. The epidemiology and control of cattle schistosomiasis. *Parasitol. Today* **1997**, *13*, 255–262. [CrossRef]
54. Olson, M.E.; O'Handley, R.M.; Ralston, B.J.; McAllister, T.A.; Thompson, R.C.A. Update on *Cryptosporidium* and *Giardia* infections in cattle. *Trends Parasitol.* **2004**, *20*, 185–191. [CrossRef]
55. Savassi, B.A.E.S.; Mouahid, G.; Lasica, C.; Mahaman, S.D.K.; Garcia, A.; Courtin, D.; Allienne, J.F.; Ibikounlé, M.; Moné, H. Cattle as natural host for *Schistosoma haematobium* (Bilharz, 1852) Weinland, 1858 × *Schistosoma bovis* Sonsino, 1876 interactions, with new cercarial emergence and genetic patterns. *Parasitol. Res.* **2020**, 1–17. [CrossRef]
56. Sene-Wade, M.; Marchand, B.; Rollinson, D.; Webster, B.L. Urogenital schistosomiasis and hybridization between *Schistosoma haematobium* and *Schistosoma bovis* in adults living in Richard-Toll, Senegal. *Parasitology* **2018**, *145*, 1723–1726. [CrossRef]
57. Standley, C.J.; Stothard, J.R. DNA Barcoding of schistosome cercariae reveals a novel sub-lineage within *Schistosoma rodhaini* from Ngamba Island chimpanzee sanctuary, Lake Victoria. *J. Parasitol.* **2012**, *98*, 1049–1051. [CrossRef]
58. Catalano, S.; Sène, M.; Diouf, N.D.; Fall, C.B.; Borlase, A.; Léger, E.; Bâ, K.; Webster, J.P. Rodents as natural hosts of zoonotic schistosoma species and hybrids: An epidemiological and evolutionary perspective from West Africa. *J. Infect. Dis.* **2018**, *218*, 429–433. [CrossRef]
59. Steinauer, M.L.; Hanelt, B.; Mwangi, I.N.; Maina, G.M.; Agola, L.E.; Kinuthia, J.M.; Mutuku, M.W.; Mungai, B.N.; Wilson, W.D.; Mkoji, G.M.; et al. Introgressive hybridization of human and rodent schistosome parasites in western Kenya. *Mol. Ecol.* **2008**, *17*, 5062–5074. [CrossRef] [PubMed]
60. Huyse, T.; Webster, B.L.; Geldof, S.; Stothard, J.R.; Diaw, O.T.; Polman, K.; Rollinson, D. Bidirectional introgressive hybridization between a cattle and human schistosome species. *PLoS Pathog.* **2009**, *5*, e1000571. [CrossRef] [PubMed]
61. World Health Organisation. *Research Priorities for Helminth Infections*; WHO Technical Report Series No. 972; World Health Organisation: Geneva, Switzerland, 2012; Available online: https://apps.who.int/iris/bitstream/handle/10665/75922 (accessed on 30 June 2020).
62. Katz, N.; Chaves, A.; Pellegrino, J. A simple device for quantitative stool thick-smear technique in *Schistosomiasis mansoni*. *Rev. Inst. Med. Trop. Sao Paulo* **1972**, *14*, 397–400. [PubMed]

63. Lamberton, P.H.L.; Kabatereine, N.B.; Oguttu, D.W.; Fenwick, A.; Webster, J.P. Sensitivity and specificity of multiple Kato-Katz thick smears and a circulating cathodic antigen test for *Schistosoma mansoni* diagnosis pre- and post-repeated-praziquantel treatment. *PLoS Negl. Trop. Dis.* **2014**, *8*. [CrossRef]
64. Adeyemo, F.E.; Singh, G.; Reddy, P.; Stenström, T.A. Methods for the detection of *Cryptosporidium* and *Giardia*: From microscopy to nucleic acid based tools in clinical and environmental regimes. *Acta Trop.* **2018**, *184*, 15–28. [CrossRef] [PubMed]
65. Zahan, N. A Comparison of microscopy and enzyme linked immunosorbent assay for diagnosis of *Giardia lamblia* in human faecal specimens. *J. Clin. Diagn. Res.* **2014**, *8*, 10–12. [CrossRef] [PubMed]
66. Barda, B.D.; Rinaldi, L.; Ianniello, D.; Zepherine, H.; Salvo, F.; Sadutshang, T.; Cringoli, G.; Clementi, M.; Albonico, M. Mini-FLOTAC, an innovative direct diagnostic technique for intestinal parasitic infections: Experience from the field. *PLoS Negl. Trop. Dis.* **2013**, *7*, e2344. [CrossRef]
67. Barda, B.; Ianniello, D.; Zepheryne, H.; Rinaldi, L.; Cringoli, G.; Burioni, R.; Albonico, M. Parasitic infections on the shore of Lake Victoria (East Africa) detected by Mini-FLOTAC and standard techniques. *Acta Trop.* **2014**, *137*, 140–146. [CrossRef]
68. Hooshyar, H.; Rostamkhani, P.; Mohsen Arbabi, M.D. Giardia lamblia infection: Review of current diagnostic strategies. *Gastroenterol. Hepatol.* **2019**, *95*, 347–349. [CrossRef]
69. Glinz, D.; Silué, K.D.; Knopp, S.; Lohourignon, L.K.; Yao, K.P.; Steinmann, P.; Rinaldi, L.; Cringoli, G.; N'Goran, E.K.; Utzinger, J. Comparing diagnostic accuracy of Kato-Katz, Koga agar plate, ether-concentration, and FLOTAC for *Schistosoma mansoni* and soil-transmitted helminths. *PLoS Negl. Trop. Dis.* **2010**, *4*, e754. [CrossRef]
70. Taye, S. Comparison of Kato-Katz and formol-ether concentration methods for the diagnosis of intestinal helminthic infections among school children of Wonji Shoa town, Eastern Ethiopia: A school based cross-sectional study. *Am. J. Heal. Res.* **2014**, *2*, 271. [CrossRef]
71. Utzinger, J.; Becker, S.L.; van Lieshout, L.; van Dam, G.J.; Knopp, S. New diagnostic tools in schistosomiasis. *Clin. Microbiol. Infect.* **2015**, *21*, 529–542. [CrossRef] [PubMed]
72. Archer, J.; Lacourse, E.J.; Webster, L.B.; Stothard, J.R. An update on non-invasive urine diagnostics for human-infecting parasitic helminths: What more could be done and how? *Parasitology* **2019**, *147*, 873–888. [CrossRef] [PubMed]
73. Colley, D.G.; Binder, S.; Campbell, C.; King, C.H.; Tchuenté, L.A.T.; N'Goran, E.K.; Erko, B.; Karanja, D.M.S.; Kabatereine, N.B.; Van Lieshout, L.; et al. A five-country evaluation of a point-of-care circulating cathodic antigen urine assay for the prevalence of *Schistosoma mansoni*. *Am. J. Trop. Med. Hyg.* **2013**, *88*, 426–432. [CrossRef] [PubMed]
74. Weerakoon, K.G.; Gordon, C.A.; McManus, D.P. DNA diagnostics for schistosomiasis control. *Trop. Med. Infect. Dis.* **2018**, *3*, 81. [CrossRef]
75. Minetti, C.; LaCourse, E.J.; Reimer, L.; Stothard, J.R. Focusing nucleic acid-based molecular diagnostics and xenomonitoring approaches for human helminthiases amenable to preventive chemotherapy. *Parasitol. Open* **2016**, *2*. [CrossRef]
76. Mwangi, I.N.; Agola, E.L.; Mugambi, R.M.; Shiraho, E.A.; Mkoji, G.M. Development and evaluation of a loop-mediated isothermal amplification assay for diagnosis of *Schistosoma mansoni* infection in faecal samples. *J. Parasitol. Res.* **2018**, *2018*. [CrossRef]
77. Poulton, K.; Webster, B. Development of a lateral flow recombinase polymerase assay for the diagnosis of *Schistosoma mansoni* infections. *Anal. Biochem.* **2018**, *546*, 65–71. [CrossRef]
78. Koehler, A.V.; Jex, A.R.; Haydon, S.R.; Stevens, M.A.; Gasser, R.B. *Giardia*/giardiasis—A perspective on diagnostic and analytical tools. *Biotechnol. Adv.* **2014**, *32*, 280–289. [CrossRef]
79. Alexander, L.C.; Niebel, M.; Jones, B. The rapid detection of *Cryptosporidium* and *Giardia* species in clinical stools using the Quik Chek immunoassay. *Parasitol. Int.* **2013**, *62*, 552–553. [CrossRef]
80. Silva, R.K.N.R.; Pacheco, F.T.F.; Martins, A.S.; Menezes, J.F.; Costa-Ribeiro, H.; Ribeiro, T.C.M.; Mattos, Â.P.; Oliveira, R.R.; Soares, N.M.; Teixeira, M.C.A. Performance of microscopy and ELISA for diagnosing *Giardia duodenalis* infection in different pediatric groups. *Parasitol. Int.* **2016**, *65*, 635–640. [CrossRef] [PubMed]
81. Gonzalez, S.J.M.; Bhattacharyya, T.; Alshehri, H.R.; Poulton, K.; Allen, S.; Miles, M.A.; Arianitwe, M.; Tukahebwa, E.M.; Webster, B.; Stothard, J.R. Application of a recombinase polymerase amplification (RPA) assay and pilot field testing for *Giardia duodenalis* at Lake Albert, Uganda. *Parasit. Vectors* **2020**, *13*, 1–9. [CrossRef]

82. Crannell, Z.A.; Cabada, M.M.; Castellanos-Gonzalez, A.; Irani, A.; White, A.C.; Richards-Kortum, R. Recombinase polymerase amplification-based assay to diagnose *Giardia* in stool samples. *Am. J. Trop. Med. Hyg.* **2015**, *92*, 583–587. [CrossRef]
83. Plutzer, J.; Karanis, P. Rapid identification of *Giardia duodenalis* by loop-mediated isothermal amplification (LAMP) from faecal and environmental samples and comparative findings by PCR and real-time PCR methods. *Parasitol. Res.* **2009**, *104*, 1527–1533. [CrossRef] [PubMed]
84. De Dood, C.J.; Hoekstra, P.T.; Mngara, J.; Kalluvya, S.E.; Van Dam, G.J.; Downs, J.A.; Corstjens, P.L.A.M. Refining diagnosis of *Schistosoma haematobium* infections: Antigen and antibody detection in urine. *Front. Immunol.* **2018**, *9*, 1–9. [CrossRef]
85. Weerakoon, K.G.A.D.; Gobert, G.N.; Cai, P.; McManus, D.P. Advances in the diagnosis of human schistosomiasis. *Clin. Microbiol. Rev.* **2015**. [CrossRef]
86. Amoah, A.S.; Hoekstra, P.T.; Casacuberta-Partal, M.; Coffeng, L.E.; Corstjens, P.L.A.M.; Greco, B.; van Lieshout, L.; Lim, M.D.; Markwalter, C.F.; Odiere, M.R.; et al. Sensitive diagnostic tools and targeted drug administration strategies are needed to eliminate schistosomiasis. *Lancet Infect. Dis.* **2020**, *3099*, 1–8. [CrossRef]
87. Pennance, T.; Person, B.; Muhsin, M.A.; Khamis, A.N.; Muhsin, J.; Khamis, I.S.; Mohammed, K.A.; Kabole, F.; Rollinson, D.; Knopp, S. Urogenital schistosomiasis transmission on Unguja Island, Zanzibar: Characterisation of persistent hot-spots. *Parasites Vectors* **2016**, *9*, 1–13. [CrossRef]
88. Stothard, J.R.; Archer, J.; Gyapong, M.; Tchuem-Tchuenté, L.A.; Bustinduy, A.L.; Kabatereine, N.B.; Al-Shehri, H. A centenary of Robert T. Leiper's lasting legacy on schistosomiasis and a COUNTDOWN on control of neglected tropical diseases. *Parasitology* **2016**, *144*, 1602–1612. [CrossRef]
89. King, C.H.; Sturrock, R.F.; Kariuki, H.C.; Hamburger, J. Transmission control for schistosomiasis-why it matters now. *Trends Parasitol.* **2006**, *22*, 575–582. [CrossRef]
90. Allan, F.; Ame, S.M.; Tian-Bi, Y.-N.T.; Hofkin, B.V.; Webster, B.L.; Diakité, N.R.; N'Goran, E.K.; Kabole, F.; Khamis, I.S.; Gouvras, A.N.; et al. Snail-related contributions from the Schistosomiasis Consortium for Operational Research and Evaluation program including xenomonitoring, focal mollusciciding, biological control, and modeling. *Am. J. Trop. Med. Hyg.* **2020**. [CrossRef] [PubMed]
91. Abbasi, I.; King, C.H.; Muchiri, E.M.; Hamburger, J. Detection of *Schistosoma mansoni* and *Schistosoma haematobium* DNA by loop-mediated isothermal amplification: Identification of infected snails from early prepatency. *Am. J. Trop. Med. Hyg.* **2010**, *83*, 427–432. [CrossRef] [PubMed]
92. Gandasegui, J.; Fernández-Soto, P.; Hernández-Goenaga, J.; López-Abán, J.; Vicente, B.; Muro, A. Biompha-LAMP: A new rapid loop-mediated isothermal amplification assay for detecting *Schistosoma mansoni* in *Biomphalaria glabrata* snail host. *PLoS Negl. Trop. Dis.* **2016**, *10*, 1–14. [CrossRef] [PubMed]
93. Bartley, P.M.; Roehe, B.K.; Thomson, S.; Shaw, H.J.; Peto, F.; Innes, E.A.; Katzer, F. Detection of potentially human infectious assemblages of *Giardia duodenalis* in fecal samples from beef and dairy cattle in Scotland. *Parasitology* **2019**, *146*, 1123–1130. [CrossRef]
94. Sawitri, D.H.; Wardhana, A.H.; Martindah, E.; Ekawasti, F.; Dewi, D.A.; Utomo, B.N.; Shibahara, T.; Kusumoto, M.; Tokoro, M.; Sasai, K.; et al. Detections of gastrointestinal parasites, including *Giardia intestinalis* and *Cryptosporidium* spp., in cattle of Banten province, Indonesia. *J. Parasit. Dis.* **2020**, *44*, 174–179. [CrossRef]
95. DiGiorgio, C.L.; Gonzalez, D.A.; Huitt, C.C. *Cryptosporidium* and *Giardia* recoveries in natural waters by using environmental protection agency method 1623. *Appl. Environ. Microbiol.* **2002**, *68*, 5952–5955. [CrossRef]
96. EPA United States Environmental Protection Agency. Method 1623: Cryptosporidium and Giardia in Water by filtration/IMS/FA. Available online: https://www.epa.gov/sites/production/files/2015-07/documents/epa-1623.pdf (accessed on 24 July 2020).
97. Bass, D.; Stentiford, G.D.; Littlewood, D.T.J.; Hartikainen, H. Diverse applications of environmental DNA methods in parasitology. *Trends Parasitol.* **2015**, *31*, 499–513. [CrossRef]
98. Sengupta, M.E.; Hellström, M.; Kariuki, H.C.; Olsen, A.; Thomsen, P.F.; Mejer, H.; Willerslev, E.; Mwanje, M.T.; Madsen, H.; Kristensen, T.K.; et al. Environmental DNA for improved detection and environmental surveillance of schistosomiasis. *Proc. Natl. Acad. Sci. USA* **2019**, *116*, 8931–8940. [CrossRef]
99. Baque, R.H.; Gilliam, A.O.; Robles, L.D.; Jakubowski, W.; Slifko, T.R. A real-time RT-PCR method to detect viable *Giardia lamblia* cysts in environmental waters. *Water Res.* **2011**, *45*, 3175–3184. [CrossRef]

100. Alzaylaee, H.; Collins, R.A.; Rinaldi, G.; Shechonge, A.; Ngatunga, B.; Morgan, E.R.; Genner, M.J. *Schistosoma* species detection by environmental DNA assays in african freshwaters. *PLoS Negl. Trop. Dis.* **2020**, *14*, 1–19. [CrossRef]
101. Lass, A.; Szostakowska, B.; Korzeniewski, K.; Karanis, P. Detection of *Giardia intestinalis* in water samples collected from natural water reservoirs and wells in northern and north-eastern Poland using LAMP, real-time PCR and nested PCR. *J. Water Health* **2017**, *15*, 775–787. [CrossRef] [PubMed]
102. Alzaylaee, H.; Collins, R.A.; Shechonge, A.; Ngatunga, B.P.; Morgan, E.R.; Genner, M.J. Environmental DNA-based xenomonitoring for determining *Schistosoma* presence in tropical freshwaters. *Parasites Vectors* **2020**, *13*, 1–11. [CrossRef] [PubMed]
103. Mulero, S.; Boissier, J.; Allienne, J.; Quilichini, Y.; Foata, J.; Pointier, J.; Rey, O. Environmental DNA for detecting *Bulinus truncatus*: A new environmental surveillance tool for schistosomiasis emergence risk assessment. *Environ. DNA* **2020**, *2*, 161–174. [CrossRef]
104. Coulibaly, G.; Ouattara, M.; Dongo, K.; Hürlimann, E.; Bassa, F.K.; Koné, N.; Essé, C.; Yapi, R.B.; Bonfoh, B.; Utzinger, J.; et al. Epidemiology of intestinal parasite infections in three departments of south-central Côte d'Ivoire before the implementation of a cluster-randomised trial. *Parasite Epidemiol. Control* **2018**, *3*, 63–76. [CrossRef] [PubMed]
105. Fofana, H.K.M.; Schwarzkopf, M.; Doumbia, M.N.; Saye, R.; Nimmesgern, A.; Landouré, A.; Traoré, M.S.; Mertens, P.; Utzinger, J.; Sacko, M.; et al. Prevalence of *Giardia intestinalis* infection in schistosomiasis-endemic areas in south-central Mali. *Trop. Med. Infect. Dis.* **2019**, *4*, 86. [CrossRef]
106. Stothard, J.R.; Sousa-Figueiredo, J.C.; Betson, M.; Bustinduy, A.; Reinhard-Rupp, J. Schistosomiasis in African infants and preschool children: Let them now be treated! *Trends Parasitol.* **2013**, *29*, 197–205. [CrossRef]
107. Al-Shehri, H.; James LaCourse, E.; Klimach, O.; Kabatereine, N.B.; Stothard, J.R. Molecular characterisation and taxon assemblage typing of giardiasis in primary school children living close to the shoreline of Lake Albert, Uganda. *Parasite Epidemiol. Control* **2019**, *4*, e00074. [CrossRef]
108. Levitz, S.; Standley, C.J.; Adriko, M.; Kabatereine, N.B.; Stothard, J.R. Environmental epidemiology of intestinal schistosomiasis and genetic diversity of *Schistosoma mansoni* infections in snails at Bugoigo village, Lake Albert. *Acta Trop.* **2013**, *128*, 284–291. [CrossRef]
109. Tchuem Tchuenté, L.A.; Momo, S.C.; Stothard, J.R.; Rollinson, D. Efficacy of praziquantel and reinfection patterns in single and mixed infection foci for intestinal and urogenital schistosomiasis in Cameroon. *Acta Trop.* **2013**, *128*, 275–283. [CrossRef]
110. Stothard, J.R.; Sousa-Figueiredo, J.C.; Navaratnam, A.M.D. Advocacy, policies and practicalities of preventive chemotherapy campaigns for African children with schistosomiasis. *Expert Rev. Anti. Infect. Ther.* **2013**, *11*, 733–752. [CrossRef]
111. Park, S.K.; Marchant, J.S. The journey to discovering a flatworm target of praziquantel: A long TRP. *Trends Parasitol.* **2020**, *36*, 182–194. [CrossRef]
112. Lo, N.C.; Addiss, D.G.; Hotez, P.J.; King, C.H.; Stothard, J.R.; Evans, D.S.; Colley, D.G.; Lin, W.; Coulibaly, J.T.; Bustinduy, A.L.; et al. A call to strengthen the global strategy against schistosomiasis and soil-transmitted helminthiasis: The time is now. *Lancet Infect. Dis.* **2017**, *17*, e64–e69. [CrossRef]
113. Wang, W.; Wang, L.; Liang, Y.S. Susceptibility or resistance of praziquantel in human schistosomiasis: A review. *Parasitol. Res.* **2012**, *111*, 1871–1877. [CrossRef]
114. Bustinduy, A.L.; Friedman, J.F.; Kjetland, E.F.; Ezeamama, A.E.; Kabatereine, N.B.; Stothard, J.R.; King, C.H. Expanding praziquantel (PZQ) access beyond mass drug administration programs: Paving a way forward for a pediatric PZQ formulation for schistosomiasis. *PLoS Negl. Trop. Dis.* **2016**, *10*, 1–7. [CrossRef]
115. Bergquist, R.; Utzinger, J.; Keiser, J. Controlling schistosomiasis with praziquantel: How much longer without a viable alternative? *Infect. Dis. Poverty* **2017**, *6*, 1–10. [CrossRef] [PubMed]
116. Doenhoff, M.J.; Cioli, D.; Utzinger, J. Praziquantel: Mechanisms of action, resistance and new derivatives for schistosomiasis. *Curr. Opin. Infect. Dis.* **2008**, *21*, 659–667. [CrossRef]
117. Hill, D.R.; Timothy, B.G. Treatment of giardiasis. *Curr. Treat. Options Gastroenterol.* **2005**, *8*, 13–17. [CrossRef]
118. Ce, G.; Reveiz, L.; Lg, U.; Cp, C. Drugs for treating giardiasis. *Cochrane Database Syst. Rev.* **2012**, *12*. [CrossRef]
119. Carter, E.R.; Nabarro, L.E.; Hedley, L.; Chiodini, P.L. Nitroimidazole-refractory giardiasis: A growing problem requiring rational solutions. *Clin. Microbiol. Infect.* **2018**, *24*, 37–42. [CrossRef] [PubMed]

120. Vercruysse, J.; Behnke, J.M.; Albonico, M.; Ame, S.M.; Angebault, C.; Bethony, J.M.; Engels, D.; Guillard, B.; Hoa, N.T.V.; Kang, G.; et al. Assessment of the anthelmintic efficacy of albendazole in school children in seven countries where soil-transmitted helminths are endemic. *PLoS Negl. Trop. Dis.* **2011**, *5*, e948. [CrossRef] [PubMed]
121. Hoerauf, A.; Pfarr, K.; Mand, S.; Debrah, A.Y.; Specht, S. Filariasis in Africa-treatment challenges and prospects. *Clin. Microbiol. Infect.* **2011**, *17*, 977–985. [CrossRef]
122. Solaymani-Mohammadi, S.; Genkinger, J.M.; Loffredo, C.A.; Singer, S.M. A meta-analysis of the effectiveness of albendazole compared with metronidazole as treatments for infections with *Giardia duodenalis*. *PLoS Negl. Trop. Dis.* **2010**, *4*, e682. [CrossRef]
123. Pickering, A.J.; Njenga, S.M.; Steinbaum, L.; Swarthout, J.; Lin, A.; Arnold, B.F.; Stewart, C.P.; Dentz, H.N.; Mureithi, M.; Chieng, B.; et al. Effects of single and integrated water, sanitation, handwashing, and nutrition interventions on child soil-transmitted helminth and *Giardia* infections: A cluster-randomized controlled trial in rural Kenya. *PLoS Med.* **2019**, *16*, 1–21. [CrossRef]
124. Aw, J.Y.H.; Clarke, N.E.; McCarthy, J.S.; Traub, R.J.; Amaral, S.; Huque, M.H.; Andrews, R.M.; Gray, D.J.; Clements, A.C.A.; Vaz Nery, S. *Giardia duodenalis* infection in the context of a community-based deworming and water, sanitation and hygiene trial in Timor-Leste. *Parasites Vectors* **2019**, *12*, 4–13. [CrossRef]
125. Roche, R.; Bain, R.; Cumming, O. A long way to go-Estimates of combined water, sanitation and hygiene coverage for 25 sub-Saharan African countries. *PLoS ONE* **2017**, *12*, 1–24. [CrossRef]
126. World Health Organization (WHO). Water, Sanitation & Hygiene for Accelerating and Sustaining Progress on Neglected Tropical Diseases. Available online: https://www.who.int/water_sanitation_health/publications/wash-and-ntd-strategy/en/ (accessed on 2 July 2020).
127. World Health Organisation. *Integrating Neglected Tropical Diseases into Global Health and Development*; World Health Organisation: Geneva, Switzerland, 2017; Available online: https://apps.who.int/iris/bitstream/handle/10665/255011/9789241565448-eng.pdf (accessed on 17 June 2020).
128. Campbell, S.J.; Savage, G.B.; Gray, D.J.; Atkinson, J.A.M.; Soares Magalhães, R.J.; Nery, S.V.; McCarthy, J.S.; Velleman, Y.; Wicken, J.H.; Traub, R.J. Water, sanitation, and hygiene (WASH): A critical component for sustainable soil-transmitted helminth and schistosomiasis control. *PLoS Negl. Trop. Dis.* **2014**, *8*, 1–5. [CrossRef]
129. Spear, R.C. Commentary by Spear, R. on "Integration of water, sanitation, and hygiene for the prevention and control of Neglected Tropical Diseases: A rationale for inter-sectoral collaboration:" Can the control of NTDs profit from a good WASH? *PLoS Negl. Trop. Dis.* **2013**, *7*, e2473. [CrossRef]
130. Rollinson, D.; Knopp, S.; Levitz, S.; Stothard, J.R.; Tchuem Tchuenté, L.A.; Garba, A.; Mohammed, K.A.; Schur, N.; Person, B.; Colley, D.G.; et al. Time to set the agenda for schistosomiasis elimination. *Acta Trop.* **2013**, *128*, 423–440. [CrossRef]
131. Reed, S.L.; Mckerrow, J.H. Why funding for Neglected Tropical Diseases should be a global priority. *Clin. Infect. Dis.* **2018**, *18*, 323–326. [CrossRef]
132. Van den Berg, H.; Kelly-Hope, L.A.; Lindsay, S.W. Malaria and lymphatic filariasis: The case for integrated vector management. *Lancet Infect. Dis.* **2013**, *13*, 89–94. [CrossRef]
133. Kelly-Hope, L.A.; Molyneux, D.H.; Bockarie, M.J. Can malaria vector control accelerate the interruption of lymphatic filariasis transmission in Africa; Capturing a window of opportunity? *Parasites Vectors* **2013**, *6*, 1–12. [CrossRef]
134. Knipes, A.K.; Lemoine, J.F.; Monestime, F.; Fayette, C.R.; Direny, A.N.; Desir, L.; Beau de Rochars, V.E.; Streit, T.G.; Renneker, K.; Chu, B.K.; et al. Partnering for impact: Integrated transmission assessment surveys for lymphatic filariasis, soil transmitted helminths and malaria in Haiti. *PLoS Negl. Trop. Dis.* **2017**, *11*, e0005387. [CrossRef]
135. Bronzan, R.N.; Dorkenoo, A.M.; Agbo, Y.M.; Halatoko, W.; Layibo, Y.; Adjeloh, P.; Teko, M.; Sossou, E.; Yakpa, K.; Tchalim, M.; et al. Impact of community-based integrated mass drug administration on schistosomiasis and soil-transmitted helminth prevalence in Togo. *PLoS Negl. Trop. Dis.* **2018**, *12*, e0006551. [CrossRef]

13

Polymerase Chain Reaction (PCR) as a Potential Point of Care Laboratory Test for Leprosy Diagnosis

Sushma Tatipally [1], Aparna Srikantam [1,*] and Sanjay Kasetty [2]

1 LEPRA Society, Blue Peter Public Health and Research Centre, Cherlapally, Hyderabad 501301, Telangana, India; sushma@leprahealthinaction.in
2 Formerly at LEPRA Society, Blue Peter Public Health and Research Centre, Cherlapally, Hyderabad 501301, Telangana, India; sanjay.kasetty@gmail.com
* Correspondence: aparna@leprahealthinaction.in;

Abstract: Leprosy is an infectious disease caused by *Mycobacterium leprae* and mainly affects skin, peripheral nerves, and eyes. Suitable tools for providing bacteriological evidence of leprosy are needed for early case detection and appropriate therapeutic management. Ideally these tools are applicable at all health care levels for the effective control of leprosy. This paper presents a systematic review analysis in order to investigate the performance of polymerase chain reaction (PCR) vis-à-vis slit skin smears (SSS) in various clinical settings and its potential usefulness as a routine lab test for leprosy diagnosis. Records of published journal articles were identified through PubMed database search. Twenty-seven articles were included for the analysis. The evidence from this review analysis suggests that PCR on skin biopsy is the ideal diagnostic test. Nevertheless, PCR on SSS samples also seems to be useful with its practical value for application, even at primary care levels. The review findings also indicated the necessity for improving the sensitivity of PCR and further research on specificity in ruling out other clinical conditions that may mimic leprosy. The *M. leprae*-specific repetitive element (RLEP) was the most frequently-used marker although its variable performance across the clinical sites and samples are a matter of concern. Undertaking further research studies with large sample numbers and uniform protocols studied simultaneously across multiple clinical sites is recommended to address these issues.

Keywords: leprosy; leprosy diagnosis; PCR; slit skin smears; point of care test; skin biopsy; early diagnosis

---

1. Introduction

Leprosy is an infectious disease caused by *Mycobacterium leprae* and mainly affects skin, peripheral nerves, and eyes [1–3]. Leprosy has long-term consequences on the structure and function of the peripheral nerves leading to disabilities in limbs, which impact on the socioeconomic well-being of the affected individuals [4]. Despite three decades of effective treatment with multidrug therapy (MDT), leprosy persists as a public health problem in many regions of the world [5]. Each year 300,000 people are newly diagnosed with leprosy worldwide; half are reported from India [6]. Despite the World Health Organization (WHO) declaring the elimination of leprosy as a public health problem in the year 2000, new leprosy cases still continue to occur in India with an annual incidence of around 135,000 cases [7]. There is evidence that many more patients still go undetected due to various reasons including social stigma attached to the disease, which hinders health-care-seeking behavior among affected persons [8]. Hence it is imperative to widen the scope and accuracy of leprosy detection for early identification before the consequences of nerve damage have set in [9]. The current standard diagnosis of leprosy is mostly based on clinical evaluation of patients, except in a few settings where the microscopy of slit skin smears (SSS) for acid-fast bacilli and/or histopathological examination (HPE) of skin biopsies are being used as additional tests [10]. Clinical manifestations of leprosy are determined by patient immune responses to *Mycobacterium leprae*. Leprosy patients are classified by the Ridley–Jopling classification on the basis of the morphology, type, and number of skin lesions, as well as nerve involvement supplemented by the bacterial index (BI) and histopathological examination. The Ridley–Jopling types are tuberculoid (TT), borderline tuberculoid (BT), borderline (BB), borderline lepromatous (BL), lepromatous leprosy (LL), pure neural (PN) and indeterminate (I) [11].

The current operational classification of leprosy used by WHO is based on number of skin lesions; patients with less than five lesions are classified as paucibacillary (PB) and more than five as multibacillary (MB) leprosy. However, this classification, merely based on the number of lesions, may not always hold good for specific treatment strategies, as it has been frequently demonstrated that acid-fast bacilli (AFB) are present in cases clinically classified as PB. Such PB patients with active lesions may potentially be transmitting *M. leprae* to their contacts unless they are treated appropriately [12]. Hence there has been an emphasis on bringing back the laboratory diagnostic component into routine practice [13]. The two traditional tests *viz.* SSS and HPE of biopsies, though still holding well in terms of convenience of usage, have their own inherent limitations. SSS is relatively low in sensitivity and includes the risk of subjective errors of microscopic examination, whereas the HPE has the limitations of long turnaround time and technically demanding laboratory procedures [14]. Hence it is very important to develop diagnostic strategies involving highly sensitive laboratory tests for early detection of leprosy. Suitable tools for providing bacteriological evidence of leprosy are needed for early case detection and appropriate therapeutic management of leprosy. Ideally these tools are applicable at all health care levels for effective control of leprosy.

Molecular diagnosis by nucleic acid amplification test (NAAT) is an emerging science in the clinical management of infectious diseases. Polymerase chain reaction (PCR) is one of the most popular NAAT currently being used for the diagnosis of infectious diseases [15]. Routine clinical use of NAAT has been well established in tuberculosis and other mycobacterial diseases. NAAT has almost replaced the conventional lab diagnostic tests in TB and has become the most widely used test at all levels of health care [16]. Such molecular diagnosis has not yet been practiced in the case of leprosy. PCR nevertheless has been popularly used for drug resistance testing and molecular typing of leprosy but never so far for the routine clinical diagnosis [17,18]. Given the potential use of this very important test, there is a need for a scientific analysis of the effectiveness of PCR for lab diagnosis of leprosy in correlation with the current standards. This evidence is envisaged to help the formulation of better policies for diagnosis and treatment of leprosy. With this background, the present systematic review analysis has been conducted in order to investigate the performance of PCR vis-à-vis SSS in various clinical settings and its potential usefulness as a routine lab test for leprosy diagnosis.

2. Materials and Methods

2.1. Study Design

The study is a systematic review analysis to assess the usefulness of PCR for the laboratory diagnosis of leprosy. The review has been carried out with the purpose of accruing evidence on the performance of PCR in correlation with clinical classification of leprosy and standard laboratory diagnostic tests. The highlights from the review are envisaged to be useful in addressing the gaps in the existing systems and recommending better strategies for the future application of PCR during routine clinical diagnosis of leprosy. The protocol has been prepared based on Preferred Reporting Items for Systematic reviews and Meta-Analyses (PRISMA) guidelines for systematic review analysis [19].

2.2. Data Search

Records of published journal articles were identified through searching the PubMed database [20]. Journal articles published until April 2018 were included. The data search was conducted between 15 March 2018 to 4 May 2018. All field searches for PCR and leprosy yielded 924 articles, which were filtered to 812 with Medical Subject Heading (MeSH) terms *Mycobacterium leprae*, leprosy, Hansen's disease, laboratory diagnosis, biomarkers, PCR, SSS examination, and biopsies (protocol furnished as Figure 1). Out of 924, 715 full text articles were shortlisted. Twenty-seven of the 715 articles were included for the analysis based on these inclusion criteria: the study should have involved PCR as one of the tests for leprosy diagnosis or confirmation along with one other standard test such as SSS or biopsy and PCR tests conducted on (any) biological (clinical) samples. Exclusion criteria included articles published in a language other than English, articles which did not have free full text available, PCR used for purposes other than leprosy diagnosis, such as PCR used as a test for drug resistance, molecular typing, or where the PCR test was not used on clinical samples.

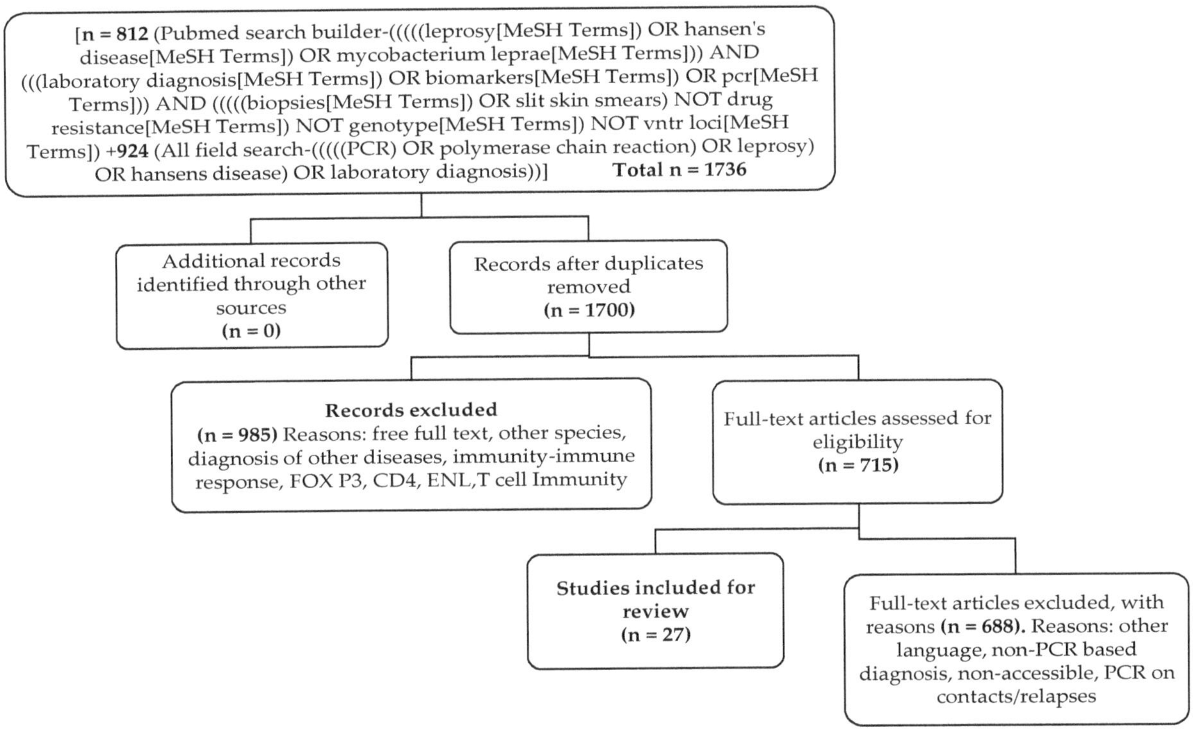

Figure 1. Flow chart detailing review steps (PRISMA guidelines).

2.3. Data Extraction

Each study was reviewed for the number of patients screened for leprosy diagnosis, mode of diagnosis including clinical examination and lab tests. Laboratory tests were further stratified into bacteriological examination by microscopy (AFB) and molecular tests (PCR) or histopathological examination (biopsy/HPE), clinical characteristics of the patients screened including PB/MB and nature of the clinical samples collected for lab diagnosis. Data on PCRs conducted on contacts/treated relapsed patients were excluded from the analysis. Percentage of positive results (sensitivity) for AFB microscopy and PCR were tabulated with reference to the clinical class of leprosy, AFB, and type of clinical sample used. Mean PCR positivity vis-à-vis genetic markers and the method of PCR used were also calculated.

2.4. Definitions of Some of the Data Terms Used in the Review

Report: Each individual paper included in the analysis is considered as one report;

Assay: PCR on each sample type and/or each gene marker from each report was considered as an independent assay;

Gene Marker: each genetic marker used for specific amplification of *M. leprae* DNA from clinical specimens;

PCR Method: laboratory technique of PCR used for amplifying the DNA targeting the *M. leprae* genetic markers.

2.5. Data Analysis

Data extraction has been carried out in such a way that PCR on each sample type and/or each gene marker was considered as an independent assay. Some of the papers reported PCR in one or more samples and/or one or more gene targets. Hence there were 38 assay resulting from the total of 27 papers that were reviewed. The matrix of published articles with types of lab tests conducted, types of samples used for testing, % PCR positivity, % AFB positivity on various samples, gene markers and/or PCR methods are tabulated for comparative analysis (Table 1). Mean and range are extracted for number of samples tested, percentage positivity of AFB, PCR for each clinical class, clinical specimen, PCR marker used, and PCR method used.

3. Results

3.1. Basic Clinical and Geographical Information

The review included published papers on PCR in new leprosy cases, along with clinical and conventional lab diagnostic tests. Out of 1700 papers screened, 27 papers qualified for the criteria of inclusion (flow chart, Figure 1). Out of the 27, nine were on leprosy patients from India, seven from Brazil, five from Bangkok, two from Philippines and one each from China, Ethiopia, Nepal, and Vietnam. Most of the reports included testing on clinically-diagnosed leprosy cases for confirming the laboratory test findings, limiting the scope of analysis for estimating only the sensitivity of the diagnostic tests. Most of those analyzed were reported based on either AFB microscopy on SSS or biopsies as the conventional lab standard test for comparing the PCR results.

3.2. Analysis

The average number of study subjects across the reports was 96 (range 20–439). Eighteen out of the 27 reports classified patients as PB and MB leprosy. Twenty-four (63%) out of 38 assays studied were less than 100 patients and 14 (37%) included more than 100 patients (Table 1). Seventeen out of 27 reports (62.9%) were based on a single PCR marker and nine (33%) used more than one marker; one (3.7%) used four markers. Three (8%) studies reported PCR results of a single marker on multiple samples (data not shown).

3.3. Clinical Classification vs. Sensitivity of AFB and PCR

Twenty-eight of the 38 of the total assays reported PCR on PB cases (six included data on AFB microscopy) (data not shown). Mean positivity for PCR was 48% (range 07–81) and AFB microscopy was 23% (range 1.7–35). Out of 38 assays, 26 reported PCR on MB leprosy cases and data on AFB was available for 17/26. Mean positivity for PCR was 77% (range 17–100) and AFB microscopy 59% (range 15–100) in reports on MB leprosy cases. Mean positivity for PCR was 44% (range 13–93) and AFB microscopy was 30% (range 10–86), if the total number of cases was not segregated as PB and MB (Table 2), indicating that PCR has only an incremental value over microscopy for bacteriological diagnosis of leprosy. Our observation on positivity of microscopy and PCR in PB leprosy cases reiterates the necessity to revise the current leprosy classification and treatment criteria. This also indicates that on an average 19% of cases were wrongly classified as PB (if only skin lesions were considered) and would have been missed treatment, had they not been tested with AFB and 10% more if PCR had not been used.

As expected, PCR turned out to be the most sensitive test for bacteriological confirmation on MB cases. Given the fact that MB leprosy lesions most frequently contain *M. leprae*, the mean PCR positivity in MB cases should have been more; however, the data suggests a lower average. This could have been due to technical bias due to errors in clinical sample collection and/or laboratory testing. These issues need to be addressed through development of robust clinical and lab protocols based on evidence from large multicentric studies through uniform study methodology.

A few reports included PCR results stratified for Ridley-Jopling classes of leprosy. Azevedo et al., 2017 [13] reported PCR across the spectrum, with percentage of PCR positivity as TT-21/38 (55.2%); BT-20/21 (95.2%); BB-18/18 (100%); BL-12/12 (100%); LL-13/13 (100%). In another recent report Chaitanya et al., 2017, reported the results for a multiplex PCR as indeterminate 31/41 (75.6%) TT-03/03 (100%); BT- 40/42 (95.2%); BB-03/03 (100%); BL-58/59 (98%); LL-70/72 (97%). PCR showed a good additional value in diagnosing TT and indeterminate cases, which are traditionally known to be negative for AFB on microscopy. This indicates that PCR could be a better test in classifying bacillary-positive cases than smear and microscopy [21].

3.4. Clinical Specimens and PCR

De Wit et al. (1993) reported on the utility of PCR for detection of *M. leprae* in nasal swab specimens amplifying the 531-bp *pra* gene, demonstrating 79.6% positivity of PCR [22]. Kyeong-Han Yoon reported PCR on slit skin samples, which was subsequently reported by many others [23–28]. PCR on biopsies has been reported by Wichitwechkarn et al. (1995), with a mean PCR positivity of 66% and subsequently by many others. We found that biopsy was the most common specimen to have been tested for PCR of *M. leprae* [13,21,29–37] (Table 1).

Out of 38 protocols studied, the majority (20) were based on skin biopsy (53%) followed by SSS (13, 34%); the rest of the samples included nerve biopsy, blood, and urine. AFB positivity in SSS has been 36% (range 18–69) and skin biopsy 44% (range 10–85). Likewise, PCR positivity on slit skin and biopsy was 61% (range 18–93) and 70% (range 46–93), respectively (Table 2). Since the skin biopsy and SSS happen to be the most frequent clinical samples collected for leprosy diagnosis, we tried to analyze the usefulness of PCR in the two samples. PCR seems to be more sensitive than microscopy in both the type of samples (SSS and biopsies), although skin biopsies have demonstrated significantly higher sensitivity to both microscopy and PCR as compared to SSS (Table 2). The reason could be the presence of a lesser number of bacilli in SSS than those in biopsy. The data suggests that PCR on skin biopsy seems to be the most sensitive test for demonstrating *M. leprae* bacilli. Nevertheless, with 62% sensitivity, PCR on SSS seems to be a better test when compared to microscopy (36%). Given the inherent limitations of skin biopsy such as the invasive nature of collection and technical expertise needed for test reporting, PCR on SSS samples with an average sensitivity of 62% seems to be more practical for application at primary care levels.

Apart from these two conventional specimens, researchers also studied *M. leprae* PCR on other unconventional samples. Caleffi et al. (2012) used PCR, amplifying a 151-bp PCR fragment of the *M. leprae pra* gene in urine samples. Thirty four of the 73 (46.58%) leprosy patients studied were positive for PCR [38]. Tiwari et al. (2017) evaluated PCR in nerve biopsy specimens of 35 pure neuritic leprosy cases. AFB was positive in 13 (37.14%) cases and PCR positivity was observed in 22 (62.86%) cases [39]. A study involved 43 newly-diagnosed leprosy patients, where quantitative PCR was carried out on whole blood samples (PCR positivity—13.95%) in comparison with SSS of the ear lobe (microscopy—30.23%; PCR positivity—41.86%) [40]. It is interesting to note that even urine and blood samples could be used for PCR testing. These reports suggest that blood and urine, although less sensitive on PCR than SSS, may still be considered as potential specimens, owing to the convenience of sample collection at all levels of health care. Future research for generating more evidence on usefulness of PCR on urine and blood, both in terms of sensitivity and feasibility for a point of care test would be promising.

Table 1. Data showing different studies involving conventional and molecular diagnosis of leprosy using different samples.

Sl. No.	Type of Sample	PCR Type	Marker/Gene	No. of Patients Studied	Smear Microscopy			PCR			*p* Value	First Author	Study Location/Country	Reference No.
					No. Tested	No. Positive	%	No. Tested	No. Positive	%				
1	Skin biopsy	Conventional PCR	RLEP	102	102	63	61.76	102	59	57.84	NA	Michelle de Campos Soriani Azevedo	Brazil	[13]
2	Skin biopsy	Multiplex PCR	RLEP	220	220	122	55.45	220	164	74.55	$p < 0.05$	V Sundeep Chaitanya	India	[21]
3	Skin biopsy	Multiplex PCR	M- PCR	220	220	122	55.45	220	205	93.18	NA	V Sundeep Chaitanya	India	[21]
4	Nasal swabs	Conventional PCR	531 bp fragment	103	0	0	0	103	82	79.61	NA	Madeleine Y. L. de Wit	Philippines	[22]
5	SSS	Conventional PCR	372 bp fragment	102	102	62	60.78	102	95	93.14	NA	Kyeong-Han Yoon	Philippines	[23]
6	Skin biopsy	Conventional PCR	372 bp	102	102	87	85.29	102	95	93.14	NA	Kyeong-Han Yoon	Philippines	[23]
7	SSS	in situ PCR	530 bp fragment	25	25	5	20	25	18	72	$p = 0.01$	R Kamal	India	[24]
8	SSS	Conventional PCR	RLEP	73	73	17	23.29	73	56	76.71	$p < 0.001$	R Kamal	India	[25]
9	SSS	Multiplex PCR	372&201 bp	439	439	223	50.8	439	371	84.51	NA	Surajita Banerjee	India	[26]
10	SSS	Conventional PCR	RLEP	50	50	9	18	50	36	72	NA	Shraddha Siwakoti	Nepal	[27]
11	SSS	Conventional PCR	PCR-LP	91	91	21	23.08	91	22	24.18	NA	Flaviane Granero Maltempe	Brazil	[28]
12	SSS	Conventional PCR	PCR-P	91	91	21	23.08	91	17	18.68	$p > 0.05$	Flaviane Granero Maltempe	Brazil	[28]
13	SSS	Conventional PCR	*pra* gene	53	0	0	0	53	17	32.08	NA	Jesdawan Wichitwechkaran	Bangkok	[29]
14	Skin biopsy	Conventional PCR	*pra* gene	53	0	0	0	53	35	66.04	NA	Jesdawan Wichitwechkaran	Bangkok	[29]
15	Skin biopsy	RT-PCR	16S rRNA	50	50	33	66	50	41	82	NA	Mekonnen Kurabachew	Ethiopia	[30]

Table 1. *Cont.*

Sl. No.	Type of Sample	PCR Type	Marker/Gene	No. of Patients Studied	Smear Microscopy			PCR			p Value	First Author	Study Location/Country	Reference No.
					No. Tested	No. Positive	%	No. Tested	No. Positive	%				
16	Nasal mucosal biopsies	RT-PCR	16S rRNA	60	60	24	40	60	47	78.33	NA	Benjawan Phetsuksiri	Bangkok	[31]
17	Skin biopsy	Conventional PCR	RLEP	110	110	43	39.09	110	81	73.64	NA	Isabela Maria Bernardes Goulart	Brazil	[32]
18	Skin biopsy	Conventional PCR	372 bp	110	110	43	39.09	110	58	52.73	NA	Isabela Maria Bernardes Goulart	Brazil	[32]
19	Skin biopsy	qPCR	16S rRNA	69	69	0	0	69	53	76.81	NA	Pham Dang Bang	Vietnam	[33]
20	Skin biopsy	qPCR	RLEP	47	0	0	0	47	38	80.85	NA	Alejandra Nóbrega Martinez	Brazil	[34]
21	Skin biopsy	qPCR	16S rRNA	47	0	0	0	47	24	51.06	NA	Alejandra Nóbrega Martinez	Brazil	[34]
22	Skin biopsy	qPCR	*sodA*	47	0	0	0	47	22	46.81	NA	Alejandra Nóbrega Martinez	Brazil	[34]
23	Skin biopsy	qPCR	85B	47	0	0	0	47	26	55.32	NA	Alejandra Nóbrega Martinez	Brazil	[34]
24	Skin biopsy	Multiplex PCR	372bp &201 bp	165	165	84	50.91	165	111	67.27	NA	Abu Hena Hasanoor Reja	India	[35]
25	Skin biopsy	qPCR	RLEP & 372 bp fragment	51	51	18	35.29	51	38	74.51	$p > 0.05$	Wen Yan	China	[36]
26	Skin biopsy	Nested PCR	RLEP &372 bp fragment	51	51	18	35.29	51	37	72.55	NA	Wen Yan	China	[36]
27	Skin biopsy	Conventional PCR	530 bp fragment	55	55	9	16.36	55	40	72.73	NA	Mohammad Shah Alam	Bangladesh	[37]
28	Urine	Conventional PCR	*pra* gene	73	73	0	0	73	34	46.58	$p > 0.05$	K.R. Caleffi	Brazil	[38]

Table 1. *Cont.*

Sl. No.	Type of Sample	PCR Type	Marker/Gene	No. of Patients Studied	Smear Microscopy			PCR			p Value	First Author	Study Location/Country	Reference No.
					No. Tested	No. Positive	%	No. Tested	No. Positive	%				
29	Nerve biopsy	Conventional PCR	375 bp fragment	35	35	13	37.14	35	22	62.86	NA	Vandana Tiwari	India	[39]
30	SSS	qPCR	16S rRNA	43	43	13	30.23	43	18	41.86	NA	Rafael Silva Gama	Brazil	[40]
31	blood	qPCR	16S rRNA	43	0	0	0	43	6	13.95	NA	Rafael Silva Gama	Brazil	[40]
32	SSS	Multiplex PCR	372 bp fragment	164	164	65	39.63	164	135	82.32	$p < 0.0001$	Surajita Banerjee	India	[41]
33	SSS	qPCR	16S rRNA	66	66	36	54.55	66	52	78.79	NA	Janisara Rudeeaneksin	Bangkok	[42]
34	Skin biopsy	in situ PCR	530 bp fragment	20	20	2	10	20	12	60	NA	R. Dayal	India	[43]
35	SSS	Conventional PCR	*pra* gene	122	122	49	40.16	122	86	70.49	$p < 0.001$	Kowit Kampirapap	Bangkok	[44]
36	Skin biopsy	Conventional PCR	RLEP	180	180	122	67.78	180	114	63.33	$p < 0.0001$	V Sundeep Chaitanya	India	[45]
37	Skin biopsy	Conventional PCR	ML1545	180	180	122	67.78	180	164	91.11	NA	V Sundeep Chaitanya	India	[45]
38	SSS	Conventional PCR	372 bp fragment	52	52	36	69.23	52	36	69.23	NA	Lucas Gomes Patrocínio	Brazil	[46]

Table 2. Details of assay—clinical classification, clinical sample vs. smear microcopy and polymerase chain reaction (PCR) positivity.

Classification	No. of Assay (Reports) Studied	Average Number of Patients/Samples Tested (Range)	No. of Assay Reported the AFB Microscopy	%AFB Positivity Mean (Range)	No. of Assay Reported PCR Tests	%PCR Positivity
Bacillary Load						
Paucibacillary	28	37.07 (7–234)	6	25.18 (1.75–35.29)	28	48.63 (7.69–81)
Multibacillary	27	61.40 (12–205)	17	62.25 (15.38–100)	27	79.65 (17.39–100)
Clinical samples						
Slit skin samples	14	101 (25–439)	12	37.73 (18–69.23)	14	60.71 (18.68–93.14)
Skin biopsy	20	96.3 (20–220)	14	48.96 (10–85.29)	20	70.27 (46.81–93.18)

3.5. Gene Markers—PCR Sensitivity

Various published reports on PCR in leprosy diagnosis studied a spectrum of gene markers as PCR targets on various clinical samples by multiple laboratory methods. There were twelve different markers used for PCR testing (Table 1). RLEP and 16S rRNA are the most frequent markers used, with PCR sensitivity ranging between 57% and 80% for RLEP and from 13% to 82% for 16S rRNA. RLEP seems to be the most sensitive marker for detecting *M. leprae* DNA, although its variable performance across the assays needs to be further addressed (Table 3). The sensitivity of RLEP PCR varied between samples, between clinical settings, and also between studies of the same authors. Martinez et al. (2011) reported highest RLEP sensitivity (81%) as compared to other three PCR markers [34]. Maltempe et al. (2016) reported RLEP PCR on SSS to be equally sensitive as AFB smear microscopy (24%) [28], which is the lowest (data not shown). Yan et al. (2014) reported at least 72% of RLEP PCR positivity as compared to 35% on smear microscopy of paraffin-embedded biopsies among PB leprosy cases [36]. The observations paved the way for exploring more evidence on RLEP PCR, the most frequently used and promising marker, for reasons of its variable performance and opportunities for improving its effectiveness. It was also observed that multiplexing RLEP with other markers yielded better results (data not shown), indicating the necessity for undertaking more studies in this direction, with large sample numbers and uniform protocols simultaneously studied across multiple clinical sites. The data also suggested that the highest mean positivity with any of the markers so far reported seems to be only 71%, which needs to be improved if PCR is to be used as a robust test for diagnosing leprosy. Since DNA extraction is one of the critical steps in any PCR-based diagnosis, it is logical to look into impact of role of DNA extraction procedures on PCR outcomes. We observed that most of the assays reviewed were based on the standard DNA extraction protocols such as phenol:chloroform method. We did not find any specific protocol associated with a higher PCR sensitivity (data not shown). None of the assays had reported the use of DNA extraction controls, which could have validated the sample processing procedure.

Table 3. PCR markers and methods vs. sensitivity.

	Number of Assays Studied (n = 38)	Highest Positivity (%PCR)	Lowest Positivity (%PCR)
		Gene markers	
RLEP	9	80.85	57.84
16S rRNA	10	82	13.95
		Method of PCR	
Conventional	19	93.14	18.68
Multiplex	6	93.18	67.27
Q-PCR	6	80.85	13.95
RT-PCR	5	74.5	82

There should be more research exploring better markers and suitable lab protocols for increasing the sensitivity of PCR for detecting *M. leprae*. Advancing scientific knowledge and an omics approach should throw some light on identifying such novel markers and developing them into robust PCR test modules for point-of-care diagnostic testing in leprosy.

3.6. Method of PCR vs. PCR Sensitivity

Out of 27 reports reviewed, 19 were based on conventional PCR, 6 were on quantitative real time PCR (qPCR), 4 on multiplex PCR and 2 were on reverse transcriptase PCR (RT-PCR) assays. Researchers have employed various PCR techniques for molecular diagnosis of *M. leprae* from SSS, skin biopsy, blood and urine samples. Conventional PCR targeting a single gene has been found to be the most frequently reported method. Several authors have used conventional PCR on slit skin, biopsy, urine, blood [27,37–40]. On the other hand, few studies have utilized multiplex PCR on slit skin and biopsies, amplifying more than one target sequence, at the same level of laboratory settings as conventional PCR [21,26,35,41]. There are also reports on methods such as quantitative PCR, RT-PCR and in situ PCR, which are based on advanced laboratory facility and studies have reported RT-PCR on skin biopsies, SSS and nasal biopsies [30,31,33,36,42]. Real-time quantitative (q-PCR) PCR technique was used by Martinez et al. (2011) and Gama et al. (2018) [34,40]. Yan et al. (2014) studied the nested PCR technique using two sets of primers to apply two different *M. leprae*-specific gene fragments from paraffin-embedded skin biopsy specimens [36]. Dayal et al. (2005) and Kamal et al. (2010) reported in situ PCR [24,43].

From the above analyzed assay, the highest percentage of PCR sensitivity was observed using multiplex PCR technique (82%) followed by RT-PCR (78%) and conventional PCR (63%). These two techniques seem to be very useful PCR techniques in the rapid diagnosis of *M. leprae*. This observation indicates that even a simple PCR but with more than one marker and appropriate technical protocol could do better in picking up *M. leprae* DNA from clinical samples. This in turn indicates the usefulness of simple PCR-based tests for bacteriological diagnosis of leprosy even with a modestly-equipped laboratory facility, although RT-PCR carries a technical advantage over simple PCR by providing quantitative estimate.

The review analysis found that no individual *M. leprae* gene marker has been associated with higher sensitivity. However, using more than one marker in a multiplex format of conventional PCR seem to have yielded significantly higher mean positivity and hence could be a better choice (Table 3). Almost all studies reported in this review have studied techniques based on traditional laboratory-based PCRs, since the evidence gathered through this review suggests that it is more important to have appropriate protocols and robust markers for PCR sensitivity than sophisticated technology. Recent advancements in molecular methods has enhanced the capability of detection and characterization of infectious diseases. PCR is one of the techniques of molecular diagnosis that has great benefits and enhances advancements in rapid diagnosis. There are many simple point of care (POC) PCRs such as the LAMP test and Xpert TB available for diseases like TB, HIV, and malaria etc. [47–52]. Developing one or more of the existing markers into such POC platforms should be the goal of future research in molecular diagnosis of leprosy. Developing such point-of-care, easy-to-use PCR modules could have potential application at all healthcare levels. This addresses the issue of access to healthcare for persons affected by leprosy or those at risk of developing leprosy. Increasing access to healthcare leads to early detection of leprosy and prevention of consequences—the most important aspects of leprosy control. Hence it is envisaged that further research on PCR in leprosy include investigating various markers for the usefulness of point-of-care testing.

4. Conclusions

The evidence from this review analysis suggests that PCR on a skin biopsy is the ideal diagnostic test. Nevertheless, PCR on SSS samples also seems to be useful with its practical value for application at primary healthcare levels. Future research for better evidence on the usefulness of PCR on other samples such as urine and blood are recommended to avoid collecting slit skin/biopsy samples, which are relatively more invasive. Our observation on positivity of AFB microscopy and PCR in PB leprosy cases reiterates the necessity to revise the current leprosy classification and treatment criteria based merely on the number of skin lesions. PCR could be a better test in classifying bacillary positive cases than smear microscopy. Having said that, our review findings indicate the necessity for improving the sensitivity of PCR and further research on specificity is required in ruling out other clinical conditions that may mimic leprosy. Development of robust clinical and lab protocols based on evidence from large multicenter studies through uniform study methodology might be of great help in addressing the sensitivity and specificity issues. We found that no individual *M. leprae* gene marker has been associated with higher PCR sensitivity, indicating the need for more evidence for robust markers. However, using more than one marker in a multiplex format of conventional PCR seems to have yielded significantly higher PCR positivity and hence could be a better choice. RLEP, although the most frequent marker used, showed variable performance across the clinical sites, and samples are a matter of concern. Combining it with other markers in a multiplex PCR format might work. Multiplexing more than one target *M. leprae* gene might also help to address this issue. Undertaking more studies of this nature, with large sample numbers and uniform protocols simultaneously studied across multiple clinical sites would be useful. In addition, there should be more research exploring better markers for increasing sensitivity of PCR for detecting *M. leprae*. Advancing scientific knowledge and omics approach should throw some light on the identification of such novel markers and developing them into robust PCR test modules for point-of-care diagnostic testing in leprosy.

Limitations of This Systematic Review Analysis

The present review has been mainly based on the reports available on the PubMed database and did not include any other databases due to the time and resource constraints. This might have led to a selection bias of papers published only on PubMed. We did not gather any other types of information sources such as unpublished data, data from ongoing studies from various researchers, which could perhaps have made our observations stronger. The data from records mainly comprising clinically-diagnosed leprosy cases, except one record, meant that we were unable to estimate test specificity. Analysis included data only on new patients. However, the authors would like to address the other two important applications of PCR, namely for contact screening and treatment monitoring through separate independent reviews. We limited the analysis to systematic review only and did not attempt meta-analysis due to heterogeneity of the data. This review could not elicit any significant evidence on usefulness of any specific marker for PCR, due to either limited number of studies or limited number of samples. Further studies with large sample sizes with existing or new markers are warranted to enhance evidence on this particular aspect.

Author Contributions: A.S.: Conceived the idea, formed the review group, prepared the review protocols, data analysis, manuscript writing, review, approval of the manuscript; S.T.: Data collection, manuscript writing, reading of individual review papers; S.K.: reading of individual review papers, manuscript writing.

Acknowledgments: LEPRA-Blue Peter Public Health and Research Center is core funded by Lepra, UK. S.T. is supported under ICMR grant No. AMR/IN/113/2017-ECD-II. Authors are thankful for the assistance provided by Pramilesh Suryavanshi for his initial contributions during the protocol preparation and Chakrapani Chatla for his assistance during data analysis and critical review.

References

1. Noordeen, S.K. The epidemiology of leprosy. In *Leprosy*; Hastings, R.C., Ed.; Churchill Livingstone, Produced by Longman Group Ltd.: Hong Kong, China, 1985; pp. 15–30.
2. Dockrell, H.M. *Leprosy*, 3rd ed.; Bryceson, A.D.M., Pfaltzgraff, R.E., Eds.; Churchill Livingstone: Edinburgh, UK, 1990; p. 240, ISBN 0-443-03373-0.
3. Lockwood, D.N.J. Leprosy. *Medicine* **2005**, *33*, 26–29. [CrossRef]
4. Van Brakel, W.H.; Sihombing, B.; Djarir, H.; Beise, K.; Kusumawardhani, L.; Yulihane, R.; Kurniasari, I.; Kasim, M.; Kesumaningsih, K.I.; Wilder-Smith, A. Disability in people affected by leprosy: The role of impairment, activity, social participation, stigma and discrimination. *Glob. Health Action.* **2012**, *5*. [CrossRef] [PubMed]
5. World Health Organization. *Global Target Attained, Remaining Endemic Countries Pose Greatest Challenge*; Press Release, WHA/2; WHO: Geneva, Switzerland, 2002.
6. World Health Organization. *The Global Leprosy Strategy 2016–2020: Accelerating towards a Leprosy-Free World*; WHO: Geneva, Switzerland, 2016.
7. World Health Organization. Global leprosy update, 2016: Accelerating reduction of disease burden. *Wkly. Epidemiol. Rec.* **2017**, *92*, 501–520.

8. Sermrittirong, S.; van Brakel, W.H. Stigma in leprosy: Concepts, causes and determinants. *Lepr. Rev.* **2014**, *85*, 36–47. [PubMed]
9. Duthie, M.S.; Truman, R.W.; Goto, W.; O'Donnell, J.; Hay, M.N.; Spencer, J.S.; Carter, D.; Reed, S.G. Insight toward early diagnosis of leprosy through analysis of the developing antibody responses of *Mycobacterium leprae*-infected armadillos. *Clin. Vaccine Immunol.* **2011**, *18*, 254–259. [CrossRef] [PubMed]
10. Veena, S.; Kumar, P.; Shashikala, P.; Gurubasavaraj, H.; Chandrasekhar, H.R. Significance of histopathology in leprosy patients with 1–5 skin lesions with relevance to therapy. *J. Lab. Physicians* **2011**, *3*, 21–24. [CrossRef] [PubMed]
11. Lockwood, D.N.; Nicholls, P.; Smith, W.C.; Das, L.; Barkataki, P.; van Brakel, W.; Suneetha, S. Comparing the clinical and histological diagnosis of leprosy and leprosy reactions in the INFIR cohort of Indian patients with multibacillary leprosy. *PLoS Negl. Trop. Dis.* **2012**, *6*, e1702. [CrossRef] [PubMed]
12. Fischer, M. Leprosy—An overview of clinical features, diagnosis, and treatment. *J. Dtsch. Dermatol. Ges.* **2017**, *15*, 801–827. [CrossRef] [PubMed]
13. Lastória, J.C.; Abreu, M.A. Leprosy: A review of laboratory and therapeutic aspects—Part 2. *An. Bras. Dermatol.* **2014**, *89*, 389–401. [CrossRef] [PubMed]
14. Azevedo, M.C.; Ramuno, N.M.; Fachin, L.R.; Tassa, M.; Rosa, P.S.; Belone, A.F.; Diorio, S.M.; Soares, C.T.; Garlet, G.P.; Trombone, A.P. qPCR detection of *Mycobacterium leprae* in biopsies and slit skin smear of different leprosy clinical forms. *Braz. J. Infect. Dis.* **2017**, *21*, 71–78. [CrossRef] [PubMed]
15. Speers, D.J. Clinical applications of molecular biology for infectious diseases. *Clin. Biochem. Rev.* **2006**, *27*, 39–51. [PubMed]
16. Niemz, A.; Boyle, D.S. Nucleic acid testing for tuberculosis at the point-of-care in high-burden countries. *Expert Rev. Mol. Diagn.* **2012**, *12*, 687–701. [CrossRef] [PubMed]
17. Martinez, A.N.; Talhari, C.; Moraes, M.O.; Talhari, S. PCR-based techniques for leprosy diagnosis: From the laboratory to the clinic. *PLoS Negl. Trop. Dis.* **2014**, *8*, e2655. [CrossRef] [PubMed]
18. Male, M.M.; Rao, B.G.; Chokkakula, S.; Kasetty, S.; Rao, P.V.R.; Jonnalagada, S.; Reddy, A.M.; Srikantam, A. Molecular screening for primary drug resistance in *M. leprae* from newly diagnosed leprosy cases from India. *Lepr. Rev.* **2016**, *87*, 322–331.
19. Moher, D.; Liberati, A.; Tetzlaff, J.; Altman, D.G.; Group, P. Preferred reporting items for systematic reviews and meta-analyses: The PRISMA statement. *Ann. Intern. Med.* **2009**, *151*, 264–269. [CrossRef] [PubMed]
20. Canese, K.; Weis, S. PubMed: The Bibliographic Database. In *The NCBI Handbook [Internet]*, 2nd ed.; National Center for Biotechnology Information (US): Bethesda, MD, USA, 2013.
21. Chaitanya, V.S.; Cuello, L.; Das, M.; Sudharsan, A.; Ganesan, P.; Kanmani, K.; Rajan, L.; Ebenezer, M. Analysis of a novel multiplex polymerase chain reaction assay as a sensitive tool for the diagnosis of indeterminate and tuberculoid forms of leprosy. *Int. J. Mycobacteriol.* **2017**, *6*, 1–8. [CrossRef] [PubMed]
22. De Wit, M.Y.; Douglas, J.T.; McFadden, J.; Klatser, P.R. Polymerase chain reaction for detection of *Mycobacterium leprae* in nasal swab specimens. *J. Clin. Microbiol.* **1993**, *31*, 502–506. [PubMed]
23. Yoon, K.H.; Cho, S.N.; Lee, M.K.; Abalos, R.M.; Cellona, R.V.; Fajardo, T.T., Jr.; Guido, L.S.; Dela Cruz, E.C.; Walsh, G.P.; Kim, J.D. Evaluation of polymerase chain reaction amplification of mycobacterium leprae-specific repetitive sequence in biopsy specimens from leprosy patients. *J. Clin. Microbiol.* **1993**, *31*, 895–899. [PubMed]
24. Kamal, R.; Natrajan, M.; Katoch, K.; Katoch, V.M. Evaluation of diagnostic role of in situ PCR on slit-skin smears in pediatric leprosy. *Indian J. Lepr.* **2010**, *82*, 195–200. [PubMed]
25. Kamal, R.; Dayal, R.; Gaidhankar, K.; Biswas, S.; Gupta, S.B.; Kumar, N.; Kumar, R.; Pengoria, R.; Chauhan, DS.; Katoch, K.; et al. RLEP PCR as a definitive diagnostic test for leprosy from skin smear samples in childhood and adolescent leprosy. *Indian J. Lepr.* **2016**, *88*, 193–197.
26. Banerjee, S.; Sarkar, K.; Gupta, S.; Mahapatra, P.S.; Gupta, S.; Guha, S.; Bandhopadhayay, D.; Ghosal, C.; Paine, S.K.; Dutta, R.N.; et al. Multiplex PCR technique could be an alternative approach for early detection of leprosy among close contacts—A pilot study from India. *BMC Infect. Dis.* **2010**, *10*, 252. [CrossRef] [PubMed]
27. Siwakoti, S.; Rai, K.; Bhattarai, N.R.; Agarwal, S.; Khanal, B. Evaluation of polymerase chain reaction (PCR) with slit skin smear examination (SSS) to confirm clinical diagnosis of leprosy in eastern Nepal. *PLoS Negl. Trop. Dis.* **2016**, *10*, e0005220. [CrossRef] [PubMed]

28. Maltempe, F.G.; Baldin, V.P.; Lopes, M.A.; Siqueira, V.L.D.; de Lima Scodro, R.B.; Cardoso, R.F.; Caleffi-Ferracioli, K.R. Critical analysis: Use of polymerase chain reaction to diagnose leprosy. *Braz. J. Pharm. Sci.* **2016**, *52*. [CrossRef]
29. Wichitwechkarn, J.; Karnjan, S.; Shuntawuttisettee, S.; Sornprasit, C.; Kampirapap, K.; Peerapakorn, S. Detection of *Mycobacterium leprae* infection by PCR. *J. Clin. Microbiol.* **1995**, *33*, 45–49. [PubMed]
30. Kurabachew, M.; Wondimu, A.; Ryon, J.J. Reverse transcription-PCR detection of *Mycobacterium leprae* in clinical specimens. *J. Clin. Microbiol.* **1998**, *36*, 1352–1356. [PubMed]
31. Phetsuksiri, B.; Rudeeaneksin, J.; Supapkul, P.; Wachapong, S.; Mahotarn, K.; Brennan, P.J. A simplified reverse transcriptase PCR for rapid detection of *Mycobacterium leprae* in skin specimens. *FEMS Immunol. Med. Microbiol.* **2006**, *48*, 319–328. [CrossRef] [PubMed]
32. Goulart, I.M.; Cardoso, A.M.; Santos, M.S.; Goncalves, M.A.; Pereira, J.E.; Goulart, L.R. Detection of *Mycobacterium leprae* DNA in skin lesions of leprosy patients by PCR may be affected by amplicon size. *Arch. Dermatol. Res.* **2007**, *299*, 267–271. [CrossRef] [PubMed]
33. Bang, P.D.; Suzuki, K.; Phuong le, T.; Chu, T.M.; Ishii, N.; Khang, T.H. Evaluation of polymerase chain reaction-based detection of *Mycobacterium leprae* for the diagnosis of leprosy. *J. Dermatol.* **2009**, *36*, 269–276. [CrossRef] [PubMed]
34. Martinez, A.N.; Ribeiro-Alves, M.; Sarno, E.N.; Moraes, M.O. Evaluation of qPCR-based assays for leprosy diagnosis directly in clinical specimens. *PLoS Negl. Trop. Dis.* **2011**, *5*, e1354. [CrossRef] [PubMed]
35. Reja, A.H.; Biswas, N.; Biswas, S.; Dasgupta, S.; Chowdhury, I.H.; Banerjee, S.; Chakraborty, T.; Dutta, P.K.; Bhattacharya, B. Fite-Faraco staining in combination with multiplex polymerase chain reaction: A new approach to leprosy diagnosis. *Indian J. Dermatol. Venereol. Leprol.* **2013**, *79*, 693–700. [CrossRef] [PubMed]
36. Yan, W.; Xing, Y.; Yuan, L.C.; De Yang, R.; Tan, F.Y.; Zhang, Y.; Li, H.Y. Application of RLEP real-time PCR for detection of *M. leprae* DNA in paraffin-embedded skin biopsy specimens for diagnosis of paucibacillary leprosy. *Am. J. Trop. Med. Hyg.* **2014**, *90*, 524–529. [CrossRef] [PubMed]
37. Alam, M.S.; Shamsuzzaman, S.M.; Mamun, K.Z. Demography, clinical presentation and laboratory diagnosis of leprosy by microscopy, histopathology and PCR from Dhaka city in Bangladesh. *Lepr. Rev.* **2017**, *88*, 122–130.
38. Caleffi, K.R.; Hirata, R.D.; Hirata, M.H.; Caleffi, E.R.; Siqueira, V.L.; Cardoso, R.F. Use of the polymerase chain reaction to detect *Mycobacterium leprae* in urine. *Braz. J. Med. Biol. Res.* **2012**, *45*, 153–157. [CrossRef] [PubMed]
39. Tiwari, V.; Malhotra, K.; Khan, K.; Maurya, P.K.; Singh, A.K.; Thacker, A.K.; Husain, N.; Kulshreshtha, D. Evaluation of polymerase chain reaction in nerve biopsy specimens of patients with Hansen's disease. *J. Neurol. Sci.* **2017**, *380*, 187–190. [CrossRef] [PubMed]
40. Gama, R.S.; Gomides, T.A.R.; Gama, C.F.M.; Moreira, S.J.M.; de Neves Manta, F.S.; de Oliveira, L.B.P.; Marcal, P.H.F.; Sarno, E.N.; Moraes, M.O.; Garcia, R.M.G.; et al. High frequency of *M. leprae* DNA detection in asymptomatic household contacts. *BMC Infect. Dis.* **2018**, *18*, 153. [CrossRef] [PubMed]
41. Banerjee, S.; Biswas, N.; Kanti Das, N.; Sil, A.; Ghosh, P.; Hasanoor Raja, A.H.; Dasgupta, S.; Kanti Datta, P.; Bhattacharya, B. Diagnosing leprosy: Revisiting the role of the slit-skin smear with critical analysis of the applicability of polymerase chain reaction in diagnosis. *Int. J. Dermatol.* **2011**, *50*, 1522–1527. [CrossRef] [PubMed]
42. Rudeeaneksin, J.; Srisungngam, S.; Sawanpanyalert, P.; Sittiwakin, T.; Likanonsakul, S.; Pasadorn, S.; Palittapongarnpim, P.; Brennan, P.J.; Phetsuksiri, B. LightCycler real-time PCR for rapid detection and quantitation of *Mycobacterium leprae* in skin specimens. *FEMS Immunol. Med. Microbiol.* **2008**, *54*, 263–270. [CrossRef] [PubMed]
43. Dayal, R.; Singh, S.P.; Mathur, P.P.; Katoch, V.M.; Katoch, K.; Natrajan, M. Diagnostic value of in situ polymerase chain reaction in leprosy. *Indian J. Pediatr.* **2005**, *72*, 1043–1046. [CrossRef] [PubMed]
44. Kampirapap, K.; Singtham, N.; Klatser, P.R.; Wiriyawipart, S. DNA amplification for detection of leprosy and assessment of efficacy of leprosy chemotherapy. *Int. J. Lepr. Other Mycobact. Dis.* **1998**, *66*, 16–21. [PubMed]
45. Sundeep Chaitanya, V.; Das, M.; Eisenbach, T.L.; Amoako, A.; Rajan, L.; Horo, I.; Ebenezer, M. *Mycobacterium leprae* specific genomic target in the promoter region of probable 4-alpha-glucanotransferase (ML1545) gene with potential sensitivity for polymerase chain reaction based diagnosis of leprosy. *Int. J. Mycobacteriol.* **2016**, *5*, 135–141. [CrossRef] [PubMed]

46. Patrocínio, L.G.; Goulart, I.M.; Goulart, L.R.; Patrocinio, J.A.; Ferreira, F.R.; Fleury, R.N. Detection of *Mycobacterium leprae* in nasal mucosa biopsies by the polymerase chain reaction. *FEMS Immunol. Med. Microbiol.* **2005**, *44*, 311–316. [CrossRef] [PubMed]
47. Boehme, C.C.; Nabeta, P.; Henostroza, G.; Raqib, R.; Rahim, Z.; Gerhardt, M.; Sanga, E.; Hoelscher, M.; Notomi, T.; Hase, T.; et al. Operational feasibility of using loop-mediated isothermal amplification for diagnosis of pulmonary tuberculosis in microscopy centers of developing countries. *J. Clin. Microbiol.* **2007**, *45*, 1936–1940. [CrossRef] [PubMed]
48. Boehme, C.C.; Nabeta, P.; Hillemann, D.; Nicol, M.P.; Shenai, S.; Krapp, F.; Allen, J.; Tahirli, R.; Blakemore, R.; Rustomjee, R.; et al. Rapid molecular detection of tuberculosis and rifampin resistance. *N. Engl. J. Med.* **2010**, *363*, 1005–1015. [CrossRef] [PubMed]
49. Mori, Y.; Notomi, T. Loop-mediated isothermal amplification (LAMP): A rapid, accurate, and cost-effective diagnostic method for infectious diseases. *J. Infect. Chemother.* **2009**, *15*, 62–69. [CrossRef] [PubMed]
50. Lawn, S.D.; Nicol, M.P. Xpert® MTB/RIF assay: Development, evaluation and implementation of a new rapid molecular diagnostic for tuberculosis and rifampicin resistance. *Future Microbiol.* **2011**, *6*, 1067–1082. [CrossRef] [PubMed]
51. Arora, D.R.; Maheshwari, M.; Arora, B. Rapid point-of-care testing for detection of HIV and clinical monitoring. *ISRN AIDS* **2013**, *2013*, 287269. [CrossRef] [PubMed]
52. Kim, S.; Nhem, S.; Dourng, D.; Ménard, D. Malaria rapid diagnostic test as point-of-care test: Study protocol for evaluating the VIKIA® Malaria Ag Pf/Pan. *Malar. J.* **2015**, *14*, 114. [CrossRef] [PubMed]

14

Infection of Rodents by *Orientia tsutsugamushi*, the Agent of Scrub Typhus, in Relation to Land Use in Thailand

Kittipong Chaisiri [1], Jean-François Cosson [2]and Serge Morand [3,*]

1 Department of Helminthology, Faculty of Tropical Medicine, Mahidol University, Bangkok 10400, Thailand; kittipong.cha@mahidol.ac.th
2 NRA, Biologie Moléculaire et Immunologie Parasitaires et Fongiques, BIPAR, Ecole Nationale Vétérinaire d'Alfort, 94704 Maisons-Alfort Cedex, France; cosson@supagro.inra.fr
3 CNRS ISEM-CIRAD ASTRE, Faculty of Veterinary Technology, Kasetsart University, Bangkok 10220, Thailand
* Correspondence: serge.morand@umontpellier.fr or serge.morand@cirad.fr;

Abstract: The relationship between land use structures and occurrence of the scrub typhus agent, *Orientia tsutsugamushi*, in small wild mammals was investigated in three provinces of Thailand: Buriram, Loei, and Nan. *O. tsutsugamushi* detection was performed using 16S ribosomal DNA (rDNA) amplicon sequencing approach using Miseq Illumina platform. In total, 387 animals (rodents and shrews) were examined for the infection. The 16S rDNA sequences of the bacterium were found in nine animals, namely *Bandicota savilei*, *Berylmys bowersi*, *Leopoldamys edwardsi*, *Rattus exulans*, *R. tanezumi*, and *Rattus* sp. phylogenetic clade 3, yielding 2.3% infection rate, with two new rodent species found infected by the bacterium in Thailand: *B. bowersi* and *L. edwardsi*. Using a generalized linear mixed model (GLMM) and Random Forest analyses for investigating the association between human-land use and occurrence of the bacterium, forest habitat appeared as a strong explicative variable of rodent infection, meaning that *O. tsutsugamushi*-infected animals were more likely found in forest-covered habitats. In terms of public health implementation, our results suggest that heterogenous forested areas including forest-converted agricultural land, reforestation areas, or fallows, are potential habitats for *O. tsutsugamushi* transmission. Further understanding of population dynamics of the vectors and their hosts in these habitats could be beneficial for the prevention of this neglected zoonotic disease.

Keywords: *Orientia tsutsugamushi*; scrub typhus; 16S rDNA amplicon sequencing; rodents; land use land cover; Thailand

1. Introduction

The obligate intracellular bacterium *Orientia tsutsugamushi* (Rickettsiales: Rickettsiaceae) is the causative agent of scrub typhus in humans, mainly reported in the Asia-Pacific region, and sporadically in some other regions of the world [1,2]. Approximately one million cases of scrub typhus occur annually in Asia, with a 7% to 10% fatality rate if the patients are not treated sufficiently and early in the course of illness [3,4]. Chiggers, the six-legged parasitic larval stage of mites belonging to the family Trombiculidae, are the disease vectors carrying and transmitting the bacterial agent through their bites. *O. tsutsugamushi* is strictly confined to this mite family [5], and potentially develops a symbiotic relationship with its mite host [6–8]. Chigger species from the genus *Leptotrombidium* are the main vectors of scrub typhus in Asia [9,10]. *O. tsutsugamushi* was also reported in other trombiculid species [11] but there is still a lack of supporting evidence to prove their vectorial role in disease transmission, or whether they attack humans. In terms of vertebrate hosts apart from humans, small terrestrial mammals such as rodents (rats, mice and ground squirrels), insectivores and tree-shrews have been reported as hosts of *Leptotrombidium* and are infected by the bacterium. They play important roles in the ecology of chigger mites and thus for the epidemiology of the disease [12,13]. In addition, some other vertebrates such as bats, birds or reptiles, can be also hosts for chigger mites [14,15]. It was hypothesized that their feeding activity on a wide range of hosts may explain the huge diversification of strains of *O. tsutsugamushi* [9,13].

A large diversity of chigger mites can infect Asian small mammals, particularly rodents [16,17] and similarly, a large number of rodent and other small mammal species have been found to be infected by *O. tsutsugamushi* [18]. In Thailand, more than 10 species of rodents (*Bandicota indica, B. savilei, Berylmys berdmorei, Menestes berdmorei, Mus caroli, Niviventer fulvescens, Rattus andamanensis, R. argentiventer, R. exulans, R. losea, R. norvegicus* and *R. tanezumi*) and one species of tree-shrew (*Tupaia glis*) have been reported to be infected by the bacterium [12,19–25]. According to these studies, *O. tsutsugamushi* was detected using serological methods (i.e., fluorescence antibody assay), or by detecting the genetic material of the bacterium via specific gene target polymerase chain reaction (PCR) assays (i.e., the 56-kD type-specific antigen gene).

With the advent of modern molecular tools in bacteriology, high throughput sequencing provides affordable costs, effective detection, and rapid generation of microbial profiling using two main approaches: 16S rDNA amplicon sequencing (sequencing the genome of particular gene targets) and microbiome metagenomics (sequencing the whole particular genome in a sample) [26]. Here in the present study, 16S rDNA amplicon sequencing was conducted to screen the 16S rDNA gene of *O. tsutsugamushi* alongside other bacterial profiles in wild rodents from Thailand.

Environmental factors, including land cover and land use, are known to influence the reproduction and survival of both trombiculid mites [27,28] and rodents [29], and ultimately the spatial heterogeneity of infection risk. The increasing incidence of scrub typhus in South China was associated with habitats characterized by forested areas and climate factors such as relative humidity [30]. In Taiwan, a significant correlation was observed between scrub typhus incidence and habitats characterized by a mosaic of cropland and vegetation [28], which represent transitional land cover use. Scrub typhus occurs in transitional habitats such as forest edges, fallows along streams or abandoned agricultural lands [9]. These habitats favor both chigger mites, because of soil moisture, and their rodent hosts, by providing food and shelters [31].

The present study proposes to investigate the relationships between the structure of landscape and *O. tsutsugamushi* incidence in rodents captured from human-dominated habitats in Thailand. The structure of landscapes may promote *O. tsutsugamushi* transmission in rodents, and consequently the risk of transmission to humans [32,33]. Heterogenic landscape affects the distribution and abundance of rodent species regarding their specialization to habitat [29]. We explored the relationship between the structure of the landscape at a fine environmental scale and individual rodents investigated for infection by *O. tsutsugamushi*. For this, we used the land covers developed for investigating other rodent-borne diseases for each locality investigated in this study [29]. Specifically, we hypothesized that heterogeneous habitats with high forest cover may favor the transmission ecology of *O. tsutsugamushi* among rodents and mites, and its potential transmission to humans.

2. Materials and Methods

2.1. Ethical Statement

Rodent species included in the study are neither on the Convention on International Trade in Endangered Species of Wild Fauna and Flora (CITES) list, nor the Red List (IUCN). Animals were treated in accordance with the guidelines of the American Society of Mammologists, and within the European Union legislation guidelines (Directive 86/609/EEC). Each trapping campaign was validated by the national and local health authorities. Approval notices for trapping and investigation of rodents were provided by the Ethical Committee of Mahidol University, Bangkok, Thailand, number 0517.1116/661 (see [29] for more details), based on the CERoPath protocols for field and laboratory rodent studies [34].

2.2. Study Sites and Rodent Trappings

Three different sites in Thailand were investigated for the presence of *O. tsutsugamushi*. Rodents were trapped in the provinces of Buriram (14.89 N, 103.01 E), Loei (17.39 N, 101.77 E) and Nan (19.15 N, 100.83 E) in 2008 and 2009 (Figure 1). These sampling sites were part of the CERoPath project (www.ceropath.org). Reported human cases of scrub typhus were obtained from national statistics [35]. Reported cases of scrub typhus per 100,000 from 2003–2007 were 72.5 in Nan, 23.3 in Loei and less than 12.2 in Buriram. Nan and Loei belonged to the 10 leading provinces in the incidence rate of scrub typhus [35] (Bureau of Epidemiology, 2007).

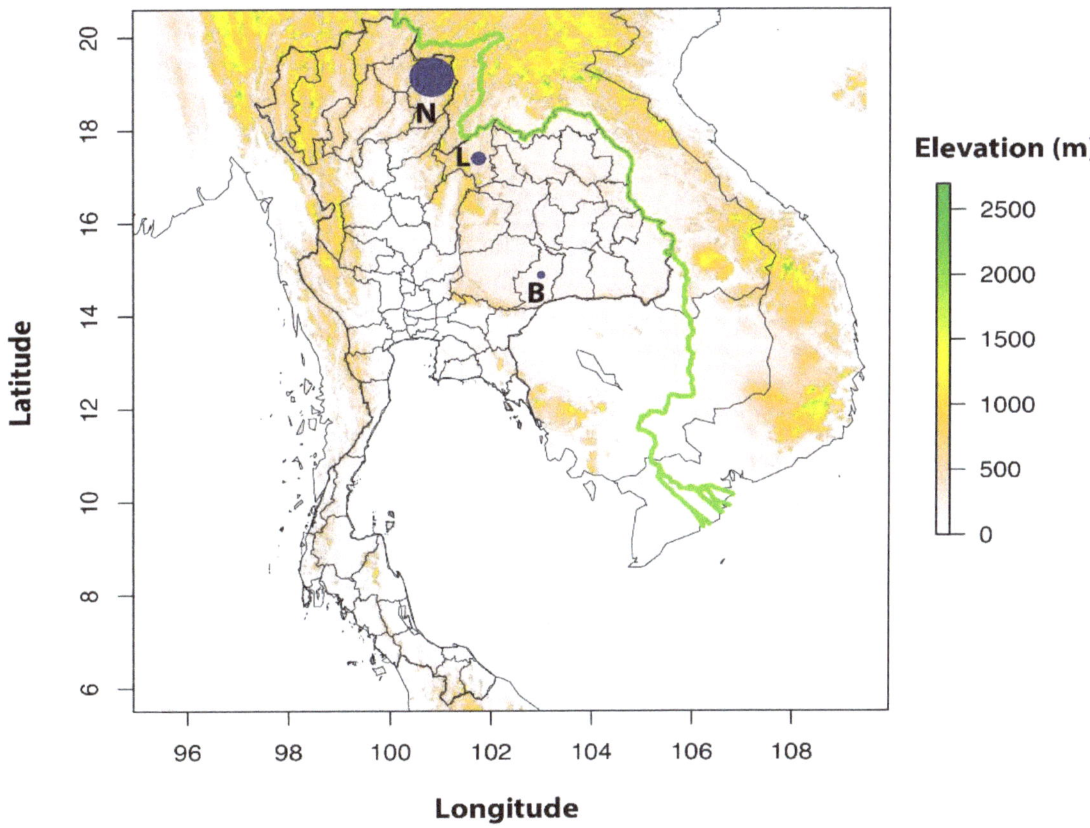

Figure 1. Map of Thailand with locations of the three sample sites in the provinces of Buriram (B), Loei (L) and Nan (N), with reported cases of scrub typhus per 100,000 from 2003–2007: 72.5 in Nan, 23.3 in Loei and <12.2 in Buriram. The relative size of the blue circles indicates average scrub typhus case numbers at each site. Nan and Loei belonged to the 10 leading provinces in the incidence rate of scrub typhus [35].

The methodology was described in Morand et al. [29]. Trapping sessions were conducted in each locality in both wet and dry seasons during 2008–2009. At each locality, the same trap-lines were trapped over a four-night period during each trapping session, with 30 lines of 10 traps (10 m between each trap) placed in three different habitats, namely: (1) forests and mature plantations (rubber trees, teak trees, palm trees, coffee trees), (2) non-flooded lands or fields (shrubby waste land, fallow, young plantations, orchards), (3) rain-fed or irrigated lowland paddy rice fields corresponding to a cultivated floodplain (irrigation allows several crop harvests per year). This corresponded to a total of 1200 night-traps per trapping session. Locally-made live cage-traps were used, and the lines were placed in the same positions during each trapping session using GPS coordinates. Villages and isolated houses, which corresponded to a fourth habitat category, human settlement, were also sampled opportunistically using cage-traps distributed to residents.

Rodent and shrew species were identified in the field using morphological criteria, but were confirmed using molecular methods if needed using a mitochondrial gene for barcoding of some rodent species [36]. Complete data on the animals used as reference specimens for the barcoding assignment are available on the 'Barcoding Tool/RodentSEA' section of the CERoPath project web site (www.ceropath.org).

2.3. *Environmental Indices and Land Use*

The methodology was described in Morand et al. [30] and Bordes et al. [33]. For each locality, recent (years 2007–2008) high spatial resolution (2.5 m in panchromatic mode and 10 m in multispectral mode) SPOT 5 satellite images were acquired (CNES 2009©, distributed by Astrium Services/Spot Image S.A., Toulouse, France). SPOT-digital elevation model (DEM) with a spatial resolution of 20 m together with SRTM (shuttle radar topography mission) was also acquired. For each locality, the SPOT scene was classified into different land-cover types using an object-based approach. The land-cover maps and the DEM were integrated into a geographic information system (GIS) in order to compute landscape metrics for each trapping site. In order to describe the landscape surrounding the trapping location of each individual rodent, landscape metrics were calculated within a 100 m radius. These metrics included: cover of agriculture on steep land, cover of agriculture on flat land, cover of irrigated agricultural land, cover of forest, cover of human settlement, cover of irrigated land, a proxy of habitat diversity (patch density), a proxy of habitat fragmentation (edge density), and all distances between each rodent trapped and each land-cover types.

2.4. *Rodent Screening for O. tsutsugamushi*

Rodent spleens were placed in RNAlater® storage solution (Sigma-Aldrich, Saint Louis, MO, USA) then stored at −20 °C until further analysis. Genomic DNA was then extracted from the spleen using the DNeasy®96 Tissue Kit (Qiagen, Germany). Spleen DNA samples were screened for the presence of bacteria using universal primers (16S-V4F [GTGCCAGCMGCCGCGGTAA] and 16S-V4R [GGACTACHVGGGTWTCTAATCC]) targeting the hypervariable region V4 of the 16S rRNA gene (251 bp) via Illumina MiSeq (Illumina) sequencing. The V4 region has been proven to have excellent taxonomic resolution at the genus level [37]. A multiplexing strategy enabled the identification of bacterial genera in each individual sample. We followed the method described in Kozich et al. [38] to perform PCR amplification, indexing, pooling, de-multiplexing and finally taxonomic identification using the SILVA SSU Ref NR 119 database as a reference [39] (http://www.arb-silva.de/projects/ssu-ref-nr/). We then used the trimming strategy of Galan et al. [39,40] in order to clean the raw data set and to estimate reliable rodent positivity for bacteria.

2.5. *Statistical Analyses*

To analyze the infection of rodents, we first modeled the probability of presence/absence of *O. tsutsugamushi* as a function of several environmental indices with logistic regression, GLMM with logit function and random effects (locality), using package 'lme4' [40,41] implemented in R freeware [41,42]. The binomial variable, infected or non-infected individual rodent, was used in the logistic regression. The initial model included the environmental indices related to the habitat structure, and calculated for a buffer of 100 m for each individual rodent trapped: cover of agriculture on steep land, cover of agriculture on flat land, cover of irrigated agricultural land, cover of forest, cover of human settlement, cover of irrigated land, a proxy of habitat diversity (patch density), and a proxy of habitat fragmentation (edge density). No interactions were added among the independent variables. We evaluated support for competing models, investigating the relationship between the prevalence of *O. tsutsugamushi* and all explanatory variables of interest. We used AIC adjusted for sample size (AICc) to assess the relative information content of the models. We quantified the uncertainty that the 'best' model would emerge as superior if different data were used with Akaike weights (w_r), the probability that a particular model is the best one from the available data. Selection of the best competing models was made using the package 'glmulti' (version 1.0.7 2) [42,43] implemented in R, which allows the exploration of all models using automated model selection and model-averaging procedure using a genetic algorithm.

We also modeled the probability of presence/absence of *O. tsutsugamushi* as a function of several environmental indices with statistical learning Random Forest [43,44] using the 'randomForest' package [44,45]. The measures of importance of each variable are given by values of mean decrease accuracy, i.e., the decrease of model accuracy when the variable is dropped and by values of mean decrease Gini impurity, an index measuring the importance of each variable. All statistical analyses were performed in R freeware [40,41].

3. Results

3.1. Micro-Mammal Identification and O. tsutsugamushi Screening

In total, 387 rodents and shrews were captured and identified at species level (Table 1). The 16S rDNA sequences of *O. tsutsugamushi* were found in only nine rodent individuals (representing 2.3% rate of infection of all the micro-mammals investigated), i.e., *B. savilei* (2), *B. bowersi* (1), *L. edwardsi* (1), *R. exulans* (1), *R. tanezumi* (2), and *Rattus* sp. clade 3 (2) (Table 1). Two rodent species were newly recorded in Thailand for infection by the bacterium: *B. bowersi* and *L. edwardsi*. *O. tsutsugamushi* was detected in all the three localities: Buriram (5), Loei (3), and Nan (1) (Table 1).

Table 1. List and number of host species infected by *O. tsutsugamushi* in three localities of Thailand.

Locality	Micro-Mammal Species	Number Tested	*O. tsutsugamushi* Positive
Buriram	*Bandicota indica*	2	0
	Bandicota savilei	10	2
	Menetes berdmorei	1	0
	Mus caroli	8	0
	Mus cervicolor	11	0
	Mus cookii	1	0
	Rattus argentiventer	1	0
	Rattus exulans	32	0
	Rattus sakaretensis	2	0
	Rattus tanezumi	3	1
	Rattus sp. clade 3	26	2
Loei	*Bandicota indica*	15	0
	Bandicota savilei	12	0
	Berylmys berdmorei	9	0
	Berylmys bowersi	14	1
	Cannomys badius	1	0
	Chiropodomys gliroides	2	0
	Crocidura attenuate	1	0
	Hapalomys delacouri	1	0
	Leopoldamys edwardsi	5	1
	Leopoldamys sabanus	5	0
	Maxomys surifer	15	0
	Mus caroli	5	0
	Mus cervicolor	5	0
	Mus cookii	6	0
	Mus fragilicauda	1	0
	Niviventer fulvescens	16	0
	Rattus exulans	26	1
	Rattus sakaretensis	30	0
	Rattus nitidus	1	0
	Rattus tanezumi	16	0
	R. tanezumi clade 3	2	0

Table 1. *Cont.*

Locality	Micro-Mammal Species	Number Tested	*O. tsutsugamushi* Positive
Nan	*Bandicota indica*	30	0
	Berylmys berdmorei	8	0
	Berylmys bowersi	1	0
	Mus caroli	1	0
	Mus cookiie	4	0
	Rattus exulans	24	0
	Rattus tanezumi	25	1

3.2. Individual Surrounding Habitat Characteristics and O. tsutsugamushi Infection

Infected rodents were trapped in forested and reforestation areas, fallows, cassava plantations, and rice fields.

Comparisons of models testing the effect of several surrounding habitat characteristics on individual rodent infection (GLMM with logit function) are given in Table 2 (best top 3 models) for the three sites in Thailand. Results of GLMM model-averaged importance of surrounding habitat characteristics explaining the infection of rodents by *O. tsutsugamushi* showed that only the explanatory variable forest cover is found in 100 per cent of the top best models (Figure 2).

Table 2. Comparison of models testing the effect of several surrounding habitat characteristics on individual rodent infection by *O. tsutsugamushi* [generalized linear mixed model (GLMM) with logit function] for the three localities (locality as random factor). Models are ranked from lowest to highest supported, according to corrected Akaike information criteria (AIC). Only localities with at least one individual infected rodent were kept for each analyzed dataset. The initial model included the following explanatory variables: cover of agriculture on steep land, cover of agriculture on flat land, cover of agriculture on irrigated land, cover of forest, cover of human settlement, habitat diversity (patch density), habitat fragmentation (edge density), slope, distance to agriculture on flat land, distance to agriculture on steep land, distance to forest, distance to human settlement (K is the number of estimated parameters, AICc is the selection criterion, and w_r are the Akaike weights)

Models (Best Top Three)	K	AICc	w_r
slope + cover of forest + distance to agriculture on flat land	4	84.70	0.033
slope + cover of forest	3	85.02	0.028
Slope+ cover of agriculture on steep land + cover of agriculture on flat land + cover of forest + distance to agriculture on flat land + distance to human settlement	6	85.22	0.025

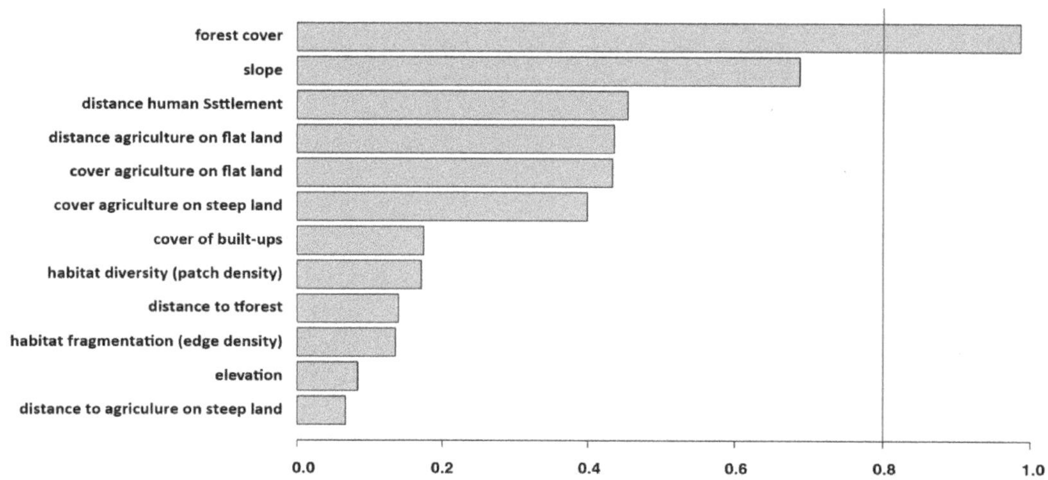

Figure 2. Results of GLMM model-averaged importance of surrounding habitat characteristics explaining the infection of rodents by *O. tsutsugamushi*. Note that only the explanatory variable forest cover is found in 100 per cent of the top best models.

Hence, the best top model selected using AICc values demonstrated that surrounding habitat characterized by large forest cover on slow slope, distant from agriculture on flat land, explained the occurrence of the bacterium in rodents (Table 2). However, forest cover was the only significant variable ($p < 0.05$, Table 3).

Table 3. Results of the best GLMM (with logit link function, and locality as random factor) explaining the occurrence of *O. tsutsugamushi* in rodents, as a function of surrounding habitat characteristics (see Table 2 for the initial models and best top 3 selected models) (estimate of the logit function with SD = standard deviation, residual deviance with DF = degree of freedom).

Explanatory Surrounding Habitat Characteristics	Estimate (SD), *p*	Log Likelihood, Deviance (DF)
Forest cover	3.87 (1.25), 0.002	
Distance to agriculture on flat land	0.003 (0.001), 0.096	
Slope	−0.22 (0.14), 0.10	−160.6, 321.1 (1360)

Using Random Forest analysis, again forest cover was selected as the best explanatory variable, followed by cover of agriculture on flat land (Figure 3). However, the values of mean decrease accuracy and mean decrease Gini dropped from cover of agriculture on flat land (Figure 2). Although the accuracy of the Random Forest was high with a value of 0.991 (with 95% CI: 0.97–0.999), the p value was not significant ($p = 0.059$), due to the low number of infected rodents (9) compared to the negative ones (378).

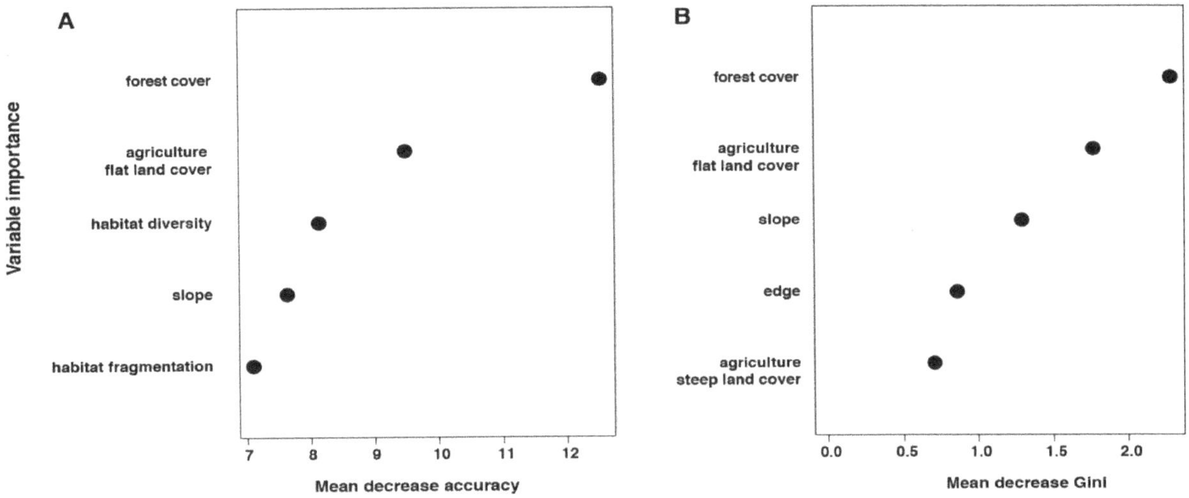

Figure 3. Results of Random Forest analysis with: (**a**) values of mean decrease accuracy; measuring the decrease of model accuracy when variables are dropped; (**b**) values of mean decrease Gini impurity index measuring the importance of each variable.

4. Discussion

The goal of this study was to investigate the relationship between the landscape structure of the three localities and the occurrence of the bacterium *O. tsutsugamushi* in wild rodents detected using the 16S rDNA amplicon sequencing approach. Our findings indicate that the prevalence of the bacterium is very low, with only nine out of the 387 micro-mammals investigated, positive (2.3%). The prevalence of bacterium in animals was higher on the site of Buriram than the sites of Nan and Loei, in contrast to the human scrub typhus incidence report, which gave higher human incidence in Nan and Loei than in Buriram [35]. However, the data were not obtained at the same scale; the whole province is represented in health surveillance, versus only a few square kilometers for the rodent survey.

We confirmed the presence of the bacterium in several known rodent host species, such as *B. savilei*, *R. exulans* and the two species of the *R. tanezumi* complex [24]. We confirmed that the *Mus* species did not appear as infected by *O. tsutsugamushi* [21]. We recorded two new infected rodent species in Thailand: *B. bowersi* and *L. edwardsi*. The positive rodents are either habitat specialists, such as the forest-dwelling *L. edwardsi*, or habitat generalists, such as *R. tanezumi* [29]. Moreover, our results showed the epidemiological importance of the two synanthropic species, *R. exulans* and *R. tanezumi*, which live in close association with humans [29,46,47].

Our results seem to support our hypotheses that rodents infected by *O. tsutsugamushi* were more likely to be found in environments with large forest cover using either GLMM or Random Forest analysis. Our results suggest that a rodent was likely infected in a habitat such as a house, a fallow, or a rice field, if these habitats were in the vicinity of a forested area. The low support values (w_r) for the overall models could be explained by the fact that the prevalence of the bacterium is very low with a low number of positive individuals for each land use land cover of the three localities. This low prevalence also explains why the accuracy of the Random Forest analysis was not significant (although close to significance).

The significance of forest cover for scrub typhus seropositivity was expected, as several studies conducted in Taiwan or in China showed that the incidence of scrub typhus is related to land use characterized by forested areas with abandonment of agriculture land and return to fallows and forests [28,30,31]. Southeast Asia is characterized by increased fragmentation and conversion of forest to agricultural land [48,49]). This new frontier of forest conversion is potentially risky habitat for scrub typhus infection.

4.1. Limitations of Our Study

There are some limitations of our study. First, we are just starting to obtain an evaluation on the sensitivity of 16S amplicon sequencing in the frame of epidemiological studies. Razzauti et al. [50] recently showed that the sensitivity of 16S rRNA amplicon sequencing on the MiSeq platform was equivalent to that of whole-RNA sequencing (RNA-seq) on the HiSeq platform for detecting bacteria in rodent samples. Galan et al. [36] revealed an excellent repeatability of bacterial detection (93%) using systematic replicates in 711 rodents. Finally, work in progress at our laboratory (unpublished result) shows that the sensitivity of the 16S rRNA amplicon sequencing approach used here is as good as the sensitivity of quantitative PCR (qPCR) performed with specific primers, the current gold standard for bacterial detection in biological samples. Thus, we are confident in our *Orientia* screening.

Second, more detailed information on human cases at high resolution, i.e., at the level of sub-district or villages, will help to accurately investigate accurately the relationship between human cases and rodent infection by *O. tsutsugamushi*.

Third, our study could not assess the impact of seasonality on the epidemiology of *O. tsutsugamushi*. Another limitation concerns the diversity and infection of chigger mites. All chigger mites were collected and preserved. Future studies are planned to explore this point.

4.2. Implications for Public Health

The incidence of scrub typhus is increasing in several countries of East Asia. Previous studies [30] showed that habitat fragmentation and extensive agriculture disrupt rodent habitats favoring generalist and synanthropic rodent species, which ultimately enhance rodent-borne transmission. The results of our study suggest that risky habitats for *O. tsutsugamushi* transmission are heterogenous forested areas, comprising conversed agriculture or reforested areas, fallow or abandoned agriculture. Surveillance of rodents' population dynamics in these habitats may help to prevent zoonotic transmission.

Acknowledgments: This study was funded by the French ANR CERoPath (www.ceropath.org) CP&ES, grant ANR 11 CPEL 002 BiodivHealthSEA project (www.biodivhealthsea.org). SM is supported by the Thailand International Cooperation Agency (TICA). Special thanks to Annelise Tran for the GIS development. We thank the CERoPath team and the drivers for their invaluable help during fieldwork.

Author Contributions: J.F.C. and S.M. conceived the trapping sampling and the design of the experiment; J.F.C. designed the screening of rodents; all authors analyzed the data; all authors contributed equally to the writing of the paper.

References

1. Kelly, D.J.; Fuerst, P.A.; Ching, W.M.; Richards, A.L. Scrub typhus: The geographic distribution of phenotypic and genotypic variants of *Orientia tsutsugamushi*. *Clin. Infect. Dis.* **2009**, *15*, S203–S230. [CrossRef] [PubMed]
2. Cosson, J.-F.; Galan, M.; Bard, E.; Razzauti, M.; Bernard, M.; Morand, S.; Brouat, C.; Dalecky, A.; Ba, K.; Charbonnel, N.; et al. Detection of *Orientia* sp. DNA in rodents from Asia, West Africa and Europe. *Parasites Vect.* **2015**, *8*, 172. [CrossRef] [PubMed]
3. Watt, G.; Parola, P. Scrub typhus and tropical rickettsioses. *Curr. Opinion Infect. Dis.* **2003**, *16*, 429–436. [CrossRef]
4. Walker, M.D. Scrub typhus—Scientific neglect, ever-widening impact. *N. Engl. J. Med.* **2016**, *375*, 913–915. [CrossRef] [PubMed]
5. Chaisiri, K.; McGarry, J.W.; Morand, S.; Makepeace, B.L. Symbiosis in an overlooked microcosm: A systematic review of the bacterial flora of mites. *Parasitology* **2015**, *142*, 1152–1156. [CrossRef] [PubMed]
6. Roberts, L.W.; Rapmund, G.; Gadigan, F.G. Sex ratios in *Rickettsia tsutsugamushi*-infected and noninfected colonies of *Leptotrombidium*. (Acari: Trombiculidae). *J. Med. Entomol.* **1977**, *14*, 89–92. [CrossRef] [PubMed]
7. Frances, S.P.; Watcharapichat, P.; Phulsuksombati, D. Vertical transmission of *Orientia tsutsugamushi* in two lines of naturally infected *Leptotrombidium deliense* (Acari: Trombiculidae). *J. Med. Entomol.* **2001**, *38*, 17–21. [CrossRef] [PubMed]
8. Phasomkusolsil, S.; Tanskul, P.; Ratanatham, S.; Watcharapichat, P.; Phulsuksombati, D.; Frances, S.P.; Lerdthusnee, K.; Linthicum, K.J. Influence of *Orientia tsutsugamushi* infection on the developmental biology of *Leptotrombidium imphalum* and *Leptotrombidium chiangraiensis* (Acari: Trombiculidae). *J. Med. Entomol.* **2012**, *49*, 1270–1275. [CrossRef]
9. Traub, R.; Wisseman, C.L.J. The ecology of chigger-borne rickettsiosis (scrub typhus). *J. Med. Entomol.* **1974**, *11*, 237–303. [CrossRef] [PubMed]
10. Stekolnikov, A.A. *Leptotrombidium* (Acari: Trombiculidae) of the world. *Zootaxa* **2013**, *3728*, zootaxa.3728.1.1. [CrossRef]
11. Santibanez, P.; Palomar, A.M.; Portillo, A.; Santibanez, S.; Oteo, J.A. The role of chiggers as human pathogens. Available online: https://www.intechopen.com/books/an-overview-of-tropical-diseases/the-role-of-chiggers-as-human-pathogens (accessed on 5 October 2017).
12. Coleman, R.E.; Monkanna, T.; Linthicum, K.J.; Strickman, D.A.; Frances, S.P.; Tanskul, P.; Kollars, T.M., Jr.; Inlao, I.; Watcharapichat, P.; Khlaimanee, N.; et al. Occurrence of *Orientia tsutsugamushi* in small mammals from Thailand. *Am. J. Trop. Med. Hyg.* **2003**, *69*, 519–524. [PubMed]
13. Paris, D.H.; Shelite, T.R.; Day, N.P.; Walker, D.H. Unresolved problems related to scrub typhus: A seriously neglected life-threatening disease. *Am. J. Trop. Med. Hyg.* **2013**, *89*, 301–307. [CrossRef] [PubMed]
14. Shatrov, A.B.; Kudryashova, N.I. Taxonomic ranking of major trombiculid subtaxa with remarks on the evolution of host-parasite relationships (Acariformes: Parasitengona: Trombiculidae). *Ann. Zool.* **2008**, *58*, 279–287. [CrossRef]
15. Zhang, M.; Zhao, Z.; Yang, H.L.; Zhang, A.H.; Xu, X.Q.; Meng, X.P.; Zhang, H.Y.; Wang, X.J.; Li, Z.; Ding, S.J.; et al. Molecular epidemiology of *Orientia tsutsugamushi* in chiggers and ticks from domestic rodents in Shandong, northern China. *Parasites Vect.* **2013**, *6*, 312. [CrossRef] [PubMed]
16. Chaisiri, K.; Stekolnikov, A.A.; Makepeace, B.L.; Morand, S. A Revised checklist of chigger mites (Acari: Trombiculidae) from Thailand, with the description of three new species. *J. Med. Entomol.* **2016**, *53*, 321–342. [CrossRef] [PubMed]
17. Peng, P.Y.; Guo, X.G.; Ren, T.G.; Song, W.Y.; Dong, W.G.; Fan, R. Species diversity of ectoparasitic chigger mites (Acari: Prostigmata) on small mammals in Yunnan Province, China. *Parasitol. Res.* **2016**, *15*, 3605–3618. [CrossRef] [PubMed]
18. Meerburg, B.G.; Singleton, G.R.; Kijlstra, A. Rodent-borne diseases and their risks for public health. *Crit. Rev. Microbiol.* **2009**, *35*, 221–270. [CrossRef] [PubMed]

19. Khuntirat, B.; Lerdthusnee, K.; Leepitakrat, W.; Kengleucha, A.; Wongkalasin, K.; Monkanna, T.; Mungviriya, S.; Jones, J.W.; Coleman, R.E. Characterization of *Orientia tsutsugamushi* isolated from wild-caught rodents and chiggers in northern Thailand. *Ann. N. Y. Acad. Sci.* **2003**, *990*, 205–212. [CrossRef]
20. Lerdthusnee, K.; Nigro, J.; Monkanna, T.; Leepitakrat, W.; Leepitakrat, S.; Insuan, S.; Charoensongsermkit, W.; Khlaimanee, N.; Akkagraisee, W.; Chayapum, K.; et al. Surveys of rodent-borne disease in Thailand with a focus on scrub typhus assessment. *Integrat. Zool.* **2008**, *3*, 267–273. [CrossRef] [PubMed]
21. Wangroongsarb, P.; Saengsongkong, W.; Petkanjanapong, W.; Mimgratok, M.; Panjai, D.; Wootta, W.; Hagiwara, T. An application of duplex PCR for detection of *Leptospira* spp. and *Orientia tsutsugamushi* from wild rodents. *Jpn. J. Inf. Dis.* **2008**, *61*, 407–409.
22. Rodkvamtook, W.; Gaywee, J.; Kanjanavanit, S.; Ruangareerate, T.; Richards, A.L.; Sangjun, N.; Jeamwattanalert, P.; Sirisopana, N. Scrub typhus outbreak, northern Thailand, 2006–2007. *Emerg. Inf. Dis.* **2013**, *19*, 774–777. [CrossRef] [PubMed]
23. Rodkvamtook, W.; Ruang-Areerate, T.; Gaywee, J.; Richards, A.L.; Jeamwattanalert, P.; Bodhidatta, D.; Sangjun, N.; Prasartvit, A.; Jatisatienr, A.; Jatisatienr, C. Isolation and Characterization of *Orientia tsutsugamushi* from rodents captured following a scrub typhus outbreak at a military training base, Bothong District, Chonburi Province, Central Thailand. *Am. J. Trop. Med. Hyg.* **2011**, *84*, 599–607. [CrossRef] [PubMed]
24. Herbreteau, V.; Bordes, F.; Jittapalapong, S.; Supputamongkol, Y.; Morand, S. Rodent-borne diseases in Thailand: Targeting rodent carriers and risky habitats. *Infect. Ecol. Epidemiol.* **2012**, *2*, 18637. [CrossRef] [PubMed]
25. Chareonviriyaphap, T.; Leepitakrat, W.; Lerdthusnee, K.; Chao, C.C.; Ching, W.M. Dual exposure of *Rickettsia typhi* and *Orientia tsutsugamushi* in the field-collected *Rattus* rodents from Thailand. *J. Vect. Ecol.* **2014**, *39*, 182–189. [CrossRef] [PubMed]
26. Hamady, M.; Knight, R. Microbial community profiling for human microbiome projects: Tools, techniques, and challenges. *Genome Res.* **2009**, *19*, 1141–1152. [CrossRef] [PubMed]
27. Muul, I.; Lim, B.L.; Walker, J.S. Scrub typhus infection in rats in four habitats in Peninsular Malaysia. *Trans. R Soc. Trop. Med. Hyg.* **1977**, *71*, 493–497. [CrossRef]
28. Wardrop, N.A.; Kuo, C.-C.; Wang, H.-C.; Clements, A.C.A.; Lee, P.-F.; Atkinson, P.M. Bayesian spatial modelling and the significance of agricultural land use to scrub typhus infection in Taiwan. *Geospatial Health* **2013**, *8*, 229–239. [CrossRef] [PubMed]
29. Morand, S.; Bordes, F.; Blasdell, K.; Pilosof, S.; Cornu, J.-F.; Chaisiri, K.; Chaval, Y.; Cosson, J.-F.; Claude, J.; Feyfant, T.; et al. Assessing the distribution of disease-bearing rodents in human-modified tropical landscapes. *J. Appl. Ecol.* **2015**, *52*, 784–794. [CrossRef]
30. Sun, Y.; Wei, Y.-H.; Yang, Y.; Ma, Y.; de Vlas, S.J.; Yao, H.W.; Huang, Y.; Ma, M.J.; Liu, K.; Li, X.N.; et al. Rapid increase of scrub typhus incidence in Guangzhou, southern China, 2006–2014. *BMC Inf. Dis.* **2017**, *17*, 13. [CrossRef] [PubMed]
31. Kuo, C.C.; Huang, J.L.; Shu, P.Y.; Lee, P.L.; Kelt, D.A.; Wang, H.C. Cascading effect of economic globalization on human risks of scrub typhus and tick-borne rickettsial diseases. *Ecol. Appl.* **2012**, *22*, 1803–1816. [CrossRef] [PubMed]
32. Bordes, F.; Morand, S.; Pilosof, S.; Claude, J.; Cosson, J.-F.; Chaval, Y.; Ribas, A.; Chaisiri, K.; Blasdell, K.; Tran, A. Habitat fragmentation alters the properties of a host-parasite network: Rodents and their helminths in South-East Asia. *J. Anim. Ecol.* **2015**, *84*, 1253–1263. [CrossRef] [PubMed]
33. Bordes, F.; Caron, A.; Blasdell, K.; de Garine Wichatitsky, M.; Morand, S. Forecasting potential emergence of zoonotic diseases in South-East Asia: Network analysis identifies key rodent hosts. *J. Appl. Ecol.* **2016**, *54*. [CrossRef]
34. Herbreteau, V.; Rerkamnuaychoke, W.; Jittapalapong, S.; Chaval, Y.; Cosson, J.-F.; Morand, S. Field and laboratory protocols for rodent studies. Kasetsart University. Available online: www.ceropath.org/FichiersComplementaires/Herbreteau_Rodents_protocols_2011.pdf (accessed on 6 October 2017).
35. Bureau of Epidemiology, Department of Disease Control, Ministry of Public Health, Thailand. Annual epidemiologic surveillance report 2007. Scrub typhus. Available online: http://www.boe.moph.go.th/Annual/ANNUAL2550/Part1/Annual_MenuPart1.html (accessed on 4 October 2017).
36. Galan, M.; Pagès, M.; Cosson, J.F. Next-generation sequencing for rodent barcoding: Species identification from fresh, degraded and environmental samples. *PLoS ONE* **2012**, *7*, e4837. [CrossRef] [PubMed]

37. Claesson, M.J.; Wang, Q.; O'Sullivan, O.; Greene-Diniz, R.; Cole, J.R.; Ross, R.P.; O'Toole, P.W. Comparison of two next-generation sequencing technologies for resolving highly complex microbiota composition using tandem variable 16S rRNA gene regions. *Nucleic Acids Res.* **2010**, *38*, e200. [CrossRef] [PubMed]
38. Kozich, J.J.; Westcott, S.L.; Baxter, N.T.; Highlander, S.K.; Schloss, P.D. Development of a dual-index sequencing strategy and curation pipeline for analyzing amplicon sequence data on the MiSeq Illumina sequencing platform. *Appl. Env. Microbiol.* **2013**, *79*, 5112–5120. [CrossRef] [PubMed]
39. Silva. Available online: http://www.arb-silva.de/projects/ssu-ref-nr/ (accessed on 6 October 2017).
40. Galan, M.; Razzauti, M.; Bard, E.; Bernard, M.; Brouat, C.; Charbonnel, N.; Dehne-Garcia, A.; Loiseau, A.; Tatard, C.; Tamisier, L.; et al. 16S rRNA amplicon sequencing for epidemiological surveys of bacteria in wildlife. *MSystems* **2016**, *1*, e00032-16. [CrossRef] [PubMed]
41. Bates, D.; Maechler, M.; Bolker, B.; Walker, S. Fitting linear mixed-effects models using lme4. *J. Stat. Software* **2015**, *67*, 1–48. [CrossRef]
42. R Development Core Team. The R project for statistical computing, R version 3.4.1, 2017. Available online: https://www.r-project.org (accessed on 4 October 2017).
43. Calcagno, V.; de Mazancourt, C. Glmulti: An R package for easy automated model selection with (generalized) linear models. *J. Stat. Software* **2010**, *34*, 12. [CrossRef]
44. Breiman, L. Random Forests. *Mach. Learn.* **2001**, *45*, 5–32. [CrossRef]
45. Liaw, A.; Wiener, M. Classification and regression by random Forest. *R News* **2002**, *2*, 18–22.
46. Bordes, F.; Blasdell, K.; Morand, S. Transmission ecology of rodent-borne diseases: New frontiers. *Integrat. Zool.* **2015**, *10*, 424–435. [CrossRef] [PubMed]
47. Kosoy, M.; Khlyap, L.; Cosson, J.-F.; Morand, S. Aboriginal and invasive rats of genus Rattus as hosts of infectious agents. *Vector-Borne Zoon Dis.* **2015**, *15*, 3–12. [CrossRef] [PubMed]
48. Wilcove, D.S.; Giam, X.; Edwards, D.P.; Fisher, B.; Koh, L.P. Navjot's nightmare revisited: Logging, agriculture, and biodiversity in Southeast Asia. *Trends Ecol. Evol.* **2013**, *28*, 531–540. [CrossRef] [PubMed]
49. Cornu, J.-F.; Lajaunie, C.; Laborde, H.; Morand, S. Landscape changes and policies for biodiversity and environment conservation in Southeast Asia. In *Biodiversity Conservation in Southeast Asia: Challenges in a Changing Environment*; Morand, S., Lajaunie, C., Satrawaha, R., Eds.; Routledge: Abingdon, UK, 2017; pp. 49–66.
50. Razzauti, M.; Galan, M.; Bernard, M.; Maman, S.; Klopp, C.; Charbonnel, N.; Vayssier-Taussat, M.; Eloit, M.; Cosson, J.F. A comparison between transcriptome sequencing and 16S metagenomics for detection of bacterial pathogens in wildlife. *PLoS Negl. Trop. Dis.* **2015**, *9*, e0003929. [CrossRef] [PubMed]

15

Cushing Syndrome due to Inappropriate Corticosteroid Topical Treatment of Undiagnosed Scabies

Guadalupe Estrada-Chávez [1], Roberto Estrada [2], Daniel Engelman [3], Jesus Molina [4] and Guadalupe Chávez-López [5,*]

1 Department of Dermatology and Dermato-Oncology, Instituto Estatal de Cancerología "Dr. Arturo Beltrán Ortega", Health Secretary Guerrero, Faculty of Medicine, Universidad Autónoma de Guerrero Mexico, Community Dermatology Mexico C.A., 39850 Acapulco, Guerrero, Mexico; estradaguadalupe@hotmail.com
2 Community Dermatology Mexico C.A.; Health Secretary Guerrero, 39355 Acapulco, Guerrero, Mexico; restrada_13@hotmail.com
3 Centre for International Child Health, University of Melbourne, Melbourne, Australia/Group A Streptococcal Research, Murdoch Children's Research Institute, 3010 Melbourne, Australia; Daniel.Engelman@rch.org.au
4 Department of Pediatrics, Acapulco General Hospital, Health Secretary Guerrero, 39901 Acapulco, Guerrero, Mexico; molinabravo@prodigy.net.mx
5 Department of Dermatology and Mycology Acapulco General Hospital, Health Secretary Guerrero, Community Dermatology Mexico C.A., 39355 Acapulco, Guerrero, Mexico
* Correspondence: chavezg13@live.com.mx;

Abstract: The uncontrolled sale of topical corticosteroids has become an important risk factor for the development of iatrogenic Cushing syndrome in children, especially in countries where medications are sold over the counter. This is exacerbated by the lack of information for both the patients and pharmacists. This report documents a series of eight cases of iatrogenic Cushing syndrome secondary to an inappropriate use of topical steroids, due to a misdiagnosis of scabies.

Keywords: scabies; Cushing syndrome; iatrogenic; topical corticosteroids

---

1. Introduction

Scabies is a highly contagious skin disease caused by the mite *Sarcoptes scabiei* var. *hominis*. Transmission mainly occurs through direct skin contact, often from family members. Scabies is estimated to affect 200 million people worldwide [1]. Reported prevalence rates vary from 0.3–46% [2], with the highest prevalence rate observed in children in tropical countries. Predisposed factors include heat, humidity, overcrowding and increased contact with exposed skin areas [3]. Common (also known as typical or classical) scabies is highly symptomatic, with an intense itch and a rash consisting of discrete to moderate disseminated papules. These are secondary to the antigen released by the parasite and subsequent immune and inflammatory reactions. Other family members frequently have similar symptoms. Crusted scabies is a rarer form of the disease, usually affecting immunosuppressed patients, and presents with hyperkeratotic skin lesions containing thousands of mites.

In Mexico, a common superstition suggests that infants can develop illness if they are not held by a person who gazes at them, as it puts the infant at risk of acquiring 'the evil eye'. Therefore, parents commonly encourage others, even complete strangers, to touch and hold their child [4]. There is also a general lack of awareness that prolonged contact with an infected person can be the cause of scabies or other infectious diseases. Instead, dogs, cats or poor quality of water are often blamed as the cause of the disease. Once a child becomes unwell, parents commonly use household remedies or medications obtained at local pharmacies, where employees may not have any medical or pharmacological training. As many inflammatory dermatological conditions will respond to topical corticosteroids, these are frequently purchased by patients without consultation with a clinician. Topical corticosteroids are known to exacerbate some conditions, particularly infections such as tinea and scabies [5,6].

Topical steroids are graded in terms of potency as either low, medium, high or very high. Whilst low potency steroids are often well tolerated, the absorption of higher potency steroids through the skin can cause Cushing syndrome due to suppression of the hypothalamic-pituitary-adrenal axis, especially if used over large areas of skin, or for prolonged periods [7,8]. In Mexico, topical steroids at all potencies are available without medical prescription over the counter. One of those most commonly sold products is a combination cream containing betamethasone (0.5%), clotrimazole, and gentamicin. The cost is approximately 1.5 USD per 25 g tube [9]. In recent times, high potency combination steroid creams have been widely promoted in Mexico on television, bus advertising, social media and on-site at pharmacies. Even though steroids are used widely in dermatology, their misuse for the treatment of scabies has become increasingly common and problematic in the last 2 to 3 years, causing severe medical problems that deserve wider recognition and prevention.

Permethrin is the most effective topical treatment for scabies, but, it is expensive, which limits its use in Mexico. Other topical treatments for scabies include benzyl benzoate (the most widely available in Mexico), sulfur cream or ointment, crotamiton and lindane [10]. Topical treatments frequently cause adverse effects, including contact dermatitis, erythema, and a worsening itch, which can lead to the early suspension of treatment, intermittent usage and a high frequency of relapse. Ivermectin is an effective oral treatment but is unavailable in many settings. Furthermore, although treatment of all close contacts is recommended, family members and other contacts may be asymptomatic or otherwise reluctant to be treated, further encouraging reinfestation [11].

2. Case Series

This report documents a series of cases involving eight infants, aged from 3 months to 1.5 years (Table A1). All patients clinical signs of Cushing syndrome, including increased adiposity, prominent cheeks, mild to moderate hirsutism on the forehead and side brows, discrete striae and telangiectasias. One patient had such significant weight gain that she lost the ability to support her own body weight. All patients also had disseminated lesions of scabies, with papules, scaling and nodules predominantly in skin folds and the soles of their feet. Two infants had the severe form of crusted scabies.

All cases had a history of continuous or discontinuous use of topical corticosteroids (betamethasone (0.5%) combined with clotrimazole and gentamicin), applied to affected lesions or used on the entire body's surface.

All scabies patients were diagnosed at the Dermatology department of the Acapulco General Hospital in Guerrero, Mexico. Diagnosis was made clinically in all patients based on the typical rash, itch and affected cohabitants. The patients with crusted scabies had extensive scaling lesions on the back, palms and soles with moderate papules and discrete nodules on the rest of the body's surface, particularly in the skin folds. Symptoms of scabies had been present for 1 to 7 months prior to diagnosis. In all cases, the mothers also had clinical lesions of scabies, and in four of eight cases, the mothers had a history that was suggestive of scabies during pregnancy. The number of family members in each household that had daily contact with the patients ranged from 3 to 12. In all cases, the use of the steroid cream was reported to have resulted in initial improvement of symptoms. However, the signs and symptoms would return and worsen whenever the usage of corticosteroid was suspended. Affected family members did not seek medical advice until symptoms worsened. None of the parents were aware that the weight gain and other physical signs of Cushing syndrome were related to the use of the steroid cream. Two patients experienced recurrent upper pulmonary infections during the use of topical steroids that required referral to a physician.

All patients were treated with sulfur cream (4%). Family contacts were treated with oral ivermectin. Twenty-four-hour urine cortisol was requested for patients, but this was often not completed in the majority of cases due to lack of financial resources. One case had the investigation performed one month after cessation of betamethasone, which was reported to be within normal limits.

Follow-up information for patients was limited by the fact that families resided in distant places. All patients were referred to the pediatric service, while two attended for a consultation, with no further complications found. The rest of the patients did not attend a consultation, possibly due to the resolution of scabies symptoms after effective treatment and cessation of steroids. A telephone contact follow-up was attempted but unsuccessful. A check of the patients' hospital files did not reveal any further visits for outpatient consultation or to the emergency department.

3. Discussion

Scabies has recently been added to the list of Neglected Tropical Diseases designated as priorities for control by the World Health Organization [12]. Organizations like the International Alliance for the Control of Scabies have focused on building the evidence base and advocacy strategy for the global control of scabies. This is because of the disease's frequency, global burden, complications and effects on already disadvantaged populations [13]. Whilst common scabies, without secondary bacterial infection, is not life threatening and can be treated simply in many patients, this case series demonstrates that the uncontrolled and chronic use of high potency steroids, including clobetasol and betamethasone, can lead to potentially harmful complications such as Cushing syndrome and other endocrine disorders as well as the development of crusted scabies [7,14]. Patients with crusted scabies have intense scaling on the palms and soles and numerous nodular lesions on axillary and inguinal folds as well as on the scrotum for boys and diaper rim on the waist [15] (Figure A3). Topical or systemic glucocorticoids should be used with caution and never as a treatment for scabies in children.

There are many factors that contribute to the development of Cushing syndrome in this case series and the many other cases we have observed in our practice. Scabies is often not accurately diagnosed, particularly as a medical opinion is not sought after by families, which leads to erroneous treatment. Scabies has recently re-emerged as a major health problem in parts of Mexico, and families are searching for effective treatments for this highly symptomatic disease. At the same time, over-the-counter creams have been promoted to pharmacies and general practitioners as low-cost treatments for a broad range of bacterial, mycotic and inflammatory skin conditions. Previously, steroid-misuse complications have been widely reported, but most reports relate to either eczema in developed countries or to skin lightening creams or fungal infections in underdeveloped countries [5,16]. Patients with scabies may consider these treatments to be cost effective due to the rapid (initial) relief of itch and desire to avoid the cost of medical consultation [17].

Parents may not recognize the rapid weight gain as one of the signs of the infant's developing health problem [4], due to the common belief that 'a fat baby is a healthy one', which leads to reassuring and positive comments on the infant's appearance from friends and family members [18,19].

The incidence of Cushing syndrome secondary from the use of topical steroids is unknown and quite likely underreported [8,20–22]. In addition to the inappropriate treatment of scabies and other skin disorders (including diaper rash, psoriasis, tineas or inflammatory diseases) causing iatrogenic Cushing syndrome, there are reports of Cushing syndrome being caused by inappropriate steroid use for ophthalmologic conditions including cataracts and glaucoma [23]. These risks reinforce the importance of reporting the steroid-related consequences and secondary effects. Further reporting and investigation of these issues may increase awareness amongst health workers and organizations which will lead to advocacy for the regulation and restriction of cortisone-containing products in Mexico and other countries experiencing this issue [24–26].

Sulfur and benzyl benzoate are the most available topical scabies treatments in Mexico. Even though they are effective if applied to the whole body for the recommended duration, they frequently cause irritation, erythema, scaling, intense pruritus or even contact dermatitis, all of which may lead to the interruption of treatment or discontinuous therapy, which ultimately reduces the effectiveness of the treatment. Alternative treatments for scabies, such as tea tree oil, are under investigation but their effectiveness is unproven [27]. Economical and effective treatments are still needed in resource-limited countries, where family income is usually reserved for food, housing and clothing which leaves non-life-threating diseases as lower priorities [28].

The education of health workers is of great importance, as they are the point of first contact. Health workers need to know how to recognize, diagnose and appropriately treat common scabies, and to avoid the use of corticosteroids, especially in children. Complicated cases, or those that do not improve with first-line treatments, should be referred for further assessment. In countries like Mexico, in which there are fewer regulations on the sale of medications, it is essential to inform the general population of the potential risks when medications are not used as intended.

We have introduced teledermatology as part of the Community Dermatology program in Mexico [29] for the education of health workers and doctors in isolated communities. This approach promotes improvements in clinical diagnosis and treatment and can be used to reduce the number of complicated cases. Greater awareness and action are needed for the widespread health problems related to the inappropriate use of steroids [30].

4. Ethical Considerations

The study protocol was approved by the Ethical Review Committee of the Community Dermatology A.C. and was supported by the Health Secretary of Guerrero State prior to the study. Informed consent was obtained from the parents or legal guardians of the minors after a detailed explanation of the study's protocol. In accordance with the ethical review committee requirements, patient information was made confidential.

Author Contributions: Conceptualization, methodology, investigation: G.E.C., R.E., G.C.L., J.M., D.E.; Writing-original draft preparation: G.E.C.; Writing-review & editing, supervision: D.E., G.E.C.

Acknowledgments: We would like to thank the students of the Faculty of Medicine of the University of Guerrero (UAGro.) as well as the team of Telemedicine of the Acapulco General Hospital for their support in identifying and referral of some of the patients. We would like to thank Hay for his review of the manuscript.

Appendix A

Table A1. Cases of scabies and iatrogenic Cushing syndrome.

	Age (Months)	Sex	Topical Steroid Treatment			Clinical Features		
			Usage Duration	Frequency	Regularity	Adiposity	Scabies	Symptom Duration
1	5	Female	1 month	4 times a day	Continuous	+++	Crusted	1 month
2	6	Female	5 months	1–2 times a day	Intermittent	+++	Common	6 months
3	7	Male	3 months	2 times a day	Continuous	++++	Common	3 months
4	7	Male	2 months	2–3 times a day	Intermittent	+++	Common	7 months
5	8	Male	8 months	Daily	Continuous	++++	Crusted	8 months
6	9	Female	1 month	3 times a day	Continuous	++++	Common	6 months
7	16	Male	5 months	Daily	Continuous	++	Common	6 months
8	17	Female	4 months	1–2 times a day	Discontinuous	++	Common	3 months

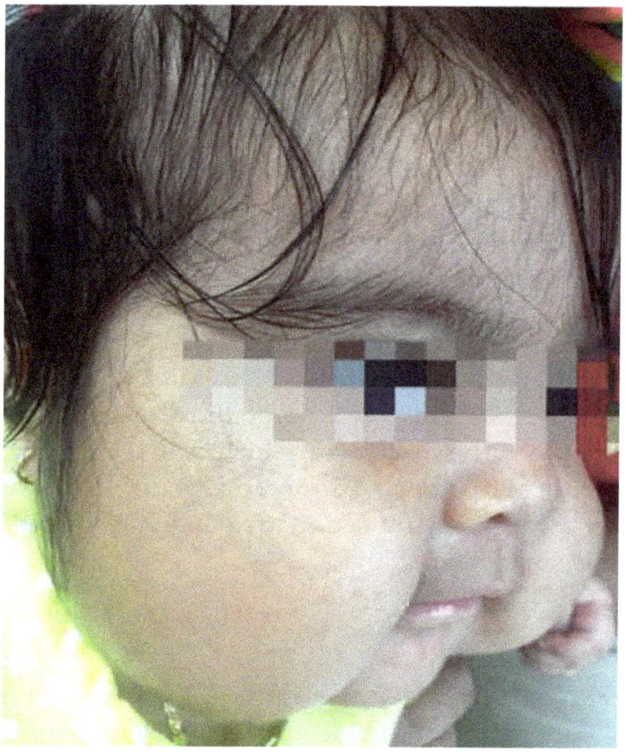

Figure A1. Infant with increased adiposity and forehead hirsutism.

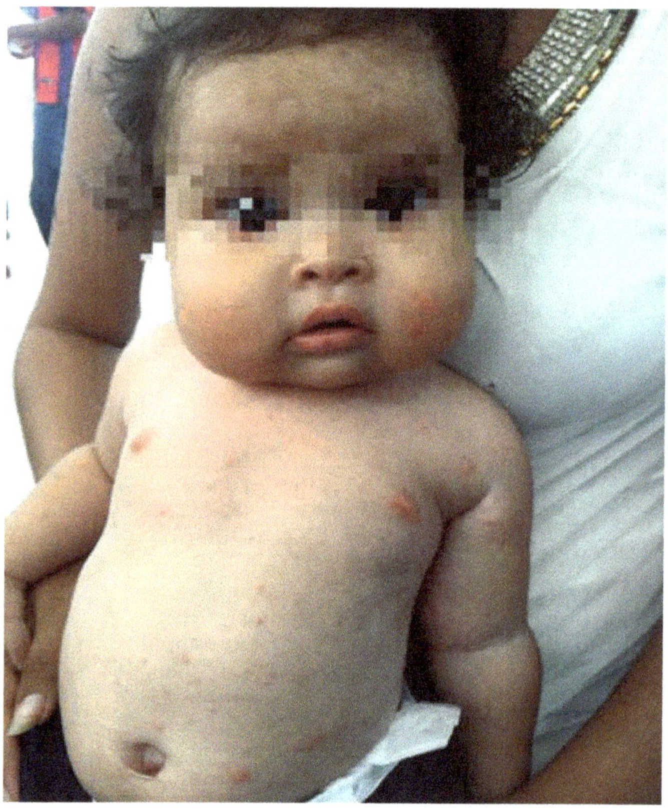

Figure A2. Prominent cheeks, mild telagiectasias and disseminated papulo-nodular lesions.

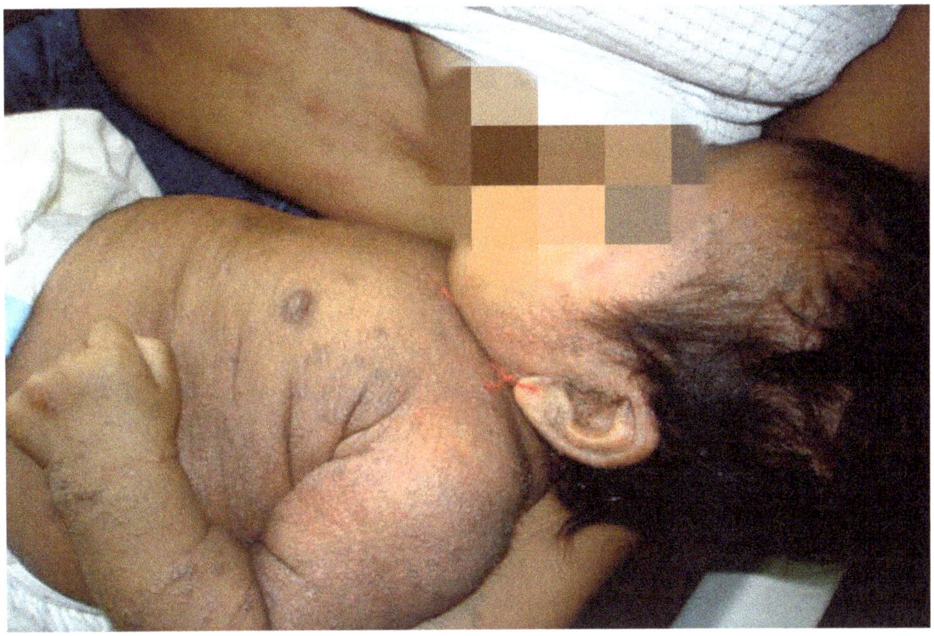

Figure A3. Crusted scabies with intense scaling and nodular lesions in child and mother with scabies.

References

1. Karimkhani, C.; Colombara, D.; Drucker, A.M.; Hay, R.; Engelman, D.; Steer, A.; Whitfield, M.; Naghavi, M.; Dellavalle, R.P. The global burden of scabies: A cross-sectional analysis from the Global Burden of Disease Study 2015. *Lancet Inf. Dis.* **2017**, *17*, 1247–1254. [CrossRef]
2. Mahe, A. Epidemiology and Management of Common Skin Diseases in Children in Developing Countries. Available online: http://whqlibdoc.who.int/hq/2005/WHO_FCH_CAH_05.12_eng.pdf (accessed on 24 July 2018).
3. Romani, L.; Steer, A.C.; Whitfield, M.J.; Kaldor, J.M. Prevalence of Scabies and impetigo worldwide: A systematic review. *Lancet Infect. Dis.* **2015**, *15*, 960–967. [CrossRef]
4. Uriostegui-Flores, A. Cultural specific syndromes treated by traditional doctors. *Rev. Salud Publica* **2015**, *17*, 277–288. [PubMed]
5. Verma, S.B.; Vasani, R. Male genital dermatophytosis- clinical features and the effects of the misuse of topical steroids and steroid combinations- an alarming problem in India. *Mycoses* **2016**, *59*, 606–614. [CrossRef] [PubMed]
6. Estrada-Chavez, G.; Estrada, R.; Chavez-López, G. Misuse of topical steroids in scabies. *Comm. Dermatol. J.* **2017**, *13*, 1–12.
7. Miller, W.L. The adrenal cortex and its disorders. In *Clinical Pediatric Endocrinology*, 4th ed.; Hindmarsh, P.C., Ed.; Oxford Blackwell Science: Oxford, UK, 2001; pp. 321–376.
8. Semiz, S.; Balci, Y.I.; Ergin, S.; Candemir, M.; Polat, A. Two cases of Cushing's syndrome due to overuse of topical steroid in the diaper area. *Pediatr. Dermatol.* **2008**, *25*, 544–547. [CrossRef] [PubMed]
9. Cómo Utilizar esta Herramienta. Available online: www.profeco.gob.mx/precios/canasta/home.aspx?th=1 (accessed on 23 February 2018).
10. Hay, R.J.; Steer, A.C.; Engelman, D.; Walton, S. Scabies in the developing world-its prevalence, complications and management. *Clin. Microbiol. Infect.* **2012**, *18*, 313–323. [CrossRef] [PubMed]
11. La-Vincente, S.; Kearns, T.; Connors, C.; Cameron, S.; Carapetis, J.; Andrews, R. Community management of endemic scabies in remote aboriginal communities of northern Australia: Low treatment uptake and high ongoing acquisition. *PLoS Negl. Trop. Dis.* **2009**, *26*, e444. [CrossRef] [PubMed]
12. Engelman, D.; Kiang, K.; Chosidow, O.; McCarthy, J.; Fuller, C.; Lammie, P.; Hay, R.; Steer, A. Members of The International Alliance For The Control of Scabies. *PLoS Negl. Trop. Dis.* **2013**, *7*, e2167.

13. Hay, R.J.; Johns, N.E.; Williams, H.C.; Bolliger, I.W.; Dellavalle, R.P.; Margolis, D.J.; Marks, R.; Naldi, L.; Weinstock, M.A.; Wulf, S.K.; et al. The global burden of skin disease in 2010: An analysis of the prevalence and impact of skin conditions. *J. Investig. Derm.* **2014**, *134*, 1527–1534. [CrossRef] [PubMed]
14. Razzaghy, A.M.; Mosalla, N.A.; Nasli, E.E. Iatrogenic Cushing's Syndrome caused by topical corticosteroid application and its life threatening complications. *J. Compr. Ped.* **2015**, *6*, e34336. [CrossRef]
15. Lima, F.C.D.R.; Cerqueira, A.M.M.; Guimaraes, M.B.S.; Padilha, C.B.S.; Craide, F.H.; Bombardelli, M. Crusted scabies due to indiscriminate use of glucocorticoid therapy in infant. *Ann. Bras. Dermatol.* **2017**, *92*, 383–385. [CrossRef] [PubMed]
16. Dlova, N.C.; Hendricks, N.E.; Martincgh, B.S. Skin-lightening creams used in Durban, South Africa. *I. J. Dermatol.* **2012**, *51* (Suppl 1), 51–53. [CrossRef] [PubMed]
17. Hay, R.J.; Estrada Castanon, R.; Alarcon Hernandez, H.; Chavez Lopez, G.; Lopez Fuentes, L.F.; Paredes Solis, S.; Andersson, N. Wastage of family income on skin disease in Mexico. *BMJ* **1994**, *309*, 848. [CrossRef] [PubMed]
18. Boscaro, M.; Giacchetti, G.; Ronconi, V. Visceral adipose tissue: Emerging role of gluco- and mineralocorticoid hormones in the setting of cardiometabolic alterations. *Ann. N. Y. Acad. Sci.* **2012**, *1264*, 87–102. [CrossRef] [PubMed]
19. Rathi, S.K.; D'Souza, P. Rational and ethical use of topical corticosteroids based on safety and efficacy. *Indian J. Dermatol.* **2012**, *57*, 251–259. [CrossRef] [PubMed]
20. Tempark, T.; Phatarakijnirund, V.; Chatproedprai, S.; Watcharasindhu, S.; Supornsilchai, V.; Wananukul, S. Exogenous Cushing's syndrome due to topical corticosteroid application: Case report and review literature. *Endocrine* **2010**, *38*, 328–334. [CrossRef] [PubMed]
21. Gen, R.; Akbay, E.; Sezer, K. Cushing syndrome caused by topical corticosteroid: A case report. *Am. J. Med. Sci.* **2007**, *333*, 173–174. [CrossRef] [PubMed]
22. Selahattin, K.; Sedat, A.; Özbek, M.N.; Ahmet, Y. Infantile Iatrogenic Cushing's Syndrome. *Indian J. Dermatol.* **2008**, *53*, 190–191.
23. Messina, M.F.; Valenzise, M.; Aversa, S.; Arrigo, T.; De-Luca, F. Iatrogenic Cushing syndrome caused by ocular glucocorticoids in a child. *BMJ Case Rep.* **2009**. [CrossRef] [PubMed]
24. West, D.P.; Micali, G. Principles of paediatric dermatological therapy. In *Textbook of Pediatric Dermatology*, 1st ed.; Harper, J., Oranje, A., Prose, N., Eds.; Blackwell Science Ltd: Oxford, UK, 2000; pp. 1731–1742.
25. Siklar, Z.; Bostancı, İ.; Atli, Ö.; Dallar, Y. An infantile Cushing syndrome due to misuse of tropical steroid. *Pediatr. Dermatol.* **2004**, *21*, 561–563. [CrossRef] [PubMed]
26. Azizi, F.; Jahed, A.; Hedayati, M.; Lankarani, M.; Bejestani, H.S.; Esfahanian, F.; Beyraghi, N.; Noroozi, A.; Kobarfard, F. Outbreak of exogenous Cushing's syndrome due to unlicensed medications. *Clin. Endocrinol.* **2008**, *69*, 921–925. [CrossRef] [PubMed]
27. Thomas, J.; Carson, C.; Peterson, G.M.; Walton, S.F.; Hammer, K.A.; Naunton, M.; Davey, R.C.; Spelman, T.; Dettwiller, P.; Kyle, G.; et al. Therapeutic potential of tea tree oil for scabies. *Am. J. Trop. Med. Hyg.* **2016**, *94*, 258–266. [CrossRef] [PubMed]
28. Hay, R.J.; Fuller, L.C. The assessment of dermatological needs in resource-poor regions. *Int. J. Dermatol.* **2012**, *50*, 552–557. [CrossRef] [PubMed]
29. Estrada, R.; Chavez-López, M.G.; Estrada-Chavez, G.; Paredes-Solis, S. specialized dermatological care for marginalized populations and education at the primary care level: Is community dermatology a feasible proposal? *Int. J. Dermatol.* **2012**, *51*, 1345–1350. [CrossRef] [PubMed]
30. Estrada-Chavez, G.E.; Estrada, C.R.; Chavez, L.G.; Paredes-Solis, S. Estudio preliminar de la prescripción indiscriminada de corticosteroides tópicos en medicina general. *Dermatol. Rev. Mex.* **2013**, *57*, 433–437.

16

Concordance between Plasma and Filter Paper Sampling Techniques for the Lymphatic Filariasis Bm14 Antibody ELISA

Jesse Masson [1,*], Jan Douglass [1], Maureen Roineau [1], Khin Saw Aye [2], Kyi May Htwe [2], Jeffrey Warner [1] and Patricia M. Graves [1]

1 College of Public Health, Medical and Veterinary Sciences, James Cook University, Cairns, QLD 4870, Australia; jan.douglass@my.jcu.edu.au (J.D.); Maureenroineau@wanadoo.fr (M.R.); jeffrey.warner@jcu.edu.au (J.W.); patricia.graves@jcu.edu.au (P.M.G.)

2 Department of Medical Research, Myanmar Ministry of Health and Sports, Nay Pyi Taw, Myanmar; ksadmr@gmail.com (K.S.A.); Kyimaywin31@gmail.com (K.M.H.)

* Correspondence: Jesse.masson@my.jcu.edu.au;

Academic Editors: Peter Leggat and John Frean

Abstract: Diagnostic testing for the antibody Bm14 is used to assess the prevalence of bancroftian and brugian filariasis in endemic populations. Using dried blood spots (DBS) collected on filter paper is ideal in resource-poor settings, but concerns have been raised about the performance of DBS samples compared to plasma or serum. In addition, two versions of the test have been used: the Bm14 CELISA (Cellabs Pty Ltd., Manly, Australia) or an in-house CDC version. Due to recent improvements in the CELISA, it is timely to validate the latest versions of the Bm14 ELISA for both plasma and DBS, especially in settings of residual infection with low antibody levels. We tested plasma and DBS samples taken simultaneously from 92 people in Myanmar, of whom 37 (40.2%) were positive in a rapid antigen test. Comparison of results from plasma and DBS samples demonstrated no significant difference in positive proportions using both the CELISA (46.7% and 44.6%) and CDC ELISA (50.0% and 47.8%). Quantitative antibody unit results from each sample type were also highly correlated, with coefficients >0.87. The results of this study demonstrate that DBS samples are a valid collection strategy and give equivalent results to plasma for Bm14 antibody ELISA testing by either test type.

Keywords: lymphatic filariasis; Bm14; filter paper; DBS; CELISA; CDC

1. Introduction

Screening assays used in The Global Program to Eliminate Lymphatic Filariasis (GPELF) are frequently performed in low resource settings where samples may be exposed to temperature changes during collection, storage and transport. Diagnostic tests that can utilise dried blood spots (DBS) collected on filter paper which do not require immediate cold storage have many advantages over plasma samples in rural communities where lymphatic filariasis (LF) occurs.

The parasite antibody Bm14 diagnostic ELISA is among the techniques used to identify bancroftian- and brugian-associated lymphatic filariasis (LF) [1–5] and is used alongside antigen detection tests to monitor and evaluate endemicity in populations [2,6,7]. However, concerns over the specificity and predictive values of the Bm14 ELISA have raised questions about its accuracy in detecting residual endemicity or resurgence [8,9]. Of the three species detected by the Bm14 antibody test, *Wuchereria bancrofti* and *Brugia malayi* contribute 90% and 9% of LF disease burden worldwide [10–12].

The Bm14 ELISA, commercially produced as the CELISA (Cellabs Pty Ltd., Manly, Australia), incorporates positive and negative control samples to check plate to plate consistency [13]. The kit recommends using an optical density cut-off value for defining a positive result (0.4) [13], although some studies use a lower cut-off of 0.25 [10]. The CDC Bm14 in-house version of the assay recommends use of a standard curve to generate antibody units, with sample antibody values greater or equal to the cut-off being considered positive [14]. For comparability in the current study, we used standard curves generated from the same positive serum for both CELISA and CDC versions. Both versions of the Bm14 ELISA recommend the application of either plasma or eluted DBS for antibody detection.

While there is not a true gold standard for LF positivity, previous studies have found that the Bm14 test with plasma or serum has high sensitivity compared to microfilaria microscopy, recorded at 98% for samples from people with *W. bancrofti* and 91% for *Brugia malayi* filariasis [10]. Gass et al. [9] found similar high specificity of 95% for plasma in anticoagulant ethylenediaminetetraacetic acid (EDTA). However, CELISA DBS sensitivity can range from 50.0% to 92.3% when compared with immunochromatographic testing and PCR testing, with consistently high negative predictive values (NPV) of >96.6% [10].

While the dried blood spot method would be an inexpensive and convenient alternative to plasma samples, Joseph and colleagues [8] have reported that specificity of DBS when using the CELISA may be as low as 77%, with a positive predictive value (PPV) of 60% when compared to plasma application. Knowledge gaps in the literature and the release of an improved CELISA kit by Cellabs require additional evaluation and comparison of these methods.

This study investigates whether results obtained using DBS are valid and comparable to results obtained using plasma with the CELISA and the CDC ELISA. These results will provide confidence in and promote appropriate application of the Bm14 ELISA for whichever collection method is available.

2. Materials and Methods

2.1. Study Population

Amarapura Township within the Mandalay Region of Central Myanmar was selected as a study site, as it was known from sentinel site records to have a high prevalence of LF infection. All young people aged 10–21 years were invited to participate in a cross-sectional study. Ethical approval for the study was given by the Myanmar Ministry of Health and Sports and James Cook University Research Human Ethics Committee, approval number H5261.

Individuals were screened for LF infection using the BinaxNOW® filariasis immunochromatographic test (ICT) card (Alere International Limited, Galway, Ireland). Young adults aged 18–21 years gave written consent to participate, while parents or guardians gave written consent for participants aged 10–17 years. An equal number of positive and negative participants were invited for a follow-up visit; however, some chose not to attend, resulting in a final collection of 37 ICT positives and 55 ICT negatives out of 92 total participants. The study sampling occurred shortly before the filariasis mass drug administration was offered in this township. Follow-up visits were done after the mass drug administration to ensure that positive participants took deworming drugs.

2.2. Preparation of Plasma and Blood Filter Paper Samples

Blood samples were collected by technical staff from the Myanmar Ministry of Health and Sports. A 10 mL sample of venous blood was collected from all participants and stored in cooled EDTA anticoagulant vacutainers (BD biosciences, Becton, Dickinson and Company, North Ryde, NSW, Australia). An amount of 10 μL of collected blood was transferred using a micropipette to each of the six protrusions of a filter paper disc (TropBio filter papers) and left to dry completely before storage in individual plastic bags. Remaining whole blood was kept on crushed ice and delivered to the Public Health Laboratory in Mandalay within four hours of collection. Plasma was separated from whole blood by centrifugation at 3000× g for 15 min and aliquoted into 2 mL tubes. Plasma samples were stored at −20 °C at the laboratory in Mandalay until transported to Yangon on dry ice and stored at −80 °C by the Department of Medical Research (DMR). One vial of each plasma sample was thawed, aliquoted and refrozen for transport to James Cook University in Cairns, Australia, where it was stored at −80 °C. Filter papers were sealed in plastic containers and kept in either 4 °C refrigeration or hand luggage during direct transport to Cairns, where they were stored at −80 °C.

2.3. Preparation of Eluates from DBS

DBS eluates were prepared for the application of the commercially available Bm14 kit (CELISA) [13] and the LF Bm14 CDC TMB-ELISA [14], using respective protocols. Sample diluent was prepared according to the instructions, with individual 495 µL and 245 µL sample diluent aliquots transferred into separate serum tubes for CELISA and CDC ELISA testing respectively, using a micropipette. Single blood-soaked filter paper protrusions were transferred to two separate serum tubes, one containing 495 µL of sample diluent to create 1:100 dilutions intended for CELISA application, and another containing 245 µL sample diluent to create a 1:50 dilution intended for CDC ELISA application. Each protrusion soaks exactly 10 µL of blood, with half of this volume estimated to be plasma and the remaining 5 µL containing all other blood products. Therefore, it is assumed that the 5 µL of plasma from each DBS added to 495 µL and 245 µL aliquots creates dilutions of 1:100 and 1:50 respectively. All samples were vortexed to ensure complete saturation of each disc and left to elute overnight at 4 °C before being warmed to room temperature (RT) of between 20 °C and 25 °C and vortexed again prior to testing.

2.4. Bm14 Filariasis Cellabs Enzyme Linked Immunosorbent Assay

Primary sample incubation was at 37 °C for 1 h before emptying and flooding wells with washing buffer three times, followed by a final emptying and upside down tapping of each plate to ensure wells were free of large droplets. Secondary IgG_4 conjugates were added and incubated for 45 min at 37 °C, before washing again and applying a final 15-min incubation with tetramethylbenzidine (TMB) substrate without light exposure. Plates were prepared for optical density reading through the addition of 50 µL of stopping solution per well.

2.5. Bm14 Filariasis CDC's Enzyme Linked Immunosorbent Assay

Antigen sensitising buffer (ASB) was created at 0.1 M using $NaHCO_3$ and dH_2O with a pH of 9.6 using NaOH. Working antigen solution (Atlanta, CDC) was prepared at 2 µg/mL using ASB. The binding of antigens to each well of Immulon 4HB plates (Thermofisher, Loughborough, UK) was achieved by adding 50 µL of 1:50 antigen solution to each well of a 96-well microplate before incubating at 4 °C overnight for at least 12 h. Working antigen solution was physically removed before the addition of 100 µL of PBS + 0.3% Tween (Life Technologies, Mulgrave, VIC, Australia), pH 7.2, to each well and incubated at 4 °C for 1 h.

Blanks were created by adding 50 µL of PBS with 0.05% Tween to intended blank wells. Dilutions of plasma or DBS eluates were added at 50 µL to each experimental well before incubating at room temperature on a rocker platform for 2 h. Washing steps between incubations were performed in an identical fashion to the CELISA, referred to earlier. Following the addition of horseradish peroxidase conjugated anti-human IgG_4 (mouse) (Life Technologies), made to a 1:500 dilution with PBS with 0.05% Tween, at 50 µL to each plate well, the plate was incubated at room temperature for 45 min. TMB substrate was added at 50 µL to each well and incubated at room temperature in the dark for 5 min before adding 50 µL of 1 M HCL.

2.6. Statistical Analysis

Optical density readings of each sample were measured at a dual wavelength of 450 nm/650 nm with a VersaMax™ ELISA microplate reader (Molecular Devices, Sunnyvale, CA, USA) using SoftMax Pro Software Version 6.4.1 (Molecular Devices, Sunnyvale, CA, USA) with background absorbance of sample diluent subtracted.A moderately-positive sample collected from an endemic area of Papua

New Guinea was used as a positive control, while negative controls were taken from Australian lab workers.

A standard curve was constructed using a single highly-positive sample from Papua New Guinea which was defined by an arbitrary high value of 1000 antibody units with subsequent 2-fold dilutions. A single cut-off point of >125 units was used to determine positive readings based on previous literature [5,9]. It should be noted that an optical density cut-off value of 0.4 is normally recommended by the CELISA manual. Relative sensitivity, specificity, positive predictive values (PPV), and negative predictive values (NPV), as well as paired *t*-tests, odds ratios, McNemar chi-square tests and correlations were performed using the IBM statistical software SPSS Version 23.0. Confidence intervals (CI) were reported at 95%.

3. Results

During October 2014, 377 young people residing in Amarapura Township were screened by ICT. Positive cases were age and gender matched to negative cases and 112 young people were invited to participate in a longitudinal study including provision of a blood sample. Not all participants returned for participation, leaving a final sample of 37 (40.2%) positive and 55 (59.8%) negative samples that were included in this study (Table 1).

Table 1. Positive proportions and chi-square results obtained when using the CELISA with plasma as a standard.

Standard	*N* Positive	% Positive (95% Confidence Interval (CI))	Comparative Test	*N* Positive	% Positive (95% CI)	McNemar Chi sq	*P* Value
CELISA Plasma 1:100	43	47 (37–57)	CELISA Dried blood spot (DBS) 1:100	41	45 (35–55)	0.5	0.7
-	-	-	CDC Plasma 1:50	46	50 (40–60)	1.3	0.5
-	-	-	CDC DBS 1:50	44	48 (38–58)	0.2	0.9

3.1. *Categorical Analysis and Comparisons of Plasma and DBS Using Cellabs and CDC ELISA Assays*

Holding all CELISA plasma samples tested at a 1:100 dilution as a standard, we compared how DBS application affects the proportion of positive results when using the CELISA at an identical dilution. We found no significant difference in positive proportions between plasma (47%) and DBS (45%) samples (Table 1).

The CELISA standard was also compared to the CDC version of the Bm14 ELISA to assess any similarity in positive proportions when using plasma or DBS at the CDC recommended 1:50 dilution. The proportions of samples classed as positive were not significantly different between the CELISA standard (47%) and CDC ELISA with plasma (50%) or DBS (48%), respectively (Table 1). These three comparisons suggest that high similarity in positive results is found between the CELISA and the CDC ELISA using either plasma or DBS.

To establish how the CDC ELISA is affected by the application method, plasma and DBS samples were compared using the 1:50 dilution. Positive proportions of 50% when using plasma, and 48% when using DBS were not significantly different (Table 2). This confirms that the CDC ELISA will yield similar results regardless of the sample application method.

Table 2. Positives proportions and chi-square results obtained when comparing plasma and DBS with the CDC ELISA.

Standard	*N* Positive	% Positive (95% CI)	Comparative Test	*N* Positive	% Positive (95% CI)	McNemar Chi sq	*P* Value
CDC Plasma 1:50	46	50 (40–60)	CDC DBS 1:50	44	48 (38–58)	1.0	0.6

3.2. *Comparing the Plasma and DBS for CELISA and CDC ELISA Samples*

To determine how application of plasma and filter paper affects CELISA agreement, relative sensitivity, specificity, PPV and NPV were calculated. When DBS was compared to plasma at a 1:100 dilution using the CELISA, results were high overall at 88.4% sensitivity, 93.9% specificity, 92.7% PPV, and 90.2% NPV (Table 3). These results suggest that the CELISA yields reliable agreement between plasma and DBS samples.

Table 3. Sensitivity, specificity, positive predictive value (PPV), negative predictive value (NPV) and odds ratio statistics comparisons of plasma and DBS application using the CELISA and CDC ELISA.

Standard	Comparative Test	Sensitivity (95% CI)	Specificity (95% CI)	PPV (95% CI)	NPV (95% CI)	Odds Ratio (95% CI)	*P* Value
CELISA Plasma 1:100	CELISA DBS 1:100	88.4% (74.9–96.1)	93.9% (83.1–98.7)	92.7% (80.8–95.5)	90.2% (80.1–95.5)	116.5 (26.15–519.4)	<0.0001
-	CDC Plasma 1:50	95.4% (84.2–99.4)	89.8% (77.8–96.6)	89.1% (78.1–95.0	95.7% (85.0–98.8)	180.4 (33.2–981.7)	<0.0001
-	CDC DBS 1:50	95.4% (84.2–99.4)	93.9% (83.1–98.7)	93.2% (82.0–97.6)	95.8% (85.6–98.9)	314.3 (50.0–1975.4)	<0.0001

Performance of the CDC ELISA using plasma and DBS at a 1:50 dilution was also compared to the CELISA 1:100 plasma standard. Relative sensitivity was high at 95.4% for both CDC plasma and DBS samples, with specificity found at 89.8% and 93.9% respectively (Table 3). Predictive values were also high for both CDC plasma and DBS samples compared to CELISA plasma, yielding 89.1% and 93.2% respectively for PPV, and 95.7% and 95.8% respectively for NPV (Table 3). Therefore, there is good agreement between the CDC ELISA using plasma and DBS when compared to results yielded by the CELISA using plasma.

Again, we compared plasma and DBS using the CDC ELISA at the recommended dilution of 1:50, to determine how test performance and relative predictive values are affected. Sensitivity and specificity were 97.7% and 93.8% respectively, while PPV and NPV were 93.5% and 97.8% respectively (Table 4). These results suggest that the CDC ELISA performs equally well when using either plasma or DBS, as confirmed by a high odds ratio value (Table 4).

Table 4. Sensitivity, specificity, PPV, NPV and odds ratio statistics comparisons of plasma and DBS application using the CDC ELISA.

Standard	Comparative Test	Sensitivity (95% CI)	Specificity (95% CI)	PPV (95% CI)	NPV (95% CI)	Odds Ratio (95% CI)	*P* Value
CDC Plasma 1:50	CDC DBS1:50	97.7% (88.0–99.9)	93.8% (82.8–98.7)	93.5% (82.7–97.7)	97.8% (86.6–99.7)	645.0 (64.6–6442.6)	<0.0001

3.3. *Comparing Difference in Bm14 Antibody Units between Cellabs and CDC Assays*

All unit concentrations, with the addition of one to include results of zero, were converted to log values to approximate a normal distribution (Figure 1). Results were compared using geometric means. When analysing CELISA samples, the mean log value for plasma at 1.66 was significantly lower than the mean log value of 2.10 for DBS ($p < 0.0001$) (Table 5). However, the mean log values for CDC ELISA plasma and DBS samples at 2.03 and 2.07 respectively were not significantly different ($p = 0.34$) (Table 5). The data suggests a rise in estimated concentration when using DBS in comparison to plasma when using the CELISA, but not when using the CDC ELISA.

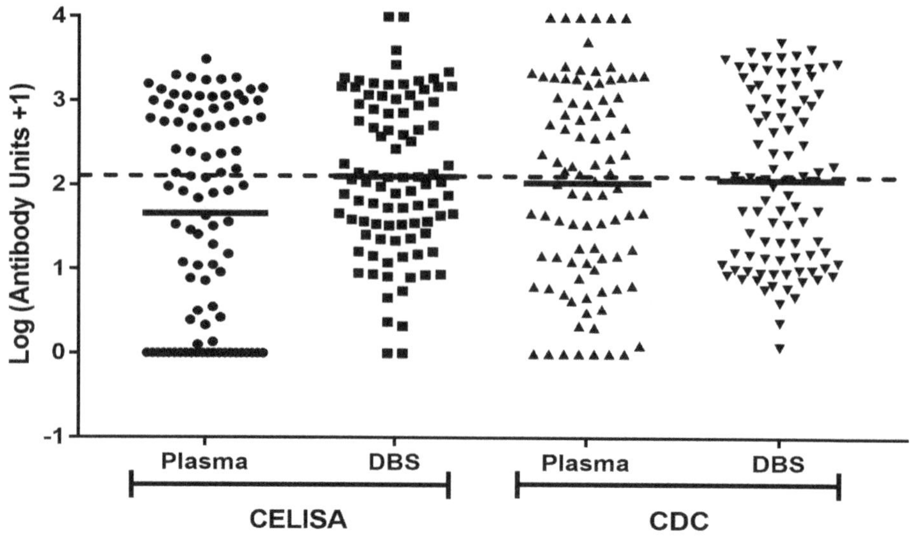

Figure 1. Filariasis Bm14 ELISA log (antibody unit concentration +1) value comparisons between plasma and DBS application of CELISA and CDC ELISA assays. Horizontal black lines refer to mean concentration of each assay, with the segmented line referring to the cut-off value at log (125 units +1). All concentrations above or equal to the defined cut-off are considered positive, while all readings below are considered negative.

Table 5. Geometric mean concentration values and *t*-test comparisons between plasma and DBS application of CELISA and CDC ELISA assays.

Group 1			Group 2			*t*-Test			
Test	**Mean log (Antibody unit +1)**	**Geometric mean**	**Test**	**Mean log (Antibody unit +1)**	**Geometric mean**	***N***	**Mean Difference**	**SD**	***p***
CELISA Plasma	1.66	45.00	CELISA DBS	2.10	124.42	92	0.44	0.63	<0.0001
CDC Plasma	2.03	105.62	CDC DBS	2.07	115.51	92	0.04	0.39	0.34

3.4. Correlation Coefficient Analysis of Bm14 Antibody Concentrations from Plasma and Eluates from Filter Paper

The log values of Bm14 unit concentrations, with the addition of one to include results of zero, between plasma and DBS application were compared to determine correlation coefficients for both CELISA and CDC ELISA assays. Strong correlations were found at 0.87 and 0.95 for CELISA (Figure 2A) and the CDC ELISA (Figure 2B) respectively when comparing plasma and DBS samples ($p < 0.0001$). This shows that quantitative values between plasma and DBS are strongly positively associated when using the CELISA and the CDC ELISA.

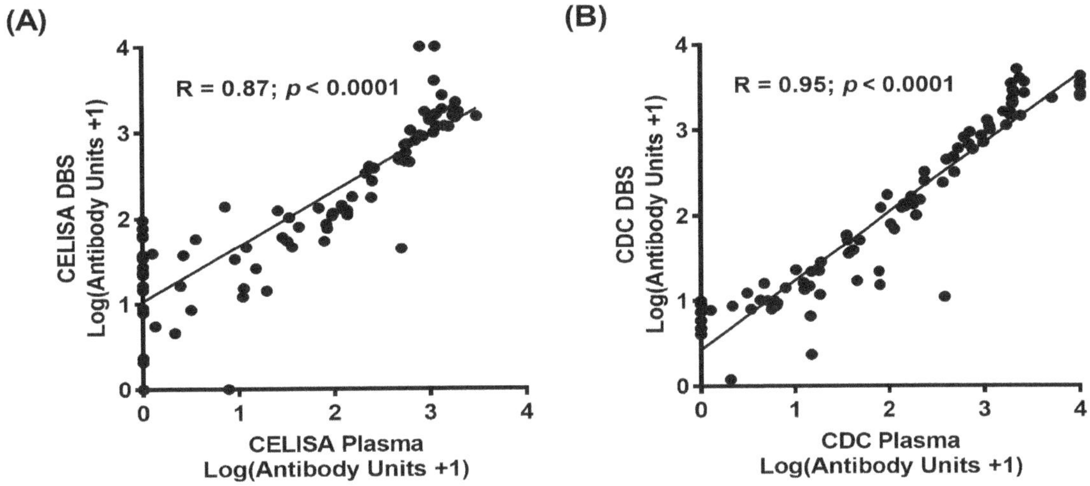

Figure 2. Filariasis Bm14 ELISA antibody unit concentration comparisons of plasma and whole blood application. (**A**) CELISA at 1:100 dilution comparisons of plasma against DBS; (**B**) CDC ELISA at 1:50 dilution comparisons of plasma against DBS.

4. Discussion

The major finding of this study is the strong agreement between plasma and DBS samples, taken from the same individuals and stored identically, when applied to either the Cellabs produced CELISA or the CDC Bm14 ELISA. In the Cellabs CELISA protocol [13], the recommended dilution is set at 1:100. According to the instructions for the in-house CDC filariasis serology assay [14], the recommended dilution is set at 1:50 dilution using serum obtained from centrifuged blood. Despite these differences in dilution optimised for the two tests, the proportions of samples classified as positive were not significantly different, with performance (relative sensitivity, specificity and predictive values) being very similar between all the tests.

High specificity and PPV values were found for comparisons of DBS against plasma using both CELISA and CDC ELISA tests. According to Joseph and Melrose [8], results obtained using the CELISA assay for DBS yielded a specificity of 77%, with 16 samples testing positive by DBS but negative by plasma, while PPV was found at 60%, suggesting that DBS sampling may result in false positives at an approximate rate of 40%. However, this work was done with an earlier version of the CELISA. Weil et al. [10] stated that blood samples with a known amount of antibody applied to DBS are not significantly different to those from serum samples under controlled conditions when using the CELISA. Our own results of 93.9% and 92.7% for specificity and PPV when comparing DBS and plasma suggest that the CELISA assay has improved in these regards.

Analysis of quantitative data showed that correlation was high between plasma and DBS for both the CELISA and CDC ELISA at >0.87. Although the mean antibody units were lower for DBS than plasma in the CDC ELISA, the difference was not significant. The significantly higher sample concentrations for DBS than plasma when using the CELISA suggests that this test gives higher background for DBS. However, the categorical results suggest no significant difference in agreement (classification of positives).If the amount of antibody present is important in future studies using DBS, it may be necessary to keep this difference in mind.

The use of DBS could facilitate more effective sample collection in endemic countries, where large-scale sampling must be undertaken with limited resources and also eliminates the risk of thawing or leaking during shipping.

Our analysis showed that both plasma and filter paper demonstrate similar results using both the CELISA and CDC ELISA. High agreement was also found when comparing the CELISA using plasma with CDC ELISA applications of either plasma or DBS. These results support the use of the

Bm14 ELISA in assessing LF prevalence in the GPELF and can be used with either plasma or DBS on filter paper.

Acknowledgments: The authors would like to thank the Myanmar Ministry of Health and Sports, for study support, specifically Tint Wai. We must also thank the Vector Borne Disease Control group (Mandalay Region) for technical support and the WHO country office in Myanmar. Special thanks go to Ye Ye and Thi Thi Lwin of the Public Health Laboratory in Mandalay for sample separation and short term samples storage, and the Department of Medical Research (Lower Myanmar) for laboratory support and long-term storage of the samples. We are grateful to Luke Becker of the Australian Institute for Tropical Medicine for his assistance with training of local research assistants in all study protocols. Thanks to Graham Burgess for comments on the manuscript. We are very grateful to Kimberly Won and Jeff Priest of CDC for advice and for provision of antigen. We would like to thank Diane Dogcio Hall and Cellabs Pty Ltd., Brookvale, New South Wales, Australia for advice and donation of kits for use in Myanmar. We must also thank the Filariasis Reagent Resource Center (FR3) (http://www.filariasiscenter.org/), who provided positive controls for the ICT cards used in initial screening of the samples. And finally, Keryn Masson and Matt Hayes for their support. This study was approved by JCU HREC number H5261 and the Myanmar Department of Health.

Author Contributions: P.M.G., J.D., J.M. and J.W. conceived of and designed the experiments; J.M., M.R., K.S.A., and K.M.H. performed the experiments; J.M. and P.M.G. analysed the data; J.M., P.M.G. and J.D. wrote the paper with input from J.W.; all authors reviewed the final draft and provided input.

References

1. Simonsen, P.E.; Pedersen, E.M.; Rwegoshora, R.T.; Malecela, M.N.; Derua, Y.A.; Magesa, S.M. Lymphatic filariasis control in Tanzania: Effect of repeated mass drug administration with ivermectin and albendazole on infection and transmission. *PLoS Negl. Trop. Dis.* **2010**, *4*, e696. [CrossRef] [PubMed]
2. Hamlin, K.L.; Moss, D.M.; Priest, J.W.; Roberts, J.; Kubofcik, J.; Gass, K.; Streit, T.G.; Nutman, T.B.; Eberhard, M.L.; Lammie, P.J. Longitudinal monitoring of the development of antifilarial antibodies and acquisition of *Wuchereria bancrofti* in a highly endemic area of Haiti. *PLoS Negl. Trop. Dis.* **2012**, *6*, e1941. [CrossRef] [PubMed]
3. Shawa, S.T.; Mwase, E.T.; Pedersen, E.M.; Simonsen, P.E. Lymphatic filariasis in Luangwa District, South-East Zambia. *Parasit. Vectors* **2013**, *6*, 299. [CrossRef] [PubMed]
4. Mwakitalu, M.E.; Malecela, M.N.; Pedersen, E.M.; Mosha, F.W.; Simonsen, P.E. Urban lymphatic filariasis in the metropolis of Dar es Salaam, Tanzania. *Parasit. Vectors* **2013**, *6*, 286. [CrossRef] [PubMed]
5. Lau, C.L.; Won, K.Y.; Becker, L.; SoaresMagalhaes, R.J.; Fuimaono, S.; Melrose, W.; Lammie, P.J.; Graves, P.M. Seroprevalence and spatial epidemiology of lymphatic filariasis in American Samoa after successful mass drug administration. *PLoS Negl. Trop. Dis.* **2014**, *8*, e3297. [CrossRef] [PubMed]
6. Weil, G.J.; Kastens, W.; Susapu, M.; Laney, S.J.; Williams, S.A.; King, C.L.; Kazura, J.W.; Bockarie, M.J. The impact of repeated rounds of mass drug administration with diethylcarbamazine plus albendazole on bancroftian filariasis in Papua New Guinea. *PLoS Negl. Trop. Dis.* **2008**, *2*, e344. [CrossRef] [PubMed]
7. Harrington, H.; Asugeni, J.; Jimuru, C.; Gwalaa, J.; Ribeyro, E.; Bradbury, R.; Joseph, H.; Melrose, W.; MacLaren, D.; Speare, R. A practical strategy for responding to a case of Lymphatic filariasis post-elimination in Pacific Islands. *Parasit. Vectors* **2013**, *6*, 218. [CrossRef] [PubMed]
8. Joseph, H.M.; Melrose, W. Applicability of the filter paper technique for detection of antifilarial IgG_4 antibodies using the Bm14 filariasis CELISA. *J.Parasitol. Res.* **2010**, *2010*, 594687. [CrossRef] [PubMed]
9. Gass, K.; Beau de Rochars, M.V.; Boakye, D.; Bradley, M.; Fischer, P.U.; Gyapong, J.; Itoh, M.; Ituaso-Conway, N.; Joseph, H.; Kyelem, D.; et al. A multicenter evaluation of diagnostic tools to define endpoints for programs to eliminate bancroftian filariasis. *PLoS Negl. Trop. Dis.* **2012**, *6*, e1479. [CrossRef] [PubMed]
10. Weil, G.J.; Curtis, K.C.; Fischer, P.U.; Won, K.Y.; Lammie, P.J.; Joseph, H.; Melrose, W.D.; Brattig, N.W. A multicenter evaluation of a new antibody test kit for lymphatic filariasis employing recombinant *Brugia malayi* antigen Bm-14. *Acta Trop.* **2011**, *120* (Suppl. 1), S19–S22. [CrossRef] [PubMed]
11. Fenwick, A. The global burden of neglected tropical diseases. *Public Health* **2012**, *26*, 233–236. [CrossRef] [PubMed]
12. World Health Organization. Global programme to eliminate lymphatic filariasis: Progress report, 2014. *Wkly. Epidemiol. Rec.* **2015**, *90*, 489–504.

13. Cellabs Pty Ltd. *Lymphatic Filariasis Bm14 Antibody CELISA*; Cellabs Pty Ltd.: Brookvale, Queensland, Australia, 2012.
14. Centers for Disease Control. *Lymphatic Filariasis Bm14CDC HRP TMB-ELISA (Modified by JCU)*; The Centers for Disease Control: Atlanta, GA, USA, 2012.

17

Rabies as a Public Health Concern in India—A Historical Perspective

Sreejith Radhakrishnan [1,2,*], Abi Tamim Vanak [3,4,5], Pierre Nouvellet [1,6] and Christl A. Donnelly [1,7]

1 MRC Centre for Global Infectious Disease Analysis, Department of Infectious Disease Epidemiology, Imperial College London, London W2 1PG, UK; Pierre.Nouvellet@sussex.ac.uk (P.N.); christl.donnelly@stats.ox.ac.uk (C.A.D.)
2 Department of Animal Husbandry, Government of Kerala, Thiruvananthapuram 695 033, India
3 Ashoka Trust for Research in Ecology and the Environment, Bengaluru 560 064, India; avanak@atree.org
4 DBT/Wellcome Trust India Alliance Fellow, Hyderabad 500 034, India
5 School of Life Sciences, University of KwaZulu-Natal, Durban 4001, South Africa
6 School of Life Sciences, University of Sussex, Brighton BN1 9QG, UK
7 Department of Statistics, University of Oxford, Oxford OX1 3LB, UK
* Correspondence: sr1614@ic.ac.uk

Abstract: India bears the highest burden of global dog-mediated human rabies deaths. Despite this, rabies is not notifiable in India and continues to be underprioritised in public health discussions. This review examines the historical treatment of rabies in British India, a disease which has received relatively less attention in the literature on Indian medical history. Human and animal rabies was widespread in British India, and treatment of bite victims imposed a major financial burden on the colonial Government of India. It subsequently became a driver of Pasteurism in India and globally and a key component of British colonial scientific enterprise. Efforts to combat rabies led to the establishment of a wide network of research institutes in India and important breakthroughs in development of rabies vaccines. As a result of these efforts, rabies no longer posed a significant threat to the British, and it declined in administrative and public health priorities in India towards the end of colonial rule—a decline that has yet to be reversed in modern-day India. The review also highlights features of the administrative, scientific and societal approaches to dealing with this disease in British India that persist to this day.

Keywords: stray dogs; Pasteur Institute; vaccination; colonial; British India; Civil Veterinary Department

---

1. Introduction

"A bite from a mad dog is more dreaded than anything I know; which arises from the horribleness of the disease, the uncertainty of the animal's being mad, or of the infection being received: The not knowing at what period to expect the effects, or to feel confident of having escaped it, keeps the person in a state of cruel suspence (sic) for months, or even years."—Daniel Johnson, Sketches of Field Sports as followed by The Natives of India with observations on the animals (1822).

The World Health Organization (WHO) identifies neglected tropical diseases (NTDs) as a group of communicable diseases affecting over a billion people globally, primarily those living in poverty in low- and middle-income countries in the tropics and subtropics [1], imposing a significant economic burden on these countries. India has the dubious distinction of bearing the largest burden of at least 11 of these NTDs [2]. This list includes rabies, a viral infection caused primarily by the bite of infected hosts belonging to the mammalian order Carnivora (although all mammals, and in exceptional circumstances birds, can be infected), and less frequently the deposition of saliva on wounds or mucous membranes. In addition, it has the highest mortality rate of all known infectious agents, with nearly all individuals who develop clinical symptoms eventually dying [3]. Rabies has been eliminated (or historically been absent) in Western Europe and several island nations such as Japan, Australia and New Zealand (except for imported cases). In North America, domestic animal rabies in dogs and cats occurs infrequently, mainly through exposure to infected wildlife reservoir hosts [4]. However, in most rabies-endemic countries in Africa and Asia including India, domestic dogs are the main rabies reservoir and source of human exposure [4,5].

Of the 59,000 annual human deaths estimated to occur globally due to dog-mediated rabies, about 35% occur in India [4]. Over three-quarters of cases in India occur in rural communities with poor access to diagnostic facilities and post-exposure prophylaxis, which are key to preventing development of disease [5]. More than 95% of cases are caused by dog bites, largely because of the approximately 60 million stray/free-ranging dogs in the country [6], and many cases of human rabies go undetected, are misdiagnosed or are under-reported [7]. A significant proportion of cases (over one-third in a recent study) are children, and despite the availability of safe and effective vaccines, awareness of and access to post-exposure prophylaxis (PEP), including rabies immunoglobulin, continue to be poor [8].

Despite the high burden of human rabies in India, the disease is not notifiable and a structured surveillance system is yet to be put in place [7]. Rabies is not included in the list of diseases for which surveillance is routinely carried out by states and reported under the Integrated Disease Surveillance Project of the Indian Ministry of Health and Family Welfare [9]. Instead, dog bites and snake bites are to be reported separately (Diseases under surveillance: Presumptive (P form)) [9]. The absence of an organised national or regional system for rabies surveillance compounds the problem of poor availability of human and animal rabies incidence data [10]. Current estimates of the burden of rabies in India (over 20,000 human deaths annually) are based on an epidemiological study conducted in 2003 [5], and even this may be an underestimate of the true disease burden. Another study estimated that 12,700 human deaths from symptomatically identifiable furious rabies occurred in India in 2005 [11]. Most recently, a multicentric survey conducted in 2017 across seven Indian states estimated an annual incidence of animal exposures (bite, scratch or lick) of 1.26%, which was reportedly lower than previous estimates from India [12]. However, the authors acknowledged that, owing to the limited scale of their study, results could not be used to generate a country-level burden of potential rabies exposures.

A perusal of the Five-Year Plans for national development in independent India (post-1947) covering the period 1951 (when the first five-year plan was unveiled) to 2002 reveals that rabies was never prioritised for control. During this period, the very term "rabies" appears only twice—once in the fourth plan (1969–1974) while listing the diseases for which research was conducted at the Central Research Institute at Kasauli and once in the sixth plan (1980–1985) in a brief description of mortality rates of environmentally linked diseases ("Diseases like TB, Gastro-intestinal infections, malaria, filaria, infectious hepatitis, rabbies (sic) and hook worm . . . ") [13]. The 10th plan (2002–2007) mentions the development of a new animal rabies vaccine "being tested for technology transfer", as well as research projects on a number of infectious diseases including rabies, although no further details are provided.

It is only in the 11th plan (2007–2012) that rabies control efforts are first mentioned in the form of pilot projects for the control of human rabies, for which 8.65 crore rupees (~2.1 million US dollars at the time) were allocated. For the first time in a Five-Year Plan, rabies control in animals, animal birth control and vaccination of stray dogs are also mentioned in this plan, as components of animal welfare to be handled by the Animal Welfare Board of India [13].

In 2014, the Ministry of Health and Family Welfare of the Government of India announced funding for a National Rabies Control Programme as part of the 12th five-year plan (2012–2017) [14]. This programme is coordinated by the National Centre for Disease Control, New Delhi, and the Animal Welfare Board of India, with the aim of halving human rabies deaths by the end of 2017. However, little information is available on the achievements of the programme, which finds no mention on the website of the national Ministry of Health and Family Welfare (https://mohfw.gov.in/) or the NITI Aayog (https://niti.gov.in/), which replaced the Planning Commission of India in 2015. A search for the term "rabies" on the Open Government Data Platform India (https://data.gov.in) returns no results [15]. The annual budget for 2018 presented by the Finance Minister of India allocated 40 crore rupees (approximately 6.13 million US dollars) for a few pilot schemes under the National Rural Health Mission, which includes control of human rabies [16]. This amount has been reduced to 25 crore rupees (approximately 3.51 million US dollars) in 2019 [17] and 2020 [18].

Given this background, it is natural to assume that rabies has always been accorded low priority in India. However, a quick glance through the literature on rabies in pre-independence India (before 1947) suggests otherwise. Rabies was one of several "tropical" afflictions, including cholera, plague, typhoid, tuberculosis, polio and snakebites, that were viewed as serious medical and public health problems, particularly for British residents in India. Consequently, it was subjected to great research and control efforts by the British colonial Government of India (hereafter referred to as GoI), frequently using native Indians as subjects for experimentation to develop and refine vaccines [19]. The effort to combat rabies and other infectious diseases was instrumental in the establishment of a wide network of research institutes in India and some important breakthroughs in development of rabies vaccines. However, the disease appears to have gradually lost priority in scientific circles and the colonial GoI, which may be the basis for its continued neglect in modern India. In this historical context, underlying reasons for the present-day underprioritisation of rabies in post-independence India need to be explored, as these may provide insights into what needs to change in order for rabies control in India to receive the priority and resources it deserves.

We used the search terms "rabies" (and variations of its spelling—"rabbies", "rabeis" and "rabes"), "hydrophobia" and "India" to review a range of historical archives and online and physical documents about rabies in pre-independence India (covering the period from the early 1800s to 1947, when India gained independence from British rule, and the few years immediately after). These included articles published in scientific journals (via PubMed and Google Scholar) and popular magazines, historical documents held at the India Office Records and Private Papers of the British Library and the Wellcome Library at the Wellcome Collection, online archives of the Medical History of British India maintained by the National Library of Scotland (https://digital.nls.uk/indiapapers/), British Parliamentary Papers available via ProQuest UK Parliamentary Papers, historical newspapers available via ProQuest Historical Newspapers and documents available online at the Hathi Trust (www.hathitrust.org) and libraries of the universities of Oxford and Cambridge.

2. Rabies Documentation in Pre-Independence India

As one of the oldest diseases known to man, rabies was widely documented by the earliest human civilisations [20]. A disease akin to rabies was recognised in ancient Indian treatises on health and medicine. The *Susruta Samhita* (*Susruta's Compendium*) is an ancient Indian text of Ayurveda (written between 1000 BCE and the first or second century CE), the Indian system of traditional medicine still practised in most parts of the country. This text details various medical conditions and surgical procedures and discusses in detail the symptoms of rabies in humans bitten by rabid dogs or wildlife, recognising that once symptoms develop in human bite victims, the disease is inevitably fatal [21]. The Mughal emperor Jahangir (1569–1627) is recorded to have noted the symptoms of rabies in an elephant that he owned [22]. It is also highly likely that rabies was documented extensively in the numerous vernacular languages on the Indian subcontinent.

Accounts of British medical and military personnel who worked in India during the 1800s highlight the fact that rabies, also referred to as hydrophobia, was widespread throughout India, responsible for the deaths of numerous Indian, British and European citizens [23–25]. The disease also caused extensive mortality in livestock and pet animals such as purebred dogs owned by British officials [23,26]. These accounts identified the occurrence of large populations of free-roaming ("stray") dogs and to a lesser extent wildlife, predominantly jackals, as the main source of infection [23,25,27]. A collection of observations on life in India by a former surgeon of the East India Company (1822) includes a chapter titled "Observations on hydrophobia and rabid animals" that describes symptoms in humans in graphic detail [23]. The same chapter and other reports provide detailed descriptions of the progress of rabies in infected pet dogs and wildlife, recounting behavioural changes as symptoms began to manifest [23,26,27]. These symptoms included changes in temperament with increased displays of affection or misdirected aggression, changes in vocalisation which were often noticed by Indian caretakers and changes in appetite, varying from voracious consumption of food to eventual rejection. In one instance, a rabid pup that was bitten by a (presumably rabid) hyena interrupted a dance party, resulting in the party having to be broken up and the pup being killed immediately [23].

These accounts also detail the experiences of British military doctors who often had to treat patients with symptoms of rabies and their agony at having to witness progression of the disease and inevitable death [23]. Much effort was put into discovering ways to treat infected individuals and potential modes of treatment, including traditional Indian cures, were keenly discussed in medical circles [24,28,29]. Even at this time, it was well recognised that treating bite wounds as soon as possible after bites occurred was key to preventing disease progression [23,24]. A letter to the editor *of The Lancet* in 1829 discusses the symptoms of rabies, disputing whether it should also be referred to as "hydrophobia", and possible ways of treatment including bleeding of patients in India [29]. A booklet on Ayurvedic treatments for various illnesses published in 1876 from Cochin, in present-day Kerala, includes symptoms of rabies and traditional treatment methods for exposure to "peppatti visham" (poison from a rabid/mad dog) such as chants, and pills and powders made from plant parts [30]. Various other treatments including Buisson baths [31] and cauterising wounds with caustic agents (e.g., nitric acid) [24,26] have also been documented. Rabies was also a significant health concern for British military personnel stationed in India, and pensions were given to the family of military personnel who died of rabies contracted in the line of duty [32].

Various aspects of rabies also found their way into Indian and British newspapers and magazines, ranging from individual theories about how the disease occurs ("a disease engendered by the practice in England of docking the tails of so many of our sporting and household dogs.") (1861) [33]; reports of incidents of rabid dog bites [34] and outbreaks in wildlife [35]; descriptions of encounters with rabid dogs, symptoms observed and suggested control measures ("lunar caustic ... apply it well to every wound.") (1859) [36]; and an account of a former army officer who claimed to have successfully recovered from rabies after being exposed in India with a detailed description of his symptoms (1836) [37]. Indian newspapers also reprinted articles about rabies that were initially published in British newspapers [38].

Such news reports and readers' letters to editors make evident that stray dogs, dog bites and rabies were an important public concern, particularly in major cities like Bombay (present-day Mumbai), Poona (present-day Pune), Lahore and Calcutta (present-day Kolkata) where many British and European citizens lived [39–44] and where significant numbers of cases were often reported [45,46]. Public awareness about rabies among British residents would also have been high when rabies was a major threat in Britain during the Victorian era and for a long time after its elimination in 1902 [47]. Complaints about "mad dogs" in India can be found in letters published as early as 1861 [33]. In addition to humans, purebred pet dogs were frequently infected [39,43] and British residents constantly demanded action from authorities to control rabies and stray dog populations [39,48,49], even proposing that private contributions be used to fund control measures [44]. Such concerns about rabies control also need to be located within discourses of sanitation, hygiene and urban improvement that were emerging in British India since the late 1800s [50]. These discourses were a product of the burden imposed by infectious diseases on British army personnel in India [50], and in rapidly expanding cities like Bombay and Calcutta, where epidemics of plague, cholera, measles and smallpox were frequently reported, particularly among the city's poor [51,52].

3. Pasteur Institutes and Rabies Vaccination in British India

The discovery of a rabies vaccine by Louis Pasteur, Emile Roux and other colleagues in 1885 [20,53] was a ground-breaking medical milestone, resulting in the establishment of Pasteur Institutes (PIs) in various parts of the world for production of rabies vaccines [54]. Initially, individuals exposed to rabies in India had to undertake a long journey to the PI in Paris for treatment, thereby affecting their chances of survival [54]; such journeys were often reported in newspapers [27,34,55–57]. These journeys were a major financial burden for the GoI, by one estimate costing £100 per person treated in 1911 (approximately £12,000 per person in 2019 terms) [58]. Recognising the need to bring rabies treatment to India ("if only for the protection of Europeans, and especially of the troops."), AV Lingard, Imperial bacteriologist at the Imperial Bacteriological Laboratory at Poona proposed in 1891 that "anti-rabic treatment and cure" could be started in the laboratory [54]. There was a public movement in the 1890s in India to gather support for the establishment of such institutes, described in detail by Chakrabarti (2012) [19]. The first PI in India started functioning at the hill station of Kasauli in 1900 under David Semple, a medical officer of the colonial Indian Medical Service [59]. It has been argued that this shift in the choice of locations from hot and humid Pune to the colder environment of Kasauli was driven primarily by a desire to maintain a distance from the native Indian population and to avoid the hot tropical climate of the Indian plains, rather than by scientific considerations [19].

Within a short period, the PI at Kasauli served as the main destination for treating an increasing numbers of individuals, both civilians and soldiers, exposed to rabies using vaccine produced at the institute [60,61] providing significant financial savings to the GoI by avoiding the costs of travel to Paris for treatment [58]. As a result of political pressure to decentralise rabies vaccination [19], PIs (or Pasteur sections within other institutions) were established throughout British India including at Coonoor in South India (1907) [62], Rangoon (in present-day Myanmar) (1915) [63], Shillong (East India) (1917), Bombay (1922) [64], Calcutta (1924) [19] and Patna (1928) [65]. Patients who were exposed through bites would often seek medical advice by sending a telegram to the PI, before deciding on travelling to the institute for treatment [66]. These PIs served thousands of individuals exposed to rabies from all parts of British India and Ceylon (present-day Sri Lanka) [67], even after India gained independence [68,69] and many continue to serve the same function to the present day [70].

Detailed statistics were collected on bite victims presenting for treatment to record information about which species bit them (dog, jackal, etc.), location, number, category and severity of bites (bites on head or face, bites through clothing, etc.), whether they completed the full course of vaccinations and the number of deaths post-vaccination—information which greatly improved scientific understanding about rabies [71]. From 1912, statistics on the number of individuals bitten by rabid animals and not seeking treatment were also compiled at Kasauli [61,72]. Hundreds of animals were also examined every year at PIs, veterinary colleges and other institutions like the Haffkine Institute in Bombay [61,62,73] to confirm a diagnosis of rabies. Thousands of copies of a pamphlet titled "Rabies and antirabic treatment in India" were printed and sent to local governments, with suggestions to translate these into local languages [63]. Updated editions of this pamphlet were published in subsequent years [74,75]. At one point, the Kasauli institute treated more patients every year than any other PI around the world [61,76].

Kasauli also became the site for extensive research into safer and more effective rabies vaccines, since the vaccines in use at the time often resulted in serious neurological complications [77]. One of the key events in the history of rabies vaccines was the development of a phenol-inactivated nerve tissue vaccine by David Semple based on Pasteur's original work and developed through experiments and trials on patients at Kasauli [78]. Used for decades in large parts of the world, production of the Semple vaccine has now been discontinued, although it is still produced for human or animal use in a few countries in Africa [4]. The development and evolution of these and other modern rabies vaccines have been covered in detail elsewhere [19,79,80].

Eventually, post-exposure treatment was also decentralised by opening "outcentres" throughout India, though not without opposition from John Cunningham, the Director of the PI at Kasauli in the 1920s who wanted to expand research on rabies vaccines at the institute [59,81]. A 1923 news report identifies such centres "at Karachi, Allahabad, Ahmednagar, Poona, Belgaum and Karwar" as well as Parel in Bombay [42]. These outcentres made it possible to greatly reduce delays in post-bite treatment, and the mortality rate among treated individuals in 1938 was reported to be 0.52%. By 1938, the Kasauli institute had over 140 outcentres in the northern provinces and other Indian states, while the Coonoor institute had 223 outcentres in Madras Presidency and southern states [82]. While public funds and government grants initially supported the establishment and functioning of PIs at Kasauli and Coonoor, the effectiveness of and demand for rabies vaccines developed at these centres meant that by the 1920s, these institutions started to function fully as private entities, with most of their income coming from the sale of rabies vaccines to government, municipal and local bodies and state hospitals [82].

4. Rabies Control in Animals

One of the earliest documented pieces of legislation for dealing with stray and rabid dogs in British India is regulation II of 1813, which permitted the destruction of ownerless dogs in Bombay city during specific periods of the year. The strict (and often overenthusiastic) enforcement of this regulation sometimes led to the destruction of owned dogs as well and is closely associated with what has been described as the "Bombay dog riots" of 1832. These riots, which also had communal overtones, have been described in detail elsewhere [83]. Other legislation included 'section 68 of the Cantonment Code of 1912', and provisions in Municipal Acts, which authorised cantonments or municipalities to detain or destroy confirmed or suspected rabid dogs as well as stray dogs. In municipalities, officers of the Civil Veterinary Department (CVD) were authorised to carry out these functions. Some Local Self-Government Acts also permitted issuing rewards for destruction of "noxious animals" [84].

A newspaper report from 1912 describes the system in Madras where dog capture was outsourced to "low caste dog-catchers", and dogs were "painlessly destroyed in a lethal chamber" [85]. It was proposed that a similar system be implemented in Bombay. A news report from 1923 describes the efforts of the Health Department of Bombay municipality in "diminishing the number of dangerous, diseased and stray dogs in the city". This was carried out by a team of "3 sub-inspectors, 2 dog carts, 8 cart drivers, 18 dog catchers and a lethal chamber ... in which dogs are destroyed by means of carbonic acid gas". The municipality reportedly spent about 10,000 rupees a year for this purpose, destroying 6579 and 6848 "ownerless dogs" and returning 22 and 6 dogs to their owners in 1921 and 1922, respectively [42]. Similar efforts were also reported from Calcutta [40] and Poona [41]. Lethal chambers and "electrocutors" for destruction of dogs were installed in local bodies—a report of the CVD of Madras Presidency (1929–1930) describes the inspection of lethal chambers in Tiruppur, Coonoor and Pollachi, construction of additional chambers at Erode and Udamalpet and an "electrocutor" at Ootacamund (present-day Ooty) [73]. However, one letter from a reader describing empty dog carts and the number of dogs on the road [39] suggests that such measures may have been no more effective in controlling dog populations and rabies than they were in more contemporary times. These measures and the methods used to kill dogs (carbonic acid gas, strychnine poisoning, clubbing to death, electrocution) [19,86] were opposed by many Indians due to religious reasons [41,83], by Indian vernacular newspapers and many British residents [19]. In addition to dogs, wildlife [74], predominantly jackals [87] were also often destroyed.

A host of other measures targeting owned dogs were largely modelled on measures implemented in Britain in the 1800s that had proven successful in making the country rabies-free by 1902 [47]. Officials recognised that owned dogs in India were often unconfined and thus could be infected with or spread rabies—one report proposed that owned female dogs that were allowed to roam freely when in oestrus resulted in increased dog fights and thus the spread of rabies [88]. Purebred dogs were often allowed to roam freely [89] or used by European soldiers to hunt pariah (unowned mongrels) dogs [19]. Such dogs risked reintroducing rabies into Britain or introducing it into other British colonies when their owners moved around the world [47,90]. Consequently, control measures included enforcing registration of owned dogs (purebred or pariah), levying a "dog tax" [19,86] and issuing badges or discs to be fitted to the collars of owned dogs [89]. Local authorities would thus be able to round up unowned dogs for destruction after 72 h, while straying owned dogs could be returned to their owners. Such a "tax and badge" policy was implemented in Shimla and Mussoorie and reported to function satisfactorily [91], while some local bodies were reportedly not keen on implementing these measures [92]. In military cantonments, kennels were set aside to isolate suspected rabid dogs for observation and destruction [93]. Some letters to newspapers proposed a ban on importation of dogs into India [49] while others argued that the quarantine of dogs imported into India would be pointless without first controlling rabies in the country [94].

As early as 1899, an annual administration report of the CVD in India highlighted the rise in number of rabies cases presented at Bombay and Lahore veterinary colleges and recommended that the GoI issue orders to prevent its spread in India [95]. However, whether rabies could ever be effectively controlled or eliminated in India appears to have been a contentious topic [96]. At the first meeting of veterinary officers in India, held at Lahore in 1919, veterinarians discussed the challenges of controlling stray dog populations and argued for mandatory licensing of all dogs and systematic destruction of strays [97]. The following resolution was adopted at this meeting—"That it is considered that any suitable measure that can be adopted for reducing and destroying the surplus population of dogs is desirable, but that it does not appear to be possible under the conditions prevailing in India to deal more effectively with the disease. Power should be given to veterinary practitioners to order the detention and destruction of dogs suffering from rabies." Based on this resolution, the GoI appears to have advised local bodies to give veterinary officers relevant powers to perform these functions [84]. At the same time, it voiced doubts about the feasibility of implementing such control measures in rural areas and appears to have left it to municipalities and local self-governments to deal with the problem. This approach appears to have persisted throughout the period of British rule in India and there seem to have been no policies for nationwide rabies control in animals. It was also believed that rabies could not be eliminated in India as it was also maintained in wildlife [91].

After the world's first rabies vaccine for dogs was developed in Japan in 1915, Umeno and Doi developed a single-dose canine rabies vaccine suitable for mass production in 1920 [98,99]. This vaccine was used for mass vaccination of dogs in Japan from 1924–25 [80,99]. In this context, experimental studies to develop a method of veterinary PEP ("anti-rabic inoculation of dogs bitten by rabid dogs"), presumably for valuable owned dogs, had begun at the Punjab Veterinary College in Lahore from 1915, also including horses in later years. These studies were inspired by work being conducted at the PI in Kasauli, fully recognising that the control of rabies in animals would benefit people as well [100]. A report of the Principal of this college in 1922–23 determined that rabies PEP of dogs could be considered an established mode of treatment (while also including caveats about conclusively establishing whether a dog was infected or not) [101]. Similar studies to develop preventive rabies vaccination in dogs were also started at the Madras Veterinary College from 1922 using rabies vaccine from the PI, Coonoor. Initial experiments were reported to be inconclusive because following vaccination, dogs from both experimental and control arms remained healthy after being infected with rabies virus [102].

Even prior to these studies, there are frequent reports of treatment of valuable animals exposed to rabies. For instance, two elephants owned by the Raja of Nilambur that were bitten by a rabid dog were given "anti-rabic treatment" in 1919–20, of which one elephant was confirmed by microscopic examination to have subsequently died of rabies. However the first record of the use of rabies vaccines for veterinary PEP, beyond those reported from the Punjab and Madras Veterinary Colleges, is found in a Madras CVD report from 1923–24, when ten animals were "treated with anti-rabic vaccine" at the veterinary hospital, Calicut (present-day Kozhikode in Kerala) [102].

From 1923, vaccines for veterinary use were issued from the PI, Coonoor, to veterinarians in Madras Presidency and Indian states [82]. The use of PEP to treat valuable animals (owned dogs, livestock at government livestock farms, equines and even a monkey) eventually started throughout most Indian provinces [102,103]. Vaccines were sourced from regional PIs, the Haffkine Institute in Bombay and the HK Mulford drug company in the USA [104]. By the 1930s and 1940s, veterinary PEP was being commonly administered at veterinary colleges and regional veterinary centres [45,73,104,105]. In response to rabies cases in Darjeeling municipality in 1933, legislation was enacted which required dog owners to vaccinate their dogs and to keep them muzzled or on a leash when in public [106].

A letter to a newspaper in 1935 complained that vaccination had failed to prevent the onset of rabies in some owned dogs [43]. Statistics of the number of patients treated at the PIs also reported figures for the number of animals vaccinated [68,107]. Between 1923 and 1948, 14,212 animals had been "prophylactically treated" at the PI in Coonoor [108]—these are all likely to have been owned.

However, the use of veterinary PEP seems to have been restricted to treating valuable owned animals, and mass vaccination of dogs for rabies control does not appear to have been seriously considered in British India. The studies conducted in Japan and the USA on preventive rabies vaccination of dogs as well as vaccination studies conducted at the Madras Veterinary College were discussed at the second meeting of veterinary officers in India, held at Calcutta in 1923. At this meeting, the opinion that rabies could never be eradicated in India persisted, and it was opined that vaccines would be useful only to reduce case numbers [84]. A newspaper report covering the conference stated that "The control of rabies in India constitutes one of the most difficult problems confronting both medical and veterinary authorities. The Conference resolved that the results of investigations upon the prophylactic vaccination of dogs against rabies should be referred to the Central Standing Advisory Committee on Epizootic Diseases and Research with a view to advising Government upon the desirability of enforcing measures of widespread inoculation of dogs against the disease." [109]. We found no records to suggest that mass vaccination of dogs was ever considered by local authorities or the GoI. Mass culling of stray and rabid dogs and registration and, in later years, vaccination of owned dogs appear to have been the most widely implemented rabies control measures in colonial-era India. Such measures were even supported by Mahatma Gandhi, a central figure in the Indian struggle for independence, who stated that "The multiplication of dogs is unnecessary. A roving dog without an owner is a danger to society and a swarm of them is a menace to its very existence" [110].

5. Historic Animal Rabies Incidence in India

Annual administration reports of the CVD provide a detailed picture of the prevalence of animal diseases in British provinces in India. Provinces and presidencies were comprised of districts and municipalities with veterinary dispensaries and diagnostic laboratories, as well as veterinary colleges in some provinces. These institutions reported the number of cases of animal diseases treated or diagnosed. Infectious disease statistics from the earliest CVD reports (1887 onwards) focused solely on those affecting productive livestock (cattle, buffalo, sheep and goats) or equines such as rinderpest, foot-and-mouth disease, haemorrhagic septicaemia, anthrax, surra, strangles, etc. Rabies was mentioned only when it affected these species, and the disease was often included in the category "Other" diseases. It is only from 1903-04 onwards that rabies cases in livestock and dogs, most likely owned, were explicitly recorded in tables of disease summaries. Subsequently, the number of cases recorded increased significantly (Figure 1), which may have been partly driven by a number of provincial administrations framing rules for rabies prevention (e.g., Madras in 1923–1924) [111].

Figure 1 presents the total number of animal rabies cases reported in all species (domestic and wildlife) between 1887–1888 and 1950–1951 across all provinces in British India. Case numbers reported from lower administrative levels (districts and municipalities), from regional veterinary colleges and/or diagnostic laboratories have been combined to present a breakdown by province/state in Figure 2. The Supplementary Information and Table S1 within contain more details on how rabies statistics were presented and compiled [112–115]. These reports indicate that animal rabies was endemic and widespread throughout all provinces in British India, affecting all species of domestic animals, most commonly dogs, and wildlife. Officials frequently highlighted their concerns about alarming increases in rabies cases and recommended implementation of control measures [96,100]. Outbreaks were occasionally reported, necessitating PEP treatment of several animals—for instance, the spike in cases in Bengal province in 1935–1936 when 950 animal rabies cases were reported from all districts [46] (Figure 1). CVD staff were often exposed to rabies and had to undergo PEP at PIs [116].

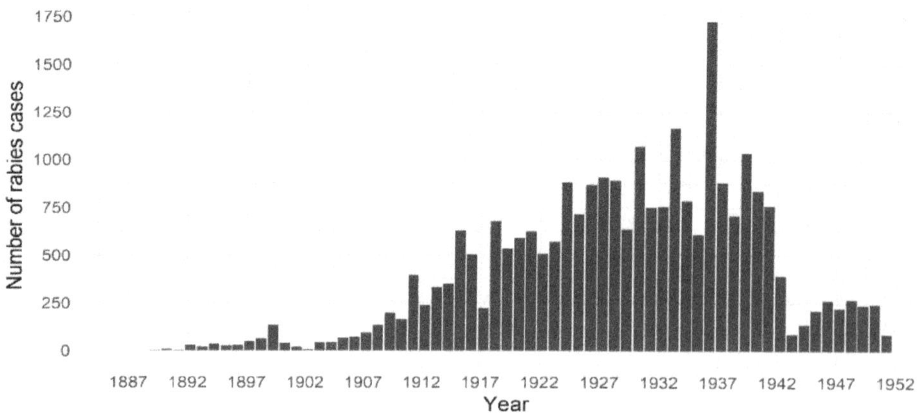

Figure 1. Total number of rabies cases reported each year in all animal species in British India between 1887 and 1951 (annual data span April to the following March, e.g., April 1887 to March 1888). Statistics were compiled from annual reports of the Civil Veterinary Department of the colonial British Government of India, available at https://digital.nls.uk/indiapapers/.

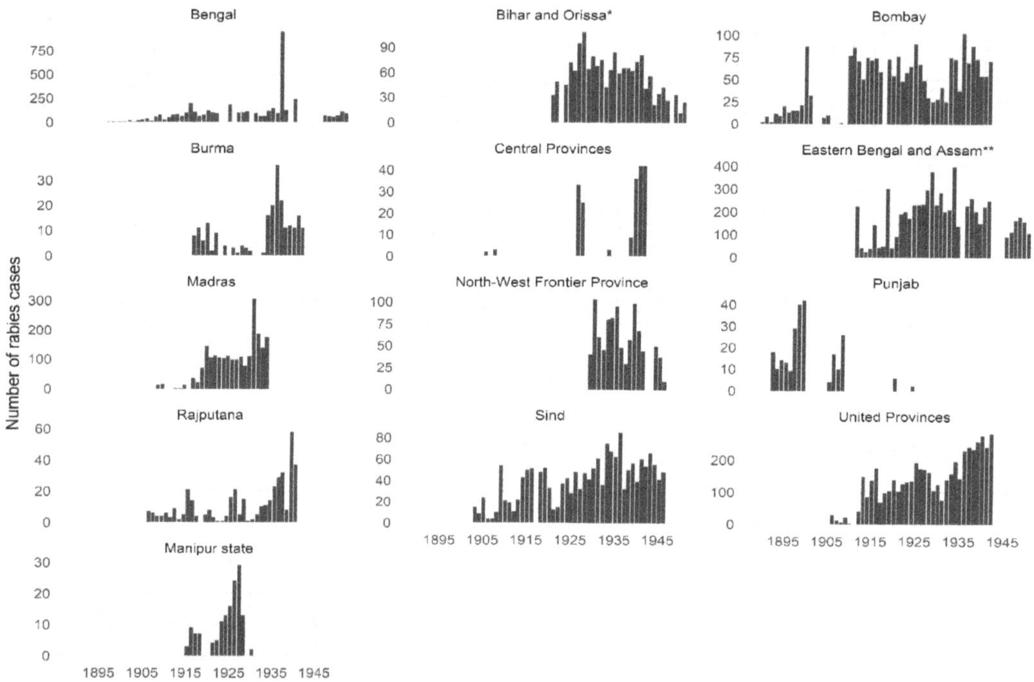

* 1911–12 to 1935–36—Bihar and Orissa provinces, 1936–37 to 1949–50—Bihar only; ** 1907–08 to 1910-11—Eastern Bengal and Assam provinces, 1912–13 to 1949-50—Assam only.

Figure 2. Annual rabies incidence in all animal species between 1887 and 1951 (annual data span April to the following March, e.g., April 1887 to March 1888) in every British province in India (except Baluchistan for which no data were available) and the princely state of Manipur. Statistics were compiled from annual reports of the Civil Veterinary Department of the colonial British Government of India, available at https://digital.nls.uk/indiapapers/. Note the different scale of the *y*-axis for each region.

CVD reports also highlight the wide variation in numbers of rabies cases reported from various provinces (Figure 2). In line with the lack of a consistent policy for rabies control in animals, there was little consistency in reporting of animal rabies cases [115]. Statistics compiled by Chakarabarti (2012) show that between 1880 and 1935 rabies caused an average of 160–170 human deaths per year in Punjab province [19]. However, the few animal rabies cases that are reported from Punjab province appear during the late 1800s and early 1900s, following which cases are reported only sporadically

(Figure 2). It was often acknowledged that reported statistics of animal rabies incidence were likely to be underestimates of the true disease burden [115,117], which was sometimes attributed to a lack of public interest in reporting cases to veterinary officials [92]. There is a marked drop in the number of recorded animal rabies cases after 1941 (Figure 1), possibly because many provinces stopped reporting cases after this period (Figure 2).

Veterinary institutions charged a fee for admission and treatment of cases [118]. Some CVD reports indicate that while there was high demand for rabies PEP, the cost of treatment was unaffordable for poor animal owners and officials were unable to provide it free of cost [45,73]. A 1928–29 CVD report from Madras Presidency describes how poor dog and livestock owners could not afford the cost of PEP for their animals and were advised to administer "indigo blue" instead [114]. In later years, PIs charged for testing brain samples (ten rupees per brain sample in 1933–34), which made this service unaffordable for poor farmers [116]. Such barriers to treatment and diagnosis are likely to have influenced estimates of the true rabies burden and efforts to limit its spread.

6. The Origins of Its Neglect?

Chakrabarti (2012) discusses in detail the various ethical, moral and political debates around scientific research and treatment for rabies in colonial India [19]. It is debatable whether the motives behind the research and development of vaccines and control efforts targeting rabies and other diseases in India were purely altruistic or driven by imperial ambitions and a scientific fascination for tropical illnesses [77,119]. However, it is evident that colonial British governments in India invested time and resources to control rabies (among other diseases) in the country and so the disease could hardly be considered "neglected" from today's perspective.

Given what has been described thus far, what might explain the neglect of rabies by public health practitioners and policymakers in modern-day India? Could it be driven by a perception that rabies had declined sufficiently to justify focusing on other more important human diseases? Dog bites and rabies clearly continued to be major public health concerns in India long after PIs started to save lives from the early 1900s. This is evident from newspaper reports and letters to newspapers from the public [35,39,40,42,93,120,121] as well as official reports and documents of the PIs and the GoI [63,77,122]. Annual reports from the PIs reveal a rapid rise in the number of patients vaccinated against rabies annually. The number of patients treated at the PI in Coonoor and its outcentres increased from under 200 in 1907 to 13,000 in 1935 [77], highlighting the high burden of animal bites in regions served by the institute. This increase was frequently attributed to wider awareness of the availability and benefits of "Pasteurian treatment" rather than any actual increase in rabies [61,63,123].

At the same time, it is not clear that human deaths from rabies reduced substantially in British India. As mentioned above, Chakarabarti (2012) found that around 160 to 170 people died of rabies every year in Punjab province between 1880 and 1935 [19]. This is despite the presence of the PI at Kasauli and the Lahore veterinary college in this province. In 1913, 243 rabies-related deaths were reported from the Central Provinces and Berar [63]. Similarly, 220 deaths were reported in India in 1922, with the report acknowledging that this figure was an underestimate of the true incidence [122]. A letter to the *Times of India* in 1911 speculated that the true number of dog bites and rabies deaths in India was likely to be much higher than those stated in reports from the PI [49]. It was recognised that not everyone completed the full course of post-exposure vaccinations and it was not possible to follow up on outcomes for all patients [122]. As human deaths from rabies in the general population outside those attending the PIs were not systematically recorded, the true death toll may have been much higher.

An examination of human disease statistics and discourses around public health in British India provides some hints about administrative and health priorities vis-à-vis rabies. Notwithstanding concerns raised by the public or officials of the CVD, provincial administrations did not consider rabies to be a concern compared to deaths from other contagious diseases or snakebites [19]. In the late 1800s, mortality statistics from British India included rabies deaths under the broad heading of "Injuries", which covered a wide variety of conditions (suicide, wounds or accidents, snakebite, injuries caused by wild beasts, etc.) [124,125]. Before the establishment of the PI in India, rabies occasionally killed several soldiers stationed in India (69 deaths in 1879–80, 146 in 1885–86), though considerably fewer than the thousands of deaths every year due to diseases like cholera or smallpox [124,125].

With the advent of PIs and the race within scientific circles around the world to develop safer and more effective rabies vaccines, detailed records began to be maintained in India of the number of people vaccinated from broad ethnic (European and Indian) or religious (Muslim, Hindu, others) groups, those developing complications or dying post-vaccination, the number of patients that completed the full course of vaccination and differences in mortality rates between European and Indian patients [71,126,127].

Such statistics were published in annual reports of PIs [71], scientific journals [91] and, during the early 1900s, regularly included in annual reports presented to the UK Houses of Parliament [61–63,123,127–130]. These efforts served to establish the safety and efficacy of different vaccines being developed at the PIs and improve scientific understanding about rabies. For instance, in a letter written in 1911, W.F. Harvey, the then Director of the PI of Kasauli, recommended the collection of statistics by local bodies on the number of people bitten by rabid animals and who subsequently die without being vaccinated. His aim in suggesting this was to prove that the true mortality rate for rabies was much lower than that reported in statistics from Europe. He stated that this would involve "two or three years' work only", within which period he expected to prove his hypothesis [72]. In several significant respects, India was at the forefront of global research on rabies and the PI at Kasauli was central to this enterprise [19].

Statistical abstracts and reports of burden of illnesses in British India were split into sections—the first dealt with morbidity and mortality in the European Army in India, followed by the Native army (later referred to as the "Indian" army), the general population and jails [61–63,67,126,127,130]. Individuals treated for rabies at PIs were categorised as Europeans (including Eurasians/Anglo-Indians) and natives/Indians and further into soldiers and civilians. The number of Europeans vaccinated against rabies did not increase substantially over the years and few ever died of rabies. The number of Indians vaccinated increased annually, as did the number of recorded deaths (Table 1).

At the same time, overall rabies-related mortality continued to be much lower than mortality from other contagious diseases. Of 22,579 patients vaccinated between 1912 and 1916, only 135 (including 4 Europeans) died. This is in marked contrast with mortality from diseases like cholera (1,259,012 deaths between 1914 and 1917) and plague (1,599,088 deaths in the same period) [131]. At the second meeting of veterinary officers in 1923, it was even remarked that the money spent on rabies control in India would prove more beneficial if diverted for the control of cholera [132]. Indeed, diseases like cholera, plague, smallpox and malaria frequently caused extensive epidemics in India (e.g., the First Cholera Pandemic (1817–1821) [133], the plague epidemic in Bombay (1896) [50]) and high human mortality requiring active interventions by the state [50]. This focus on epidemic diseases would have been in marked contrast with rabies, which was, and continues to be to this day, characterised by fewer cases and only occasional outbreaks in animals [35,46]. Such outbreaks were handled by mass culling of dogs or jackals [87,89] and, following the development of vaccines, by PEP administration to human and animal bite victims.

Table 1. Number of people given rabies post-exposure prophylaxis at various Pasteur Institutes in India. Category totals may not always match as the breakdown of the number of patients treated and the number of deaths was not always explicitly reported.

Year	Numbers Treated (Number of Deaths)			Reference
	European	Native/Indian	Total	
1900–1901 [1]	146 (1)	175 (9)	321 (10)	[130]
1901–1902 [1]	215 (2)	328 (11)	543 (13)	[130]
1902–1903 [1]	269 (1)	315 (12)	584 (12)	[130]
1903–1904 [1]	248 (0)	364 (10)	612 (10)	[130]
1904–1905 [1]	307 (0)	570 (12)	877 (12)	[130]
1905–1906 [1]	342 (2)	803 (19)	1145 (21)	[130]
1906–1907 [1]	452 (2)	846 (17)	1308 (19)	[130]
Interim, 09/08–31/12, 1907 [1]	146 (1)	373 (4)	519 (5)	[130]
1908 [2]	342 (2)	1047 (24)	1729 (26)	[128,130]
1909 [2]	675 (3)	1920 (25)	2595 (28)	[126,130]
1910 [2]	575 (0)	2325 (43)	2900 (43)	[127,130]
1911 [2]	297(1)	2911 (50)	3208 (51)	[130]
1912 [2]	400 (0)	4388 (59)	4788 (59)	[61]
1913 [2]	2 (2)	5271 (66)	5273 (68)	[129]
1914 [2]	NA (1)	NA (60)	5795 (61)	[63]
1915 [2]	468 (1)	6409 (41)	6877 (42)	[123]
1933 [1]	1356 (0)	14,582 (83)	15,938 (83)	[134]
1936 [1]	1357 (0)	NA (97)	NA (97)	[135]
1938 [3]	NA (NA)	NA (NA)	12,396 (21)	[68]

[1] Figures for Kasauli institute only; [2] figures combined for all Pasteur institutes in India, where available; [3] Coonoor institute and its subsidiary centres only; NA—not available.

As mentioned previously, there was also an emerging discourse around sanitation and urban improvement in colonial India from the late 1800s [50–52]. A range of sanitary reforms were implemented from this period, particularly aimed at improving the health of European army personnel who initially suffered significantly higher morbidity and mortality from epidemics in India when compared to Indian soldiers. Sanitary measures such as the provision of piped and filtered water, relocating barracks from swampy areas and improvements in drainage and preventive vaccination against smallpox and plague caused a remarkable and consistent decline in morbidity and mortality among British troops in India [50]. Such sanitary measures would have had little impact on rabies, which would not have been seen to be as amenable to human modification of environmental conditions. Preventive vaccination of humans against rabies, as practised for smallpox, would hardly have been considered necessary, given the sporadic nature of the disease. These epidemiological characteristics of rabies are likely to have greatly influenced colonial perceptions of what diseases could be reasonably controlled through public health interventions.

A similar situation existed with rabies in animals in India. CVD officials were more concerned with the treatment, control and prevention of diseases affecting equines and livestock, which were largely unaffected by rabies. For instance, in 1935-36, when Bengal province experienced rabies outbreaks in multiple districts and recorded 950 cases (Figure 2), the number of livestock deaths from rinderpest and haemorrhagic septicaemia was 35,281 and 3989, respectively [46]. This is unlike the situation reported in Trinidad, for instance, where between 1925 and 1958 repeated outbreaks of rabies transmitted by bats threatened the livestock industry, prompting widespread vaccination campaigns for cattle and efforts to destroy bat populations. As a result, rabies was accorded high government priority for control and elimination in Trinidad with WHO assistance, and much research was conducted on this topic [136]. Dog rabies had also been eliminated in Britain in 1902, and barring occasional outbreaks seeded by dogs brought into the country, rabies ceased to be the significant domestic public health concern it once had been for British politicians and policymakers [47]. This may also have contributed to the gradual loss of interest in investing in rabies control and prevention in British India.

The success of Semple's vaccine in reducing human rabies deaths in India was soon recognised by the global scientific community, and it began to be widely used around the world [81]. By the 1930s, statistics from the PIs continued to be published in scientific journals [108,134,135] but were no longer included in reports to the UK Parliament. During this period, one also finds a return to the practice of including rabies deaths under the head of "Injuries" [137,138]. While research to make the Semple vaccine safer did continue, the key personnel driving this research left the PI or were transferred, and research on other diseases began to take precedence. The PI at Kasauli was shut down in 1939, with work being shifted to the Central Research Institute next door [19]. Research on rabies vaccines and diagnosis continued to be conducted at the Coonoor PI after Indian independence in 1947, spearheaded by the institute's Director N. Veeraraghavan [139], but rabies no longer appears to have been accorded the same priority it once was in British India during the early 20th century.

Thus, despite the importance given to rabies in India with the advent of Pasteurism, a combination of factors is likely to have contributed to its eventual decline in administrative and public health priorities. In particular, the success of Semple's vaccines in preventing human rabies deaths will have influenced administrative officials to prioritise scarce resources towards competing and more pressing public health interventions (e.g., improving sanitation and addressing epidemics). A point to this effect is made in an anecdote in a CVD report about rabies control becoming a priority only "when the deaths amongst humans numbered some scores annually, and a genuine feeling of alarm for personal safety was felt" [140]. In this respect, rabies in British India may have become a victim of its own success, something which is recognised today in Latin America as canine rabies control has become more effective and human mortality has reduced dramatically [141].

7. Impacts on Present-Day Debates in India

Much literature exists on the medical history of a range of infectious diseases that caused major epidemics in British India, including malaria, cholera, plague and smallpox [50,51,142]. This review has examined the historical treatment in British India of rabies as a public health concern, a topic which has received relatively less attention. From being a widespread and untreatable illness, rabies rose to become a driver of Pasteurism in India and globally and a key component of British colonial scientific enterprise. The disease, however, eventually declined in administrative and public health priorities in India towards the end of colonial rule—a decline that has yet to be reversed in modern-day India. In charting this history of rabies, the review highlights features of the colonial administrative, scientific and societal approach to dealing with this disease in India that remarkably persist in the country nearly a century later.

Key among these are the interrelated issues of an absence of a rabies control policy at the national level and of systems for rabies surveillance in humans and animals [7]. Notwithstanding the existence of a National Rabies Control Programme [14], India lacks a well-considered roadmap with realistic milestones to chart progress towards effective national rabies control, let alone elimination by 2030, the target set by the WHO for global elimination of human deaths from dog-mediated rabies [4]. Policy formulation and implementation continue to be the responsibility of states and local bodies, and these are consequently inconsistent. For instance, only two states (Tamil Nadu and Sikkim) have made human rabies notifiable [143]. As was the case in colonial India, animal rabies is not seen as an economically relevant disease affecting animal production systems and hence is not prioritised for control by agriculture or animal husbandry ministries [144].

Rabies in animals was widespread in space and time across British India (Figure 2). The mean number of animal rabies cases recorded between 1903–04 and 1950–51 was 522. This is likely to be an underestimate given that reporting was unsystematic and not mandatory and reported numbers do not include cases from most princely states and territories not under direct British control. The human population of India has risen from 361 million in 1951 to over 1.2 billion in 2011 [145], and the population of dogs has increased correspondingly. In the absence of any comprehensive rabies control measures, it therefore stands to reason that the number of animal rabies cases will also have increased significantly.

Although animal rabies is notifiable in India today, disease reporting is acknowledged to be unreliable even by rabies experts in India [143], and rabies statistics such as those reported by the CVD are difficult to access. This makes the task of estimating the true prevalence in animals extremely difficult. Such gaps in knowledge of the human and animal disease burden and patchy awareness of rabies as a public health threat [146], even among medical health professionals [147], significantly hinder the development of political, scientific and societal urgency to address this burden, particularly in rural areas which bear the biggest brunt [5].

One positive change from the colonial-era approach to rabies control in India is with respect to dog population management (DPM). Although culling of dogs continued to be the mainstay of DPM and rabies control efforts for decades after independence, the Animal Birth Control (ABC) (Dogs) Rules established in 2001 outlawed this inhumane measure [148]. It was replaced by a policy of sterilisation and anti-rabies vaccination (ABC-ARV), carried out once during a dog's lifetime, after which it was returned to its original location. However, in the absence of scientifically robust methods to obtain reliable estimates of dog population sizes, ABC-ARV is implemented in a haphazard and uncoordinated manner across local bodies and states, involving various public [149,150] and private entities [151]. The policy also does not account for the need to revaccinate sterilised dogs to maintain anti-rabies immunity in the dog population and, consequently, the possibility that these dogs may continue to bite and transmit rabies to other dogs and people [152]. Rule 10 of the ABC Rules prohibits the euthanasia of dogs suspected to be rabid, instead requiring such dogs to be isolated until they die naturally of rabies [148], followed by laboratory confirmation of disease [153]. This is clearly a welfare issue for infected dogs. Enforcement of the ABC rules is also inconsistent, and culling of dogs still occurs occasionally throughout India [154], often in retaliation to incidents of injuries or deaths from dog attacks [155].

There is also a flawed perception of ABC-ARV as more than just a DPM tool. Consequently, this measure is increasingly viewed as the primary rabies control measure in India, perceived to be unsuccessful in reducing disease only because of ineffective and/or inadequate implementation [156]. This perception is despite the fact that the WHO itself recommends sterilisation of dogs only as a supportive measure to maintain levels of rabies vaccination coverage achieved through mass rabies vaccination, accepted as the most scientific method for rabies control [4]. A recent study was unable to evaluate the role of surgical sterilisation in controlling dog rabies due to poor data collection or reporting and recommended that mass vaccination should continue to be the control method of choice [157]. The ABC-ARV policy also finds support through discourses that argue for the continued existence of street dogs as "integral inhabitants of the multispecies city" [156].

Wang (2019) describes the conflict that existed in New York City from the early 20th century, between the American Society for Prevention of Cruelty to Animals and the Department of Health, over population control and muzzling of the city's free-roaming dogs [158]. No such conflict appears to have existed over dog culling in colonial India. On the contrary, there is in India today an impasse, along the lines of that which existed in New York, between two conflicting perspectives of the place of dogs on the streets, with direct impacts on rabies control efforts. On the one hand is the view that there should be a holistic approach to control stray dog populations on public health, wildlife conservation [159] and animal welfare grounds. This approach would require enforcing responsible dog ownership, civic waste and humane dog population management and a national mass rabies vaccination programme [4,152], eventually leading to the elimination of free-roaming dogs. On the other hand is the view, held primarily by animal welfare campaigners, that dogs have the right to exist on the streets and to be fed by people [160]. This latter view consequently favours ABC-ARV as the most appropriate DPM and rabies control measure, notwithstanding its drawbacks. Nadal (2020) discusses various aspects of the conflicting perspectives about DPM and rabies control, as well as the complex social, cultural and political contexts within which people and dogs interact in two major cities in North India [161].

In this respect, the ABC-ARV policy has made it difficult to adopt comprehensive measures to deal with the persistent threat of rabies posed by the large populations of unowned free-roaming dogs in

India [144], particularly implementation of mass dog vaccination. Despite evidence from the 1920s that mass vaccination of dogs successfully reduces rabies incidence and can eliminate it [98,99], there were no attempts to implement such a measure in colonial India. Instead, it was widely considered that rabies could never be effectively eliminated in India. This perception continues to hold sway at the highest levels of government to this day with the view that logistical constraints make mass vaccination of dogs unfeasible in India [162]. It is left to state administrations to implement mass vaccination policies, commonly in partnership with nongovernmental organisations [163,164].

In another unfortunate parallel with the colonial era, there is little emphasis on promoting responsible dog ownership practices such as confinement and vaccination of owned dogs in India. It is unclear how successful attempts were by colonial administrations to enforce registration and identification of owned dogs. While several local bodies have now made such measures mandatory in India, they are poorly enforced [165]. Rabies vaccination, while largely confined to owned dogs, primarily valuable pure breeds, is also not mandatory. This often results in poor compliance with vaccination regimens [165], especially in the case of owned mongrel dogs (i.e., those that do not belong to any specific breed), from poorer households who have greater difficulty accessing veterinary services. A high proportion of this latter category of dogs are also poorly confined, frequently resulting in the birth of unwanted pups and increased risk of contracting rabies from interactions with free-roaming unowned dogs [166].

8. Conclusions

Notwithstanding poor availability of disease data, the case may be made that rabies does not impose the kind of human health burden in India that diseases such as tuberculosis, malaria and HIV do. Consequently, rabies control may not be seen as a cost-effective public health investment, a view that was certainly shared by public health practitioners in British India [132]. Such a perspective, however, fails to consider the impact of rabies on individuals from rural backgrounds, particularly children [8], and the near certainty of death in the absence of access to treatment before symptoms appear. As an entirely vaccine-preventable disease disproportionately affecting the poor in low- and middle-income countries, preventing unnecessary human rabies deaths and suffering by addressing barriers to access to human PEP is an important means of achieving social justice [167]. At the same time, the cost of human PEP provision can be substantial (30 million US dollars over an unspecified timeframe in India, by one estimate) [143]. Rabies control through mass dog vaccination has been consistently shown to be more cost-effective in preventing human rabies deaths [168,169]. With the science and tools for rabies control already existing, rabies elimination is low-hanging fruit and a textbook example of the One Health approach in action. This is well recognised even in India, with zoonotic disease prioritisation exercises frequently identifying rabies as one of the main diseases for targeting control efforts [170,171]. Political will has been key to implementing effective control measures in many countries around the world [4] and is the primary factor currently hindering progress on this front in India today.

Rabies in British India was clearly not a "neglected" public health concern. Early rabies vaccines were highly effective in saving human lives, although there remained a poor understanding of the true disease burden in Indian society. These factors, combined with changing priorities of colonial British governments, in all likelihood contributed to a progressive loss of priority of rabies control in the face of the vast array of competing infectious disease and public health challenges in British India. It may be possible to argue that the current neglect of rabies in India is a legacy, albeit unintended, of British colonial rule, but this clearly is no justification for carrying on in the same vein. Current public health professionals and policy makers should look to the extensive historic and current scientific literature on evidence-based rabies control measures to formulate a strategy to achieve the lofty goal of elimination of dog-mediated human rabies deaths by 2030. Equally crucial will be measures to deal with the extensive free-roaming dog population in India, without which rabies control efforts will become unsustainable in the long run.

Author Contributions: Conceptualization, S.R.; methodology, S.R.; formal analysis, S.R.; investigation, S.R.; data curation, S.R.; writing—original draft preparation, S.R.; writing—review and editing, S.R., A.T.V., P.N. and C.A.D.; visualization, S.R.; supervision, S.R., A.T.V., P.N. and C.A.D.; project administration, S.R. and C.A.D.; funding acquisition, S.R. All authors have read and agreed to the published version of the manuscript.

Acknowledgments: We thank Vidhya Raveendranathan for her invaluable feedback on this paper. We acknowledge and appreciate the enormous effort of librarians and staff at various libraries (British Library, Wellcome library, National Library of Scotland and other libraries around the world) in preserving, maintaining and making accessible immensely valuable historical records. We are grateful for the valuable feedback from readers of the preprint of this manuscript and from the three anonymous reviewers, which greatly improved this paper.

References

1. WHO|Neglected Tropical Diseases. Available online: http://www.who.int/neglected_diseases/diseases/en/ (accessed on 21 March 2020).
2. Hotez, P.J.; Damania, A. India's neglected tropical diseases. *PLoS Negl. Trop. Dis.* **2018**, *12*, e0006038. [CrossRef] [PubMed]
3. Hanlon, C.A.; Childs, J.E. Chapter 3—Epidemiology. In *Rabies*, 3rd ed.; Jackson, A.C., Ed.; Academic Press: Boston, MA, USA, 2013; pp. 61–121, ISBN 978-0-12-396547-9.
4. WHO. *WHO Expert Consultation on Rabies: Third Report*; Abela-Ridder, B., Ed.; World Health Organization: Geneva, Switzerland, 2018; ISBN 9789241210218.
5. Sudarshan, M.K.; Madhusudana, S.N.; Mahendra, B.J.; Rao, N.S.N.; Ashwath Narayana, D.H.; Abdul Rahman, S.; Meslin, F.-X.; Lobo, D.; Ravikumar, K. Gangaboraiah Assessing the burden of human rabies in India: Results of a national multi-center epidemiological survey. *Int. J. Infect. Dis.* **2007**, *11*, 29–35. [CrossRef] [PubMed]
6. Gompper, M.E. *Free-Ranging Dogs and Wildlife Conservation*, 1st ed.; Gompper, M.E., Ed.; Oxford University Press: Oxford, UK, 2014; Volume 1, ISBN 9788578110796.
7. Mani, R.S.; Willoughby, R.E. Human Rabies in South Asia. In *Neglected Tropical Diseases—South Asia*; Singh, S.K., Ed.; Springer International Publishing: Cham, Switzerland, 2017; pp. 349–371. ISBN 9783319684932.
8. Mani, R.S.; Anand, A.M.; Madhusudana, S.N. Human rabies in India: An audit from a rabies diagnostic laboratory. *Trop. Med. Int. Heal.* **2016**, *21*, 556–563. [CrossRef] [PubMed]
9. Diseases Under Surveillance: Integrated Disease Surveillance Programme (IDSP). Available online: http://www.idsp.nic.in/index1.php?lang=1&level=1&sublinkid=5985&lid=3925 (accessed on 3 August 2020).
10. Baxter, J.M. One in a million, or one in thousand: What is the morbidity of rabies in India? *J. Glob. Health* **2012**, *2*, 1–4. [CrossRef]
11. Suraweera, W.; Morris, S.K.; Kumar, R.; Warrell, D.A.; Warrell, M.J.; Jha, P. Deaths from Symptomatically Identifiable Furious Rabies in India: A Nationally Representative Mortality Survey. *PLoS Negl. Trop. Dis.* **2012**, *6*, e1847. [CrossRef]
12. Masthi, N.R.; Pradeep, B.; Bilagumba, G. A multicentric community survey on animal exposures among humans in India. *Indian J. Public Health* **2019**, *63*, S9–S14. [CrossRef]
13. National Plans: Planning Commission, Government of India. Available online: https://niti.gov.in/planningcommission.gov.in/docs/plans/planrel/index.php?state=planbody.htm (accessed on 30 July 2020).
14. Bagcchi, S. India fights rabies. *Lancet Infect. Dis.* **2015**, *15*, 156–157. [CrossRef]

15. Search|Open Government Data (OGD) Platform India. Available online: https://data.gov.in/search/site?query=rabies (accessed on 29 July 2020).
16. *Union Budget of India 2018–2019: Notes on Demands for Grants, Demand No. 42*; Department of Health and Family Welfare: New Delhi, India, 2018; pp. 134–141.
17. *Union Budget of India 2019–2020: Notes on Demands for Grants, Demand No. 42*; Department of Health and Family Welfare: New Delhi, India, 2019; pp. 136–143.
18. *Union Budget of India 2020–2021: Notes on Demands for Grants, Demand No. 42*; Department of Health and Family Welfare: New Delhi, India, 2020; pp. 135–143.
19. Chakrabarti, P. *Bacteriology in British India: Laboratory Medicine and the Tropics*; University of Rochester Press: Rochester, NY, USA, 2012; ISBN 9781580464086.
20. Tarantola, A. Four Thousand Years of Concepts Relating to Rabies in Animals and Humans, Its Prevention and Its Cure. *Trop. Med. Infect. Dis.* **2017**, *2*, 5. [CrossRef]
21. Wasik, B.; Murphy, M. *Rabid—A Cultural History of the World's Most Diabolical Virus*; Penguin Books Ltd.: London, UK, 2012; ISBN 9780143123576.
22. Parpia, S.A. Imperial Hunting Grounds: A New Reading of Mughal Cultural History. Ph.D. Thesis, The University of Adelaide, Adelaide, SA, Australia, 20 December 2018.
23. Johnson, D. *Sketches of Field Sports as Followed by the Natives of India with Observations on the Animals*; Longman and Co.: London, UK, 1822; p. 261.
24. Fayrer, J.; Balfour, J. Hydrophobia. *Lancet* **1877**, *110*, 785–786. [CrossRef]
25. *Destruction of Life by Snakes, Hydrophobia etc. in Western India, by an Ex-Commissioner*; WH Allen and Co.: London, UK, 1880; p. 120.
26. Vaughan, J. Canine Rabies in India. *Ind. Med. Gaz.* **1896**, *31*, 273–275. [CrossRef]
27. Martin, E. Rabies in India. *J. Comp. Pathol. Ther.* **1895**, *8*, 207–212. [CrossRef]
28. Benham, F.L. A collection of cases of hydrophobia reported as successfully treated. *Lancet* **1890**, *135*, 458–460. [CrossRef]
29. Medicus. Rabies. *Lancet* **1829**, *12*, 459–461. [CrossRef]
30. [Anonymous]. *Vaidyapusthakam*; Western Star Office: Cochin, India, 1876; p. 15. (In Malayalam)
31. Pirkis, F. Results of the trial of the Buisson Bath treatment for rabies at Allahabad, Ferozepore and Sialkote 1898. India Office Records and Private Papers, British Library, IOR/P/5418 August 1898 nos 249-51: July 1898–August 1898. Available online: http://access.bl.uk/item/viewer/ark:/81055/vdc_100079495983.0x000001 (accessed on 20 October 2020).
32. *Collection 11/40—Inspection by Military Veterinary Subordinates Instead of Veterinary Officers of Dogs Suspected of Rabies*; India Office Records and Private Papers; IOR/L/MIL/7/873; British Library: London, UK, 1914–1919.
33. Mad Dogs. *Times India (1861-Current)*, 7 October 1861; p. 2.
34. A rabid dog: Four officers bitten. *The Times of India (1861-Current)*, 23 May 1907; p. 8.
35. Rabies among jackals. *The Times of India (1861-Current)*, 7 February 1930; p. 14.
36. Sirius. Hydrophobia in Dogs–Symptoms of. *The Bombay Times and Journal of Commerce*, 30 April 1859; p. 279.
37. The mad dog. *The Court Magazine and Belle Assemblee*, July 1832–January 1837, Volume 9, pp. 27–38.
38. Mad dogs. *The Times of India (1861-Current)*, 21 July 1865; p. 4.
39. Rabies in Bombay: To the editor of "The Times of India". *The Times of India (1861-Current)*, 11 September 1936; p. 20.
40. Stray dogs in Calcutta: Corporation's new plan. *The Times of India (1861-Current)*, 23 May 1925; p. 14.
41. Destruction of stray dogs in Poona. *The Times of India (1861-Current)*, 1 March 1929; p. 7.
42. Rabies in Bombay: A menace to the public. *The Times of India (1861-Current)*, 14 April 1923; p. 12.
43. Rabies in Bombay: Cases in Cumballa Hill District—To the editor of the Times of India. *The Times of India (1861-Current)*, 27 August 1935; p. 16.
44. WPP. II: To the editor of the Times of India. *The Times of India (1861-Current)*, 6 February 1911; p. 7.
45. 1895–1951—Annual Report of the Civil Veterinary Department, Bengal—Medicine—Veterinary > Civil Veterinary Departments—Medical History of British India—National Library of Scotland. Available online: https://digital.nls.uk/indiapapers/browse/archive/75719892 (accessed on 24 June 2020).
46. (185) Page 17. Annual Report of the Civil Veterinary Department, Bengal and of the Bengal Veterinary College for the year 1935–1936. Available online: https://digital.nls.uk/indiapapers/browse/archive/77010889 (accessed on 22 July 2020).

47. Pemberton, N.; Worboys, M. *Mad Dogs and Englishmen*; Palgrave Macmillan: London, UK, 2007; ISBN 978-1-349-35998-1.
48. Field, J.; Prevost, F.; McCausland, G. Rabies in Bombay: To the editor of The Times of India. *The Times of India (1861-Current)*, 4 February 1911; p. 8.
49. Cave Canem: Rabies and Plague—To the editor of The Times of India. *The Times of India (1861-Current)*, 28 February 1911; p. 8.
50. Arnold, D. *Colonizing the Body: State Medicine and Epidemic Disease in Nineteenth-Century India*; University of California Press: Berkeley, CA, USA; Los Angeles, CA, USA, 1993.
51. Kidambi, P. "An infection of locality": Plague, pythogenesis and the poor in Bombay, c. 1896–1905. *Urban History* **2004**, *31*, 249–267. [CrossRef]
52. Chattopadhyay, S. *Representing Calcutta: Modernity, Nationalism and the Colonial Uncanny*; Routledge: London, UK, 2005.
53. Rabies vaccines: WHO position paper—April 2018. *WHO Wkly. Epidemiol. Rec.* **2018**, *93*, 201–220.
54. Mackenzie, T. *Proposed establishment of a Pasteur Institute in connection with the Bacteriological Laboratory at Poona 1892*; India Office Records and Private Papers; IOR/P/4345 August 1893; British Library: London, UK, 1893; nos 79–87, pp. 327–355.
55. Clive Webb, E. Rabies and its Control in India. *Vet. J.* **1911**, *67*, 157–166. [CrossRef]
56. Patients for the Pasteur Institute. *The Times of India (1861-Current)*, 5 April 1899; p. 5.
57. Bitten by a rabid dog. *The Times of India (1861-Current)*, 15 February 1899; p. 5.
58. Fremantle, F. *Health and Empire*; John Ouseley Ltd.: London, UK, 1911.
59. Cheema, G. Historical Notes: Rabies, Anti-Rabic Vaccine and the Raj. *Indian J. Hist. Sci.* **2015**, *50*, 514–520. [CrossRef]
60. Guenther, R. Works of the East Indian Pasteur Institute for Hydrophobia in Kasauli, India. *Public Heal. Rep.* **1901**, *16*, 2446.
61. East India (Sanitary Measures). Report on Sanitary Measures in India in 1912–1913. Vol. XLVI. 20th Century House of Commons Sessional Papers. 1914, 46. Available online: https://parlipapers.proquest.com/parlipapers/docview/t70.d75.1914-018116 (accessed on 20 October 2020).
62. East India (sSanitary Measures). Report on Sanitary Measures in India in 1907–1908. Vol. XLI. 20th Century House of Commons Sessional Papers. 1909, 41. Available online: https://parlipapers.proquest.com/parlipapers/docview/t70.d75.1909-011353 (accessed on 20 October 2020).
63. East India (Sanitary Measures). Report on Sanitary Measures in India 1914–1915. Vol. XLVIII. 20th Century House of Commons Sessional Papers. 1916, 48. Available online: https://parlipapers.proquest.com/parlipapers/docview/t70.d75.1916-020132 (accessed on 20 October 2020).
64. Rabies in Bombay: To the editor of The Times of India from the Director, Bombay Bacteriological Laboratory. *The Times of India (1861-Current)*, 4 October 1924; p. 15.
65. Dutton, H. (66) Page 4. Annual Report of the Prince of Wales Medical College, Patna for the year 1928–1829. Available online: https://digital.nls.uk/indiapapers/browse/archive/74971598 (accessed on 15 July 2020).
66. (274) Page 258. Regulations for the Medical Services of the Army in India. Available online: https://digital.nls.uk/indiapapers/browse/archive/74907253 (accessed on 15 July 2020).
67. East India (Sanitary Measures). Report on Sanitary Measures in India in 1906–1907. Vol. XL. 20th Century House of Commons Sessional Papers. 1908, 40. Available online: https://parlipapers.proquest.com/parlipapers/docview/t70.d75.1908-010135 (accessed on 20 October 2020).
68. Rabies Treatment in Southern India. *Nature* **1940**, *145*, 739. [CrossRef]
69. Rabies in India. *Nature* **1961**, *190*, 678. [CrossRef]
70. Annual Report 2015–2016—Pasteur Institute of India; Coonoor, India, 2017, p. 39. Available online: http://pasteurinstituteindia.com/annual.html (accessed on 20 October 2020).
71. Pasteur Institute of India, Kasauli—The Fourteenth Annual Report of the Central Committee of the Association Together with the Report of the Directors of the Institute for the Year Ending 31st December 1914. Available online: https://digital.nls.uk/indiapapers/browse/archive/74947969 (accessed on 28 July 2020).
72. Porter, L. *Proposals for the Collection of Statistics of Persons Bitten by Rabid Animals*; India Office Records and Private Papers; IOR/P/8955 Jan 1912; British Library: London, UK, 1912; nos 14–15; pp. 3–11.

73. (1) Front Cover. Annual Administration Report of the Civil Veterinary Department, Madras Presidency, 1926–1933. Available online: https://digital.nls.uk/indiapapers/browse/archive/75692280 (accessed on 24 June 2020).
74. Webster, W. *Rabies and Anti-Rabic Treatment in India*; Govt. India Press: Simla, India, 1946; p. 17.
75. Greig, E. *Rabies and Anti-Rabic Treatment in India 1921*; Superintendent, Government Printing: Rangoon, Burma, India, 1921; p. 16.
76. Pasteur Institute in India: Most bites by dogs. *The Times of India (1861-Current)*, 5 July 1928; p. 13.
77. Pratik Chakrabarti "Living versus Dead": The Pasteurian Paradigm and Imperial Vaccine Research. *Bull. Hist. Med.* **2010**, *84*, 387–423. [CrossRef] [PubMed]
78. Semple, D. *The Preparation of a Safe and Efficient Antirabic Vaccine*; Scientific Memoirs by Officers of the Medical and Sanitary Departments of the Government of India: Calcutta, India, 1911.
79. Taylor, L.H.; Costa, P.; Briggs, D.J. Chapter 15—Public Health Management of Humans at Risk. In *Rabies*, 3rd ed.; Jackson, A.C., Ed.; Academic Press: Boston, MA, USA, 2013; pp. 543–573, ISBN 978-0-12-396547-9.
80. Rupprecht, C.E.; Nagarajan, T.; Ertl, H. Rabies Vaccines. In *Plotkin's Vaccines*; Elsevier: Philadelphia, PA, USA, 2018; pp. 918–942.e12.
81. Chakrabarti, P. Pasteurian Paradigm and Vaccine Research in India. In *Bacteriology in British India*; Chakrabarti, P., Ed.; Laboratory Medicine and the Tropics; Boydell and Brewer Limited: Suffolk, UK, 2012; Volume 22, pp. 142–178. ISBN 9781580464086.
82. Bradfield, E. (251) [Page] 239. An Indian Medical Review. Available online: https://digital.nls.uk/indiapapers/browse/archive/74941238 (accessed on 14 July 2020).
83. Palsetia, J.S. Mad Dogs and Parsis: The Bombay Dog Riots of 1832. *J. R. Asiat. Soc.* **2001**, *11*, 13–30. [CrossRef]
84. (160) Page 94. Proceedings of the Second Meeting of Veterinary Officers in India, Calcutta. 1923. Available online: https://digital.nls.uk/indiapapers/browse/archive/75515450 (accessed on 23 June 2020).
85. Bombay corporation: Destruction of stray dog. *The Times of India (1861-Current)*, 2 January 1912; p. 4.
86. The proposed dog tax: To the editor of The Times of India. *The Times of India (1861-Current)*, 6 December 1887; p. 4.
87. Simla municipality: Campaign against jackals. *The Times of India (1861-Current)*, 12 September 1907; p. 7.
88. (1) Front Cover. Annual Report of the Punjab Veterinary College and of the Civil Veterinary Department, Punjab, 1909–1919. Available online: https://digital.nls.uk/indiapapers/browse/archive/75528073 (accessed on 24 June 2020).
89. Indian notes and news: Simla electric supply, Campaign against jackals, Employment abroad, To purify water, The Mahomedan position, Calcutta ferry service. *The Times of India (1861-Current)*, 27 April 1909; p. 8.
90. McLean, F. An appeal to dog-lovers: To the editor of The Times of India. *The Times of India (1861-Current)*, 7 April 1919; p. 8.
91. Rabies in India. *Lancet* **1910**, *175*, 116–117. [CrossRef]
92. (266) Page 9. Annual Report of the Civil Veterinary Department Bihar and Orissa for the Year 1926–1927. Available online: https://digital.nls.uk/indiapapers/browse/archive/75903625 (accessed on 22 July 2020).
93. Suppression of rabies. *The Times of India (1861-Current)*, 20 May 1912; p. 8.
94. Rabies menace in India: Need for control measures. *The Times of India (1861-Current)*, 26 March 1935; p. 3.
95. (158) Page 139. Annual Administration Report of the Civil Veterinary Department of India for the Official Year 1898–1899. Available online: https://digital.nls.uk/indiapapers/browse/archive/75506674 (accessed on 21 July 2020).
96. (24) Page 17. Annual Administration Report of the Civil Veterinary Department in India for the Official Year 1908–1909. Available online: https://digital.nls.uk/indiapapers/browse/archive/75509882 (accessed on 23 July 2020).
97. (1) Front Cover—Medicine—Veterinary > Civil Veterinary Departments > Proceedings of the Meeting of Veterinary Officers in India—Medical History of British India—National Library of Scotland. Available online: https://digital.nls.uk/indiapapers/browse/archive/75514868 (accessed on 23 June 2020).
98. The etiology and prevention of rabies. *BMJ* **1924**, *1*, 1059–1063. [CrossRef]
99. Kurosawa, A.; Tojinbara, K.; Kadowaki, H.; Hampson, K.; Yamada, A.; Makita, K. The rise and fall of rabies in Japan: A quantitative history of rabies epidemics in Osaka Prefecture, 1914–1933. *PLoS Negl. Trop. Dis.* **2017**, *11*, e0005435. [CrossRef]

100. (324) Page 6. Annual Report on the Punjab Veterinary College, Civil Veterinary Department, Punjab and the Government Cattle Farm, Hissar for the year 1915–1916. Available online: https://digital.nls.uk/indiapapers/browse/archive/75532277 (accessed on 25 June 2020).
101. (300) Page 22. Annual Report of the Punjab Veterinary College, Civil Veterinary Department, Punjab, and the Government Cattle Farm, Hissar for the Year 1922–1923. Available online: https://digital.nls.uk/indiapapers/browse/archive/75536082 (accessed on 15 July 2020).
102. (1) Front Cover. Annual Administration Report of the Civil Veterinary Department, Madras Presidency, 1910–1925. Available online: https://digital.nls.uk/indiapapers/browse/archive/75692279 (accessed on 23 June 2020).
103. (1) Front cover—Medicine—Veterinary > Civil Veterinary Departments > 1911–1950—Report of the Civil Veterinary Department, Assam > Civil Veterinary Dept. Assam report 1911–1927—Medical History of British India—National Library of Scotland. Available online: https://digital.nls.uk/indiapapers/browse/archive/75722238 (accessed on 24 June 2020).
104. 1937–1946—Annual Administration Report of the Civil Veterinary Department, Sind—Medicine—Veterinary > Civil Veterinary Departments—Medical History of British India—National Library of Scotland. Available online: https://digital.nls.uk/indiapapers/browse/archive/75648798 (accessed on 24 June 2020).
105. (1) Front Cover—Medicine—Veterinary > Civil Veterinary Departments > 1914–1940—Annual administration Report of the Civil Veterinary Department, Ajmere-Merwara, British Rajputana—Medical History of British India—National Library of Scotland. Available online: https://digital.nls.uk/indiapapers/browse/archive/75645666 (accessed on 24 June 2020).
106. Pinnell, L. Order under sec. 144 CrPC about muzzling of dogs issued in 1933—Memo No. 9719 G dtd. 11/12/1944. In *Mss Eur D911: Papers of Leonard George Pinnell, Indian Civil Service, Bengal*; India Office Records and Private Papers; British Library: London, UK, 1932–1948.
107. Rabies Prevention in India. *Nature* **1938**, *141*, 72–73. [CrossRef]
108. Pasteur Institute of Southern India. *Nature* **1950**, *166*, 257. [CrossRef]
109. Animal diseases: Veterinary conference. *The Times of India (1861-Current)*, 21 March 1923; p. 12.
110. Young India, 1924–1926 by Mahatma Gandhi. Available online: https://dspace.gipe.ac.in/xmlui/handle/10973/33432 (accessed on 8 October 2020).
111. (379) Page 5. Annual Administration Report of the Civil Veterinary Department, Madras Presidency for 1923–1924. Available online: https://digital.nls.uk/indiapapers/browse/archive/75699874 (accessed on 22 July 2020).
112. (360) Page 12. Annual Administration Report of the Civil Veterinary Department, Madras Presidency for 1922–1923. Available online: https://digital.nls.uk/indiapapers/browse/archive/75699817 (accessed on 21 July 2020).
113. (48) Page 19. Report on the Operations of the Civil Veterinary Department, Madras. Recording, with Remarks, during 1911–1912. Available online: https://digital.nls.uk/indiapapers/browse/archive/75698863 (accessed on 21 July 2020).
114. (371) Page 63. Annual Administration Report of the Madras Civil Veterinary Department for the year 1928–1929. Available online: https://digital.nls.uk/indiapapers/browse/archive/75718016 (accessed on 21 July 2020).
115. (53) Page 7. Annual Report of the Civil Veterinary Department Bihar and Orissa for the year 1923–1924. Available online: https://digital.nls.uk/indiapapers/browse/archive/75900869 (accessed on 23 July 2020).
116. (59) Page 7. Report on the Civil Veterinary Department North-West Frontier Province, for the year 1933–1934. Available online: https://digital.nls.uk/indiapapers/browse/archive/75546705 (accessed on 22 July 2020).
117. (81) Page 3. Annual Administration Report of the Civil Veterinary Department in the Bombay Presidency for the Official Year 1899–1900. Available online: https://digital.nls.uk/indiapapers/browse/archive/75678945 (accessed on 23 July 2020).
118. (876) Page 23. Annual Administration Report of the Madras Civil Veterinary Department for the Year 1932–1933. Available online: https://digital.nls.uk/indiapapers/browse/archive/75719584 (accessed on 23 July 2020).
119. Chakrabarti, P. *Medicine and Empire: 1600–1960*; Palgrave Macmillan Ltd.: Basingstoke, UK, 2013; ISBN 1137374802.
120. Vaccinating Dogs. *The Times of India (1861-Current)*, 7 December 1926; p. 8.

121. Victims, O. Of the Rabid Dogs. *The Times of India (1861-Current)*, 25 November 1940; p. 6.
122. Russell, A.J.H. The Vitality of the Peoples of Southern India, its Conservation and Promotion. *Sci. Mon.* **1926**, *23*, 54–64.
123. East India (Sanitary Measures). Report of Sanitary Measures in India in 1915–1916. Vol. XLIX. 20th Century House of Commons Sessional Papers. 1918, 49. Available online: https://parlipapers.proquest.com/parlipapers/docview/t70.d75.1917-020945 (accessed on 20 October 2020).
124. Report on Sanitary Measures in India in 1879–80: Together with Miscellaneous Information up to June 1881. 19th Century House of Commons Sessional Papers. 1881, 13. 1881, 13. Available online: https://parlipapers.proquest.com/parlipapers/docview/t70.d75.1881-057412 (accessed on 20 October 2020).
125. Report on sanitary Measures in India in 1885–6: Together with Miscellaneous Information up to June 1887. 19th Century House of Commons Sessional Papers. 1887, 19. 1887, 19. Available online: https://parlipapers.proquest.com/parlipapers/docview/t70.d75.1887-063651 (accessed on 20 October 2020).
126. East India (sanitary measures). Report on Sanitary Measures in India in 1909–1910. Vol. XLIII. 20th Century House of Commons Sessional Papers. 1911, 43. Available online: https://parlipapers.proquest.com/parlipapers/docview/t70.d75.1911-013831 (accessed on 20 October 2020).
127. East India (Sanitary Measures). Report on Sanitary Measures in India in 1910–1911. Vol. XLIV. 20th Century House of Commons Sessional Papers. 1912, 44. Available online: https://parlipapers.proquest.com/parlipapers/docview/t70.d75.1912-015414 (accessed on 20 October 2020).
128. East India (Sanitary Measures). Report on Sanitary Measures in India in 1908–1909. Vol. XLII. 20th Century House of Commons Sessional Papers. 1910, 42. Available online: https://parlipapers.proquest.com/parlipapers/docview/t70.d75.1910-012721 (accessed on 20 October 2020).
129. East India (Sanitary Measures). Report on Sanitary Measures in India in 1913–1914. Vol. XLVII. 20th Century House of Commons Sessional Papers. 1915, 47. 1915, 47. Available online: https://parlipapers.proquest.com/parlipapers/docview/t70.d75.1914-019382 (accessed on 20 October 2020).
130. East India (Sanitary Measures). Report on sanitary measures in India in 1911–1912. Vol. XLV. 20th Century House of Commons Sessional Papers. 1913, 45. Available online: https://parlipapers.proquest.com/parlipapers/docview/t70.d75.1914-017723 (accessed on 20 October 2020).
131. Ministry of Health. Annual report of the Chief Medical Officer, 1919–1920. 20th Century House of Commons Sessional Papers. 1920. Available online: https://parlipapers.proquest.com/parlipapers/docview/t70.d75.1920-023861 (accessed on 20 October 2020).
132. (113) Page 47. Proceedings of the Second Meeting of Veterinary Officers in India, Calcutta. 1923. Available online: https://digital.nls.uk/indiapapers/browse/archive/75515291 (accessed on 28 July 2020).
133. Harrison, M. A Dreadful Scourge: Cholera in early nineteenth-century India. *Mod. Asian Stud.* **2020**, *54*, 502–553. [CrossRef]
134. Pasteur Institute of India, Kasauli. *Nature* **1935**, *136*, 677. [CrossRef]
135. Anti-Rabic Treatment in India. *Nature* **1939**, *144*, 148. [CrossRef]
136. Brown, K.; Gilfoyle, D. *Healing the Herds*; Brown, K., Gilfoyle, D., Eds.; Ohio University Press: Athens, Ohio, USA, 2010; ISBN 9780821443101.
137. East India (Statistical Abstract). Statistical Abstract for British India with Statistics, Where Available, Relating to Certain Indian States from 1926-27 to 1935–36 Sixty-ninth Number (Fourteenth Number of New Series). 20th Century House of Commons Sessional Papers. 1938, 69. Available online: https://parlipapers.proquest.com/parlipapers/docview/t70.d75.1937-035559 (accessed on 20 October 2020).
138. East India (Progress and Condition). Statement Exhibiting the Moral and Material Progress and Condition of India during the Year 1929–30. Sixty-fifth Number. 20th Century House of Commons Sessional Papers. 1931, 65. Available online: https://parlipapers.proquest.com/parlipapers/docview/t70.d75.1930-030809 (accessed on 20 October 2020).
139. Veeraraghavan, N.; Subrahmanyan, T. The value of duck-embryo vaccine and high-egg-passage Flury vaccine in experimental rabies infection in guinea pigs. *Bull. World Health Organ.* **1963**, *29*, 323–330.
140. (563) Page 3. Report of the Civil Veterinary Department, North-West Frontier Province for the year 1921–1922. Available online: https://digital.nls.uk/indiapapers/browse/archive/75545198 (accessed on 23 July 2020).
141. Del Rio Vilas, V.J.; Freire de Carvalho, M.J.; Vigilato, M.A.N.; Rocha, F.; Vokaty, A.; Pompei, J.A.; Molina Flores, B.; Fenelon, N.; Cosivi, O. Tribulations of the Last Mile: Sides from a Regional Program. *Front. Vet. Sci.* **2017**, *4*, 4. [CrossRef] [PubMed]

142. Polu, S.L. Malaria—India's True Plague. In *Infectious Disease in India, 1892–1940*; Palgrave Macmillan: London, UK, 2012; pp. 82–118.
143. Rahman, S.A.; Isloor, S. Rabies on the Indian subcontinent. *Rev. Sci. Tech. L'OIE* **2018**, *37*, 529–542. [CrossRef]
144. Venkataraman, L. India Is Far behind Sri Lanka and Bangladesh in Rabies Prevention. Available online: https://www.telegraphindia.com/opinion/india-is-far-behind-sri-lanka-and-bangladesh-in-rabies-prevention/cid/1690048 (accessed on 30 July 2020).
145. Census of India: Variation in Population Since 1901. Available online: https://www.censusindia.gov.in/Census_Data_2001/India_at_glance/variation.aspx (accessed on 30 July 2020).
146. Tiwari, H.K.; Robertson, I.D.; O'Dea, M.; Vanak, A.T. Knowledge, attitudes and practices (KAP) towards rabies and free roaming dogs (FRD) in Panchkula district of north India: A cross-sectional study of urban residents. *PLoS Negl. Trop. Dis.* **2019**, *13*, e0007384. [CrossRef]
147. Kakkar, M.; Ramani, S.; Menon, G.; Sankhe, L.; Gaidhane, A.; Krishnan, S. 'Zoonoses? Not sure what that is ... ' An assessment of knowledge of zoonoses among medical students in India. *Trans. R. Soc. Trop. Med. Hyg.* **2011**, *105*, 254–261. [CrossRef]
148. *Animal Birth Control (Dogs) Rules, 2001*; Animal Welfare Board of India: Chennai, India, 2001; p. 7.
149. Kudumbashree|ABC Programme. Available online: http://www.kudumbashree.org/pages/216 (accessed on 20 May 2018).
150. George, A.; Kumar, K.J.K. *ABC- ARV Program, Corporation of Koch*; Corporation of Kochi: Kerala, India, 2014.
151. Reece, J.F.; Chawla, S.K. Control of rabies in Jaipur, India, by the sterilisation and vaccination of neighbourhood dogs. *Vet. Rec.* **2006**, *159*, 379–383. [CrossRef]
152. Lenin, J.; Uniyal, M.; Vanak, A.T. Do Dogs Threaten People's Right to Safety in Public Spaces? Available online: https://thewire.in/health/dogs-rabies-neutering-safety (accessed on 4 September 2020).
153. *Revised Module for Street Dog Population Management, Rabies Eradication, Reducing Man-Dog Conflict*; Animal Welfare Board of India: Chennai, India, 2016; p. 308.
154. At Least 120 Stray Dogs Killed in Kerala's Ernakulam and Palakkad Districts in the Last Week. Available online: https://scroll.in/latest/819045/at-least-120-stray-dogs-killed-in-keralas-ernakulam-and-palakkad-districts-in-the-last-week (accessed on 7 October 2020).
155. In a Horrifying Incident, Kerala Congress Activists Kill Dogs, Hang Them on Poles—The Financial Express. Available online: https://www.financialexpress.com/india-news/in-a-horrifying-incident-kerala-congress-activists-kill-dogs-hang-them-on-poles/393946/ (accessed on 7 October 2020).
156. Srinivasan, K.; Kurz, T.; Kuttuva, P.; Pearson, C. Reorienting rabies research and practice: Lessons from India. *Palgrave Commun.* **2019**, *5*, 152. [CrossRef]
157. Collinson, A.; Bennett, M.; Brennan, M.L.; Dean, R.S.; Stavisky, J. Evaluating the role of surgical sterilisation in canine rabies control: A systematic review of impact and outcomes. *PLoS Negl. Trop. Dis.* **2020**, *14*, e0008497. [CrossRef]
158. Wang, J. *Mad Dogs and Other New Yorkers: Rabies, Medicine, and Society in an American Metropolis, 1840–1920*; Johns Hopkins University Press: Baltimore, MD, USA, 2019; ISBN 9781421409726.
159. Vanak, A.T.; Home, C. Unpacking the 'canine conundrum'. *Anim. Conserv.* **2018**, *21*, 289–290. [CrossRef]
160. Bhalla, S.; Vanak, A.T. Killing with Compassion: Why Feeding Dogs in Public Places Must Stop! Available online: https://www.downtoearth.org.in/blog/wildlife-biodiversity/killing-with-compassion-why-feeding-dogs-in-public-places-must-stop--72092 (accessed on 4 September 2020).
161. Nadal, D. *Rabies in the Streets*; Penn State University Press: University Park, PA, USA, 2020; Volume 16, ISBN 9780271085951.
162. Rabies Kills Tens of Thousands Yearly. Vaccinating Dogs Could Stop it. The New York Times. Available online: https://www.nytimes.com/2019/07/22/science/rabies-dogs-india.html (accessed on 18 October 2020).
163. Thiagarajan, K. Man bites dog: India's progress in tackling rabies. *BMJ* **2020**, *368*, l6979. [CrossRef] [PubMed]
164. Byrnes, H.; Britton, A.; Bhutia, T. Eliminating Dog-Mediated Rabies in Sikkim, India: A 10-Year Pathway to Success for the SARAH Program. *Front. Vet. Sci.* **2017**, *4*, 28. [CrossRef] [PubMed]
165. Cherian, V.; Dugg, P.; Khan, A.M. Prevalence of pet dog ownership in an urban colony of East Delhi and awareness regarding canine zoonotic diseases and responsible pet ownership among dog owners. *Indian J. Community Med.* **2020**, *45*, 89–91. [CrossRef] [PubMed]
166. Radhakrishnan, S.; Vanak, A.T.; Nouvellet, P.; Donnelly, C.A. Population characteristics of owned and unowned dogs at two urban locations in Kerala, India. 2020; unpublished; manuscript in preparation.

167. Wentworth, D.; Hampson, K.; Thumbi, S.M.; Mwatondo, A.; Wambura, G.; Chng, N.R. A social justice perspective on access to human rabies vaccines. *Vaccine* **2019**, *37*, A3–A5. [CrossRef] [PubMed]
168. Fitzpatrick, M.C.; Shah, H.A.; Pandey, A.; Bilinski, A.M.; Kakkar, M.; Clark, A.D.; Townsend, J.P.; Abbas, S.S.; Galvani, A.P. One Health approach to cost-effective rabies control in India. *Proc. Natl. Acad. Sci. USA* **2016**, *113*, 14574–14581. [CrossRef] [PubMed]
169. Mindekem, R.; Lechenne, M.S.; Naissengar, K.S.; Oussiguere, A.; Kebkiba, B.; Moto, D.D.; Alfaroukh, I.O.; Ouedraogo, L.T.; Salifou, S.; Zinsstag, J. Cost Description and Comparative Cost Efficiency of Post-Exposure Prophylaxis and Canine Mass Vaccination against Rabies in N'Djamena, Chad. *Front. Vet. Sci.* **2017**, *4*, 38. [CrossRef] [PubMed]
170. Yasobant, S.; Saxena, D.; Bruchhausen, W.; Memon, F.Z.; Falkenberg, T. Multi-sectoral prioritization of zoonotic diseases: One health perspective from Ahmedabad, India. *PLoS ONE* **2019**, *14*, e0220152. [CrossRef] [PubMed]
171. Sekar, N.; Shah, N.K.; Abbas, S.S.; Kakkar, M. Research Options for Controlling Zoonotic Disease in India, 2010–2015. *PLoS ONE* **2011**, *6*, e17120. [CrossRef]

18

Trends in *Strongyloides stercoralis* Faecal Larvae Detections in the Northern Territory, Australia: 2002 to 2012

Johanna K. Mayer-Coverdale [1], Amy Crowe [2], Pamela Smith [3] and Robert W. Baird [3,*]

1 Department of Microbiology, Pathology Queensland, Royal Brisbane and Women's Hospital, Queensland 4001, Australia; johannak.mayer@gmail.com
2 Infectious Diseases Physician, St Vincent's Hospital, 41 Victoria Pde, Fitzroy 3065, Australia; amy.crowe@svha.org.au
3 Microbiology, Territory Pathology, Royal Darwin Hospital, Tiwi 0810, Australia; pam.smith@nt.gov.au
* Correspondence: rob.baird@nt.gov.au;

Academic Editors: Patricia Graves and Peter Leggat

Abstract: *Strongyloides stercoralis* is a soil-transmitted helminth (STH) endemic to tropical and subtropical areas. We reviewed the temporal detection trends in patients with *S. stercoralis* larvae present in faecal samples, in Northern Territory (NT) Government Health facilities, between 2002 and 2012. This was a retrospective observational study of consecutive patients with microbiologically confirmed detection of *S. stercoralis* in faeces. The presence of anaemia, eosinophilia, polyparasitism, and geographic and demographic data, were included in the assessment. *S. stercoralis* larvae were present in 389 of 22,892 faecal samples (1.7%) collected across the NT over 11 years, examined by microscopy after formol ethyl acetate concentration. 97.7% of detections were in Indigenous patients. Detections, by number, occurred in a biphasic age distribution. Detections per number of faecal samples collected, were highest in the 0–5 year age group. Anaemia was present in 44.8%, and eosinophilia in 49.9% of patients. Eosinophilia was present in 65.5% of the $\leq$5 age group, compared to 40.8% of >5 year age ($p < 0.0001$). Polyparasitism was present in 31.4% of patients. There was an overall downward trend in larvae detections from 2.64% to 0.99% detections/number of faecal samples year between 2002 and 2012, consistent with the trends observed for other local STHs. *S. stercoralis* remains an important NT-wide pathogen.

Keywords: Strongyloides; anaemia; eosinophilia; polyparasitism; indigenous; Northern Territory; Australia

---

1. Introduction

Strongyloides stercoralis is a soil-transmitted helminth (STH) endemic to tropical and subtropical regions around the world. There are very wide estimates, between 3 and 100 million people [1], of the number of persons infected with *S. stercoralis* globally, because the true incidence is difficult to determine as many infections occur in regions with economic and health hardware disadvantage, and poor access to laboratory diagnostic services.

S. stercoralis infection has been estimated to occur disproportionately in Australian Indigenous people living in the northern parts of Australia, not only compared to the rest of Australia, but also to ecologically similar regions around the world [2–6]. Indigenous Australians experience substantially poorer health, social, and economic outcomes compared to other Australians, including overcrowding and poor sanitary conditions [7], both of which are of importance in the transmission of *S. stercoralis*. The Northern Territory (NT) is a large but sparsely populated area covering 1.5 million square kilometers, with numerous remote Indigenous communities. Cases of intestinal obstruction complicating *S. stercoralis* infection in children have been documented in the NT since the 1970s [2], and a 1993 study documented *S. stercoralis* endemicity in Indigenous patients over a 12-month period [3]. An association between HTLV-1 and *S. stercoralis* has been documented in central Australia where HTLV-1 is endemic [4]. *S. stercoralis* detections have been described across the tropical and subtropical areas of Western Australia and Queensland, including to latitudes below the Tropic of Capricorn (latitude 23° S) [5,6].

S. stercoralis has a complex life cycle [8]. The most common way of becoming infected is by direct contact with soil, as the filariform larvae penetrate the host skin from soil that is contaminated with *S. stercoralis* larvae. High risk activities include walking with bare feet, direct contact with human waste or sewage, as well as occupations such as farming. The larvae migrate via the venous circulation to the lungs, where they ascend the bronchial tree and eventually are swallowed, thus entering the digestive tract. Once established in the small bowel they become adults. The female worms produce eggs by parthenogenesis, which subsequently hatch in the small bowel, as rhabditiform larvae, (non-infectious), then are deposited, and develop to filariform (infectious) larvae in the soil over several days. Larvae that are not passed in the faeces have the ability to develop in the bowel to filariform larvae, that can either penetrate the bowel wall directly, or the perianal mucosa repeating the infective cycle potentially indefinitely. This process of auto-infection is characteristic of *S. stercoralis* and can lead to hyperinfection even in individuals who have not been in endemic areas for decades. Clinically, strongyloidiasis may present as a range of syndromes, ranging from asymptomatic or mild abdominal discomfort, to Crohn's-like colitis, primarily pulmonary symptoms (Loeffler's syndrome), cutaneous larva currens, and disseminated infection with high associated mortality [9]. The latter is particularly associated with immunosuppressed patients, especially those taking corticosteroids. The ability to establish ongoing, potentially life-long infection coupled with the risk of dissemination that is associated with high mortality makes screening, and in some instances empiric treatment, for *S. stercoralis* infection in people who are about to undergo immunosuppression essential, not only in endemic areas, but also in selected populations such as migrants from endemic regions and refugees [10].

Our aim was to describe the temporal trends in *S. stercoralis* larvae detection in faecal samples collected in NT Government Health facilities over a period of 11 years, and review associated demographic and laboratory features, in this population.

2. Results

Between 2002 and 2012, 22,892 faecal samples were assessed for ova, cysts, and parasites (OCP) across NT Government Health facilities. The number of annual faecal microscopy samples examined remained relatively constant throughout this time period, approximately 2000 samples/year, though 2578 and 2919 faecal microscopy and concentrates were examined in 2011 and 2012, respectively. *S. stercoralis* larvae were detected in 389 (1.7%) of all faecal samples. Eleven patients had more than one episode, with one patient having three documented episodes.

Demographic and laboratory characteristics are summarised in Table 1.

Overall 381 (97.7%) patients were Indigenous, and 164 (42.2%) were five years old or younger. In the ≤5 year-old group, 163 (99.4%) patients were Indigenous, while in the >5 year-old group 218 (96.9%) were Indigenous. In total, 216 (55.5%) patients were male and 173 (44.5%) female. The male to female ratio in the ≤5 year-old group was 79 (48.2%) male, and 85 (51.8%) female compared to 137 (60.9%) and 88 (39.1%) respectively in the older group.

Figure 1 is a cumulative graph of 11 years data presenting cases, and cases by number of faecal specimens examined. The age distribution of actual cases was biphasic (Figure 1), with the highest number of detections occurring in patients less than five years of age, with a peak in the second year of life, and a second smaller peak in the 35–50-year-old group. However, reviewing larvae detections to number of faecal specimens examined revealed the peak detection age in the 4–5 year-old age group.

Cases were detected from across the NT, with the highest detection rates coming from West Arnhem, Tiwi Islands, and the Katherine regions (Figure 2).

Table 1. Demographic and laboratory parameters of patients with *S. stercoralis* larvae detection in the Northern Territory, 2002 to 2012.

Parameter	≤ 5 Years Old (%)	> 5 Years Old (%)	All Ages (%)	*p*-Value
Number [1]	164 (42.2)	224 (57.6)	389 (100)	
Sex				
Male	79 (48.2)	137 (60.9)	216 (55.5)	0.012
Female	85 (51.8)	88 (39.1)	173 (44.5)	
Indigenous status				
Indigenous	163 (99.4)	218 (96.9)	381 (97.7)	<0.0001
Non-indigenous	1 (0.6)	7 (3.1)	8 (2.3)	
Laboratory parameters [2]				
Median haemoglobin	114 (IQR 105–122)	111 (IQR 91–134)	113 (IQR 97.8–127)	0.48
Anaemia [3]	58 (38.6)	106 (49.1)	164 (44.8)	0.04
Median eosinophil count	1 (IQR 0.2–2.4)	0.3 (IQR 0.1–0.8)	0.5 (IQR 0.1–1.3)	<0.0001
Eosinophilia [4]	95 (65.5)	89 (40.8)	184 (49.9)	<0.0001
Polyparasitism [5]	61 (37.2)	61 (27.1)	122 (31.4)	0.03
Other intestinal helminths	13 (7.9)	29 (12.9)	42 (10.8)	0.12
Hymenolepis nana	18 (11)	4 (1.8)	22 (5.6)	<0.001
Other (eg. Protozoa)	40 (24.4)	36 (16)	76 (33.8)	0.04

[1] One Indigenous male, did not have age or haematological data. [2] 23 patients (4.3%) had no haematological data, of these 14 were ≤ 5 years old. An additional 6 patients had no data for eosinophilia (5.4%), 5 were ≤ 5 years old. [3] Anaemia: Haemoglobin ≤110 g/L. [4] Eosinophilia: eosinophils > 0.5 × 10^9 /L. [5] Intestinal helminths were hookworm and *T. trichiura*. *Ascaris* species were not detected.

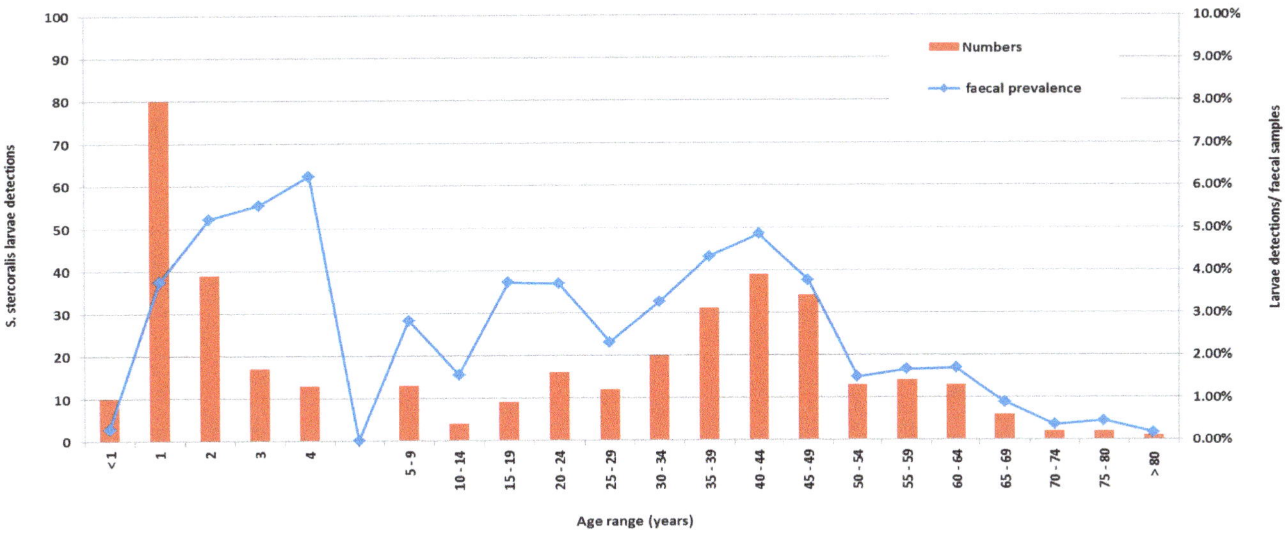

Figure 1. *S. stercoralis* larvae detections by age and diagnostic prevalence in the Northern Territory, 2002–2012.

The lowest detection rates were seen in the Darwin and the Gulf country, east of Katherine area.

Anaemia was present in 164 (44.8%) of patients, with a median Hb of 113 g/L (interquartile range (IQR) 97.8–127) across both groups, and 114 g/L (IQR 105–122) and 111 g/L (IQR 91–134) in the younger and older groups respectively ($p = 0.48$). Anaemia was present in 38.6% of the younger group, compared to 49.1% in the greater than five-year-old cohort ($p = 0.04$). 184 (49.9%) patients had eosinophilia, with a median eosinophil count of 0.5 × 10^9/L across both groups. Eosinophilia was more common in the younger group: 65.5% compared to 40.8% ($p < 0.0001$), and the median eosinophil count in $\leq$5 year-old cohort was 1×10^9/L (Figure 3), while in >5 year-old group the median was 0.3×10^9/L ($p < 0.001$).

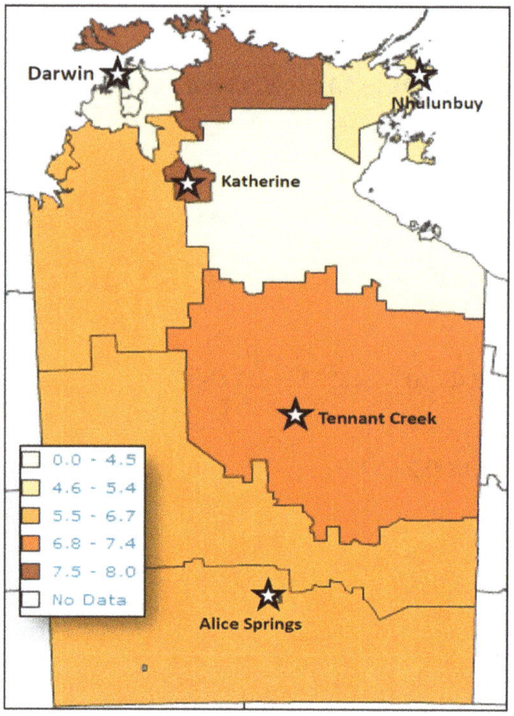

Figure 2. Geographic distribution of *S. stercoralis* larvae detection from patients in Northern Territory public healthcare facilities by geographic area of residence from 2002 to 2012. Prevalence figures are *S. stercoralis* larvae diagnostic detections in public health laboratories/10,000 Indigenous population/year.

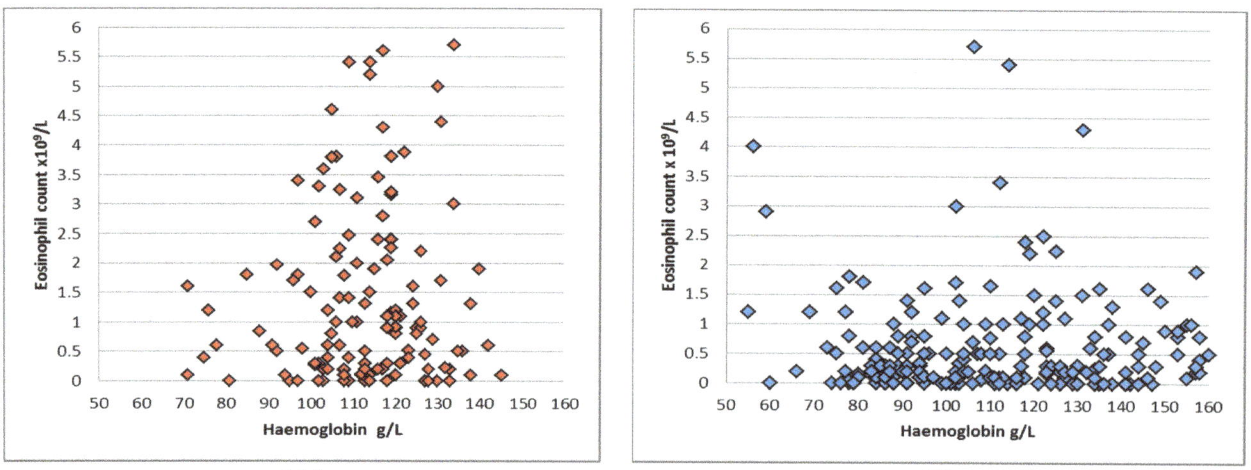

(A) **(B)**

Figure 3. Distribution of contemporaneous haemoglobin and eosinophil counts in patients with *S. stercoralis* larvae detection. **(A)** Patients five-years-old and under (red diamonds represent the individual data points). **(B)** Patients aged older than five years of age (blue diamonds represent individual data points).

A normal haemoglobin and normal eosinophil count was present in 19% of the younger group, and 29.6% of the older cohort. The combination of anaemia and eosinophilia was present in 22% of the ≤5 year-old age group, compared to 18% in the older cohort.

Polyparasitism was observed in 122 (31.4%) of all patients with *S. stercoralis* larvae detections. In the younger cohort 61 (37.2%) patients had at least one other parasite identified in their faecal specimen, while in the older group 61 (27.1%) of patients had at least one other parasite identified. Overall, 42 (10.8%) patients had co-infection with at least one other STH, 22 (5.6%) also had *Hymenolepis nana* identified, while 76 (33.8%) had co-infection with intestinal protozoa.

Over the 11 years of this study, there was a downward trend in *S. stercoralis* detections from 2.64% (in 2012) to 0.99% (in 2012) larvae detections/stool specimens examined. (Figure 4), mirroring the results for hookworm and *T. trichiura* over the same time period from the same cohort. This downward trend in detections was due to a three-fold reduction in detections in children under the age of five, while detection of larvae in patients over the age of five, remained relatively constant. 10,208 samples from children less than five were examined during this time period, with a median 882 samples/year (IQR 883–1003); with no significant variation in faecal numbers during the study period to account for the three-fold reduction.

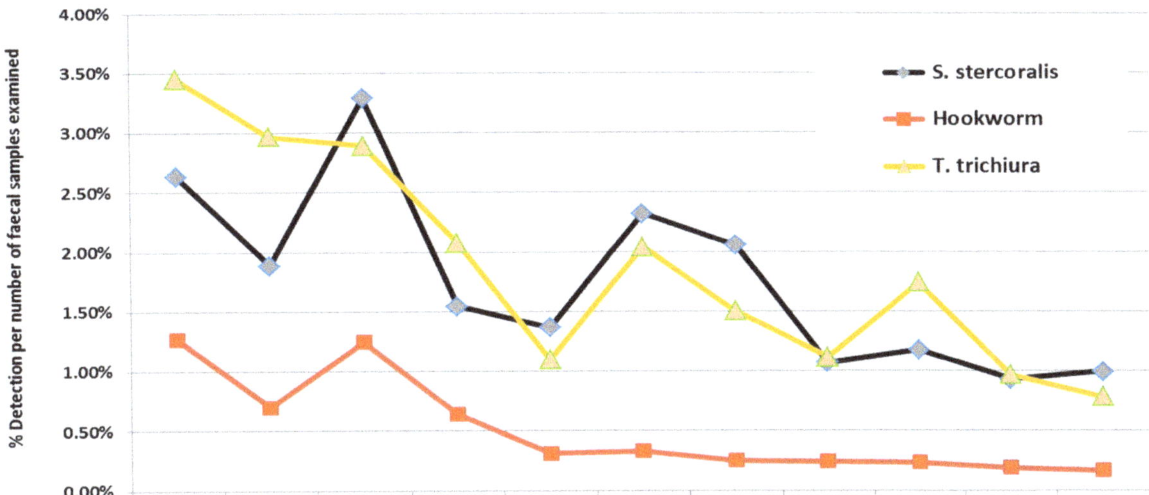

	2002	2003	2004	2005	2006	2007	2008	2009	2010	2011	2012
S. stercoralis	2.64%	1.89%	3.29%	1.55%	1.37%	2.32%	2.06%	1.07%	1.18%	0.93%	0.99%
Hookworm	1.27%	0.70%	1.25%	0.64%	0.32%	0.33%	0.25%	0.24%	0.24%	0.19%	0.17%
T. trichiura	3.46%	2.97%	2.89%	2.08%	1.10%	2.04%	1.50%	1.12%	1.75%	0.97%	0.79%

Figure 4. Comparative yearly detection of soil-transmitted helminths in the Northern Territory public laboratories, 2002 to 2012, by yearly diagnostic prevalence.

3. Discussion

The main findings of this study include: (i) the declining rate of *S. stercoralis* detection over the 11 years of this study, which mirrors the previously noted decline of two other helminths, namely, hookworm, [11] and whipworm [12]; (ii) the biphasic age distribution of the patients with larvae detection; and (iii) *S. stercoralis* infections' poor correlation with the presence of eosinophilia, particularly in detections in patients over the age of five, where eosinophilia was present in only 40.8% of patients.

Our findings are consistent with other studies of STH detection in the same time period [11,12] from the same cohort, revealing a declining detection rate in the NT. Two additional factors, possibly influencing the rates of detection of STHs in NT health care facilities have to be considered before definitely attributing the reduction to a community-wide decline in helminth infections. Firstly, hookworm has been targeted by an Indigenous community children's deworming program (CCDP) in the NT since 1995, which administers single-dose albendazole to children aged 6 months to 16 years, twice a year [11]. This is a lower albendazole dose than current recommended for *S. stercoralis* treatment therapy, but may have a partial effect. The Central Australian Rural Practitioners Association (CARPA) [13] currently recommends for *S. stercoralis* therapy: albendazole daily for three days (children ≤5 years of age), or ivermectin, for children >5 years and adults. The albendazole given as part of the CCDP may still have some effect, as noted by decreases in the detection of whipworm [12] in the same population. Dwarf tapeworm (*Hymenolepis nana*), which is common, and not susceptible to albendazole, has not shown a temporal decrease in detection in the NT [14], from the same cohort, during this time period, suggesting the CCDP may possibly be associated with some additional STH reductions outside the targeted hookworm-infected population. Secondly, hospital paediatric admissions for diarrhea have reduced Australia-wide, since the introduction of rotavirus vaccine in 2006 [15]. This may have led to a decrease in detection of asymptomatic *S. stercoralis* infection in patients admitted with acute diarrhoeal diseases. However, the decreasing trend may reflect some improvement in socio-economic and sanitary circumstances, but this is speculative until formal prevalence studies are temporally conducted in a cross-section of the many remote communities spread across the 1.5 million square kilometers of the Northern Territory.

The biphasic age distribution of patients in raw detection numbers with a secondary age peak between 35 and 50 years of age, with a male predominance across the NT, is quite different to the pattern observed with whipworm [12] in the NT from the same cohort, where conversely, women had a statistically significant higher proportion of infections. It was postulated that adult women have higher rates of infection because they care for and live in closer proximity to infected children who contaminate the nearby environment. The adult male and female population is outside the target group for CCDP, so these infections detections do represent continuing NT wide endemic disease.

This study used a standard widely-used concentration method to detect *S. stercoralis* faecal larvae as the diagnostic, allowing the demographic and laboratory parameters in patients with current *S. stercoralis* infection to be accurately correlated with actual infection, rather than implied from serological results, that can remain positive after the infection is cleared [16]. The gold standard for the diagnosis of *S. stercoralis* remains serial stool examination [17]. However, traditional stool examinations are insensitive, and require up to seven stool exams to reach a sensitivity of 100%. Specialized stool exams include Harada-Mori filter paper culture, quantitative acetate concentration technique, and nutrient agar plate cultures [17]. Detection by nucleic acid amplification of faecal strongyloides DNA, is in development, but has not as yet been demonstrated to be superior to traditional methods for *S. stercoralis* infection [18,19] and is not yet widely available.

Of note in our study was the significant difference in eosinophilia observed between the ≤5 year-old group and the >5 year-old group. This observation supports local NT and Australia-wide guidelines endorsing ivermectin prophylaxis for all Indigenous adults undergoing immunosuppression, rather than just those with eosinophilia. Eosinophilia could also be more common in the younger age group related to factors such as more recent infection, presence of other nematodes or to a lesser extent, the cestode, *H. nana*. Our study emphasises that the presence or absence of eosinophilia is not an adequate proxy test for *S stercoralis* infection in a community where the infection is prevalent, particularly in patients over the age of five years. This finding supports an earlier study where *S. stercoralis* serology results and the presence of eosinophilia, were found to correlate poorly [20] though the correlation in patients with diabetes was somewhat better. The higher rates of anaemia, we noted in the Indigenous older age group has been documented previously, as anaemia is highly prevalent in Indigenous communities. A study in an Aboriginal community of Western Australia identified anaemia among 55% of women and 18% of men [21], the causes being multifactorial, and often associated with other comorbidities, including social disadvantage [22].

Our retrospective study has several limitations and several potential biases that require consideration when interpreting this data. This was not a formal prevalence study, as systematic sampling from individual communities was not undertaken, so the actual prevalence rates are undoubtedly much higher than the laboratory microscopically-diagnosed rates found in our study population. The study population mainly reflected inpatients of NT Government health facilities, reflecting a selection bias towards patients with acute illness and comorbid conditions. Bias may have been introduced in regards to Indigenous status (as Indigenous patients are over-represented amongst admissions to NT Health Care facilities) and the bias towards inclusion of hospitalised patients may have resulted in an inflated estimate of comorbid anaemia and co-infection. Reduced recovery of parasites due to delays incurred by transport of specimens to the laboratory from remote locations, and use of routine laboratory methods rather than specialised enrichment techniques, will have led to an underestimate of the actual number of infections.

The main findings of this study of *S. stercoralis* larvae detections from NT Government health care facilities include: detections occur almost exclusively from Indigenous patients, across the entire NT; the detection of larvae in all age groups, the geographic distribution of larvae detection, and the lack of active infections being associated with eosinophilia. This last finding has important implications for patients receiving immunosuppressive therapy and their need for prophylactic *S. stercoralis* therapy. The temporal trend over the 11 years of this study, reveals declining rates of *S. stercoralis* detection, which mirrors that of the other helminths, whipworm, and hookworm, though all remain endemic in the NT, and remain markers of social disadvantage.

4. Materials and Methods

We conducted a retrospective observational review of microbiologically detected *S. stercoralis* larvae in faecal samples collected at NT Government Health facilities between 2002 and 2012 inclusive. Ethical approval for the study was obtained from both the Top End HREC-2013-1978 and Central Australian ethics committees, HREC-14-267. Cases were identified from the NT government pathology laboratory information system, Labtrak (Intersystems), which covers all NT Government Health facilities, including 5 hospitals, 2 correctional centres, and over 50 remote clinics. Previous STH studies have shown the NT public laboratories identified 94% of all documented STHs, as compared to 6% from other pathology providers, during this time period [11]. Given the intermittent shedding of *S. stercoralis* larvae, all faecal microscopy specimens (including second and third samples) were included in the analysis, but only one episode of larvae detection was recorded, even if multiple positive larvae detections were recorded in an individual episode of hospitalisation. Repeated episodes in a single patient were counted, if the temporal spacing was greater than six months. The episodes were linked to NT government electronic databases via medical record number to obtain data on age, sex, Indigenous status, geographic residence, haemoglobin level, and eosinophil count. Anaemia was defined as a haemoglobin <110 g/L and eosinophilia as a count $\geq 0.5 \times 10^9$/L. Parasite identification was done by faecal specimen examination by wet mount microscopy followed by a formol ethyl-acetate concentration method [17]. Initially manual, the lab has also changed to use a proprietary product, namely Mini Parasep SF Faecal Concentrator (Apacor, Wolkingham, England). Local standard reporting procedures were followed. Quantitative assessment of parasite numbers was not performed. Detection of larvae allowed specific correlation of current infection with the haematological parameters, but is relatively insensitive compared to research methods [17].

5. Statistical Analysis

Data was collected in a Microsoft Excel 2010 (Microsoft Corporation, Redmond, Washington, DC, USA) database and analysed using the 'Real-statistics' plug in (Zaiontz C. 2015, www.real-statistics.com). Results are presented as medians and interquartile ranges (IQRs) for non-normally distributed parameters. Age range groups, and faecal detection rates were cumulated for presentation in Figure 1. Indigenous population data from the NT were obtained from Australian Bureau of Statistics data [23]. Bivariate analyses were performed using the Chi Square or Fisher exact test (if expected frequencies were less than 5). For non-parametric data, (median haemoglobin and eosinophil counts, as well as polyparasitism in patients above and below the age of 5 years), the Mann–Whitney U test was used, with p values of <0.05 considered significant. The age cut-off of five years was chosen based on previous studies of STH in a similar population [11].

Acknowledgments: Microbiology staff of the five public hospital laboratories of the Northern Territory for helminth identification over the 11 years of this study.

Author Contributions: J.M.-C. compiled and extracted data, and prepared the submission, A.C. wrote the ethics submissions, compiled and extracted data, and prepared the submission. P.S. supervised all the laboratory components and parasite identification, and assisted with manuscript preparation. R.B. oversaw the project, assisted with data and manuscript preparation, revisions, and aspects of the discussion.

References

1. Schar, F.; Trostdorf, U.; Giardina, F.; Khieu, V.; Muth, S.; Marti, H.; Vounatsou, P.; Odermatt, P. *Strongyloides stercoralis*: Global distribution and risk factors. *PLoS Negl. Trop. Dis.* **2013**, *7*, e2288. [CrossRef] [PubMed]
2. Walker, A.C.; Blake, G.; Downing, D. A syndrome of partial intestinal obstruction due to *Strongyloides stercoralis*. *Med. J. Aust.* **1976**, *6*, 47–48.
3. Fisher, D.; McCarry, F.; Currie, B. Strongyloidiasis in the Northern Territory. Under-recognised and under-treated. *Med. J. Aust.* **1993**, *159*, 88–90. [PubMed]
4. Einsiedel, L.J.; Pham, H.; Woodman, R.J.; Pepperill, C.; Taylor, K.A. The prevalence and clinical associations of HTLV-1 infection in a remote Indigenous community. *Med. J. Aust.* **2016**, *205*, 305–309. [CrossRef] [PubMed]
5. Holt, D.C.; McCarthy, J.S.; Carapetis, J.R. Parasitic diseases of remote Indigenous communities in Australia. *Int. J. Parasitol.* **2010**, *40*, 1119–1126. [CrossRef] [PubMed]
6. Prociv, P.; Luke, R. Observations on strongyloidiasis in Queensland aboriginal communities. *Med. J. Aust.* **1993**, *158*, 160–163. [PubMed]
7. Vos, T.; Barker, B.; Begg, S.; Stanley, L.; Lopez, A.D. Burden of disease and injury in Aboriginal and Torres Strait Islander Peoples: The Indigenous health gap. *Int. J. Epidemiol.* **2009**, *38*, 470–477. [CrossRef] [PubMed]
8. WHO. Intestinal Worms Strongyloidiasis. Available online: http://www.who.int/intestinal_worms/epidemiology/strongyloidiasis/en/ (accessed on 5 January 2017).
9. Lim, L.; Biggs, B. Fatal disseminated strongyloidiasis in a previously treated patient. *Med. J. Aust.* **2001**, *174*, 355–356. [PubMed]
10. Caruana, S.R.; Kelly, H.A.; Ngeow, J.Y.; Ryan, N.J.; Bennett, C.M.; Chea, L.; Nuon, S.; Bak, N.; Skull, S.A.; Biggs, B.A. Undiagnosed and potentially lethal parasite infections among immigrants and refugees in Australia. *J. Travel Med.* **2006**, *13*, 233–239. [CrossRef] [PubMed]
11. Davies, J.; Majumdar, S.S.; Forbes, R.T.; Smith, P.; Currie, B.J.; Baird, R.W. Hookworm in the Northern Territory: Down but not out. *Med. J. Aust.* **2013**, *198*, 278–281. [CrossRef] [PubMed]
12. Crowe, A.L.; Smith, P.; Ward, L.; Currie, B.J.; Baird, R.W. Decreasing prevalence of *Trichuris trichiura* (whipworm) in the Northern Territory from 2002 to 2012. *Med. J. Aust.* **2014**, *200*, 286–289. [CrossRef] [PubMed]
13. Remote Primary Health Care Manuals. CARPA Standard Treatment Manual. Available online: http://www.remotephcmanuals.com.au/publication/stm/CARPA_STM_home_page.html (accessed on 1 February 2017).
14. Willcocks, B.; McAuliffe, G.N.; Baird, R.W. Dwarf tapeworm (*Hymenolepis. nana*): Characteristics in the Northern Territory 2002–2013. *J. Paediatr. Child. Health* **2015**, *51*, 982–987. [CrossRef] [PubMed]
15. Buttery, J.P.; Lambert, S.B.; Grimwood, K.; Nissen, M.D.; Field, E.J.; Macartney, K.K.; Akikusa, J.D.; Kelly, J.J.; Kirkwood, C.D. Reduction in rotavirus-associated acute gastroenteritis following introduction of rotavirus vaccine into Australia's national childhood vaccine schedule. *Pediatr. Infect. Dis. J.* **2011**, *30*, S25–S29. [CrossRef] [PubMed]
16. Page, W.A.; Dempsey, K.; McCarthy, J.S. Utility of serological follow-up of chronic strongyloidiasis after anthelminthic chemotherapy. *Trans. R Soc. Trop Med. Hyg.* **2006**, *100*, 1056–1062. [CrossRef] [PubMed]
17. Garcia, L.S.; Bruckner, D. *Diagnostic Medical Parasitology*, 3rd ed.; ASM Press: Washington, DC, USA, 1997; pp. 615–618.

18. Llewellyn, S.; Inpankaew, T.; Nery, S.V.; Gray, D.J.; Verweij, J.J.; Clements, A.C.; Gomes, S.J.; Traub, R.; McCarthy, J.S. Application of a multiplex quantitative PCR to assess prevalence and intensity of intestinal parasite infections in a controlled clinical trial. *PLoS Negl. Trop. Dis.* **2016**, *10*, e0004380. [CrossRef] [PubMed]
19. Verweij, J.J.; Canales, M.; Polman, K.; Ziem, J.; Brienen, E.A.; Polderman, A.M.; Lieshout, L.V. Molecular diagnosis of *Strongyloides stercoralis* in faecal samples using real-time PCR. *Trans. R. Soc. Trop. Med. Hyg.* **2009**, *103*, 342–346. [CrossRef] [PubMed]
20. Hays, R.; Thompson, F.; Esterman, A.; McDermott, R. *Strongyloides stercoralis*, eosinophilia, and type 2 diabetes mellitus: The predictive value of eosinophilia in the diagnosis of *S. stercoralis* infection in an endemic community. *Open Forum. Infect. Dis.* **2016**, *3*, ofw029. [CrossRef] [PubMed]
21. Hopkins, R.M.; Gracey, M.S.; Hobbs, R.P.; Spargo, R.M.; Yates, M.; Thompson, R.C. The prevalence of hookworm infection, iron deficiency and anaemia in an Aboriginal community in north-west Australia. *Med. J. Aust.* **1997**, *166*, 241–244. [PubMed]
22. Beknazarova, M.; Whiley, H.; Ross, K. Strongyloidiasis: A disease of socioeconomic disadvantage. *Int. J. Environ. Res. Public Health* **2016**, *13*. [CrossRef] [PubMed]
23. Australian Bureau of Statistics. *Experimental Estimates and Projections, Aboriginal and Torres Strait Islander Australians, 1991 to 2021*; (ABS Cat. No. 3238.0.); ABS: Canberra, Australia, 2009. Available online: http://www.abs.gov.au/ausstats/abs@.nsf/mf/3238.0.55.001 (accessed on 5 January 2017).

Mycetoma: The Spectrum of Clinical Presentation

Ahmed Hassan Fahal [1,*], Suliman Hussein Suliman [2] and Roderick Hay [3]

1 The Mycetoma Research Centre, University of Khartoum, Khartoum 11111, Sudan
2 Department of Surgery, Faculty of Medicine, University of Khartoum, Khartoum 11111, Sudan; sul.hus.sul@gmail.com
3 The International Foundation for Dermatology, London W1P 5HQ, UK; roderick.hay@ifd.org
* Correspondence: ahfahal@hotmail.com or ahfahal@uofk.edu;

Abstract: Mycetoma is a chronic infection, newly designated by the World Health Organization (WHO) as a neglected tropical disease, which is endemic in tropical and subtropical regions. It follows implantation of infectious organisms, either fungi (eumycetomas) or filamentous bacteria (actinomycetomas) into subcutaneous tissue, from where infection spreads to involve skin, bone and subcutaneous sites, leading to both health related and socioeconomic problems. In common with other NTDs, mycetoma is most often seen in rural areas amongst the poorest of people who have less access to health care. The organisms form small microcolonies that are discharged onto the skin surface via sinus tracts, or that can burrow into other adjacent tissues including bone. This paper describes the clinical features of mycetoma, as early recognition is a key to early diagnosis and the institution of appropriate treatment including surgery. Because these lesions are mostly painless and the majority of infected individuals present late and with advanced disease, simplifying early recognition is an important public health goal.

Keywords: mycetoma; clinical presentation; review

---

1. Introduction

Mycetoma is a unique and troubling neglected tropical disease, endemic in many tropical and subtropical areas. In addition, it is reported from different parts of the world [1,2]. It is a chronic granulomatous subcutaneous inflammatory disease that has a profound and negative impact on numerous medical, health-related and socioeconomic aspects of the lives of patients and communities in the endemic regions [3,4]. The causative organisms of mycetoma are of bacterial or fungal origin and hence these are classified as actinomycetomas and eumycetomas respectively [5,6]. Traumatic implantation of these causative organisms, which are soil and environmental inhabitants, into the subcutaneous tissue via minor trauma or injury is believed to be the route of entry in the development of mycetoma [7,8]. During the evolution of the infection, the causative organisms grow into modified localised microcolonies known as grains that are surrounded by inflammatory cells and give rise to inflammatory sinus tracts. Mycetoma is basically a localised disease; the inflammatory process usually involves the local subcutaneous tissue but it then spreads along the different tissue planes to invade the skin, deep tissues and structures and eventually the bones [9,10]. If not treated appropriately, it can lead to enormous tissue damage, disfigurement and disability that hinder the patients' normal daily activities [11,12]. Mycetoma patients are unique. They are of low socioeconomic status and health educational level, reside in remote, poor rural areas with meagre medical and health resources. Furthermore, their lesions are usually painless and hence the majority of them present late and with advanced pathology [13,14].

2. Age, Gender and Occupation in Mycetoma

No age is exempted from infection but the majority of patients are young adults in the age group of 15–30 years [15,16]. In most of the reported series, children account for 30% of the cases [17]. This has massive implications for the patients, families and communities in the endemic areas as these are the working and wage-earning members of each society and many of these drop out of education due to illness, which increases the pressure on family and community income and resources in households that are already impoverished [18,19].

Male predominance is a constant finding in mycetoma with a gender ratio of 3.7:1 [20,21]. This is commonly attributed to the greater risk of exposure to microorganisms in the soil during outdoor work-related activities. However, in mycetoma-endemic areas, females are also involved in outdoor work activities and thus other genetic or immunological factors cannot be ruled out [22,23].

Mycetoma is seen in most communities in farmers, field labourers and in herdsmen who come in contact with the land, although in endemic areas people from other occupations are affected [24,25].

The patients' photographs were all obtained following due informed consent procedure.

3. The Clinical Presentation

More than 70 microorganisms are incriminated in causing mycetoma. Nevertheless, the clinical presentation of mycetoma is almost indistinguishable regardless of the causal microorganism [26]. The triad of painless subcutaneous swelling, multiple draining sinuses and discharge that contains grains is characteristics of mycetoma. The swelling is usually firm and rounded but it may be soft, lobulated and, rarely, cystic and it is often mobile (Figure 1) [27]. Multiple secondary nodules then evolve, the nodules may suppurate and drain through multiple sinus tracts, and these sinuses may close transiently after discharge during the active phase of the disease. Prior to discharge, pustules may be visible. Fresh adjacent sinuses may open while some of the old ones may heal completely. The sinuses are connected with each other, with deep abscesses and with the skin surface (Figure 2) [28]. The discharge is usually serous, serosanguinous or purulent. During the active phase of the disease, the sinuses discharge grains, consisting of the microorganisms encapsulated in a cement-like material, melanin and other substances. The grains are believed to protect these microorganisms against host defence mechanisms, antimicrobials and antifungals [29]. The grain colour depends on the causative organism. The grains can be black, yellow, white or red and they are of variable size and consistency. In most mycetomas, they are visible to the naked eye and may be noticed by patients; the exception is actinomycetoma, due to the *Nocardia* species, in which the grains are very small and only visible under the microscope. The black grains are most commonly due to *M. mycetomatis* and related species, the red ones are due to *A. pelletierii*, the yellow to *Streptomyces somaliensis* and the white grains can be due to *A. madurae* [30]. However, black fungi may also produce grains of pale colour. Pus, exudate, the dressing gauze and biopsy material should be examined for the presence of the grains as they may give a clue to the causative organisms although the identity needs to be confirmed as visual inspection alone is not sufficiently accurate (Figure 3).

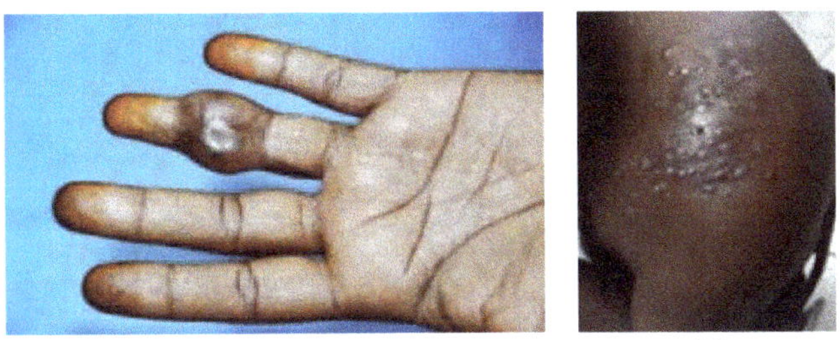

(A) (B)

Figure 1. (**A**) A small mycetoma swelling engulfing the middle part of the left ring finger with a scar of previous surgical excision. (**B**) Multiple small nodules of *Nocardia* actinomycetoma at an earlier stage.

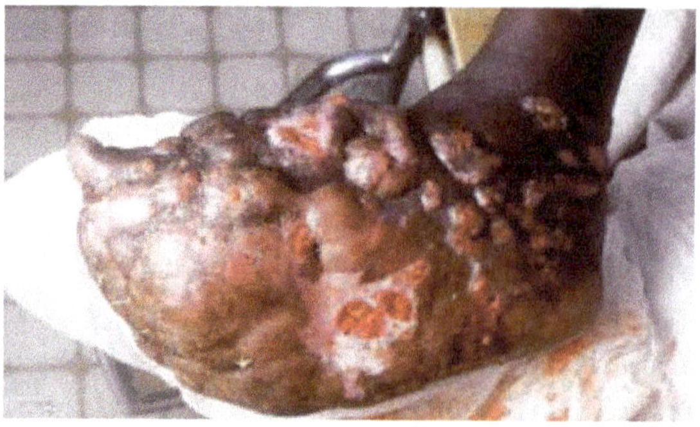

Figure 2. Massive actinomycetoma foot with multiple sinuses and discharge.

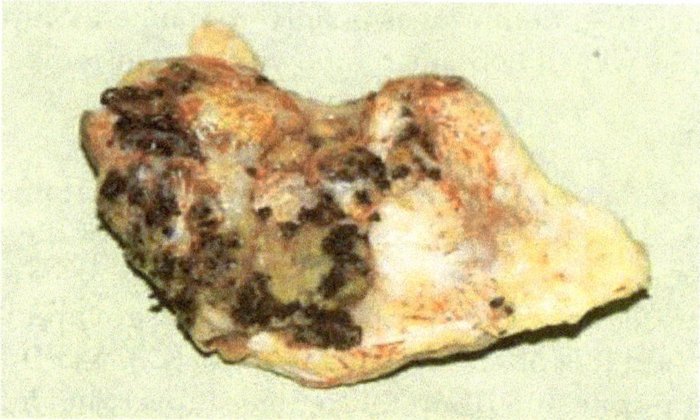

Figure 3. Surgical specimen with multiple black grains.

The onset and progress rate is more rapid with actinomycetoma than with eumycetoma. In eumycetoma, the lesion grows slowly with clearly defined margins and remains encapsulated for a long period, whereas, in actinomycetoma, the lesion is more inflammatory, more destructive and invades the bone at an earlier period; this is more evident in *A. pelletierii* actinomycetoma [31].

As the mycetoma granuloma increases in size, the skin over it becomes attached and stretched. The skin may become smooth, shiny and areas of hypo or hyperpigmentation may develop (Figure 4) [32]. In some patients, there may be areas of local hyperhidrosis confined to the mycetoma lesion itself and the skin around it. This is commonly seen with massive lesions in patients with active disease and the cause is unclear but increased local temperature due to brisk arterial circulation may a cause (Figures 5 and 6). In *Nocardia* actinomycetomas the chest wall or back is often affected and here the edges of the lesions are unclear and hard to define.

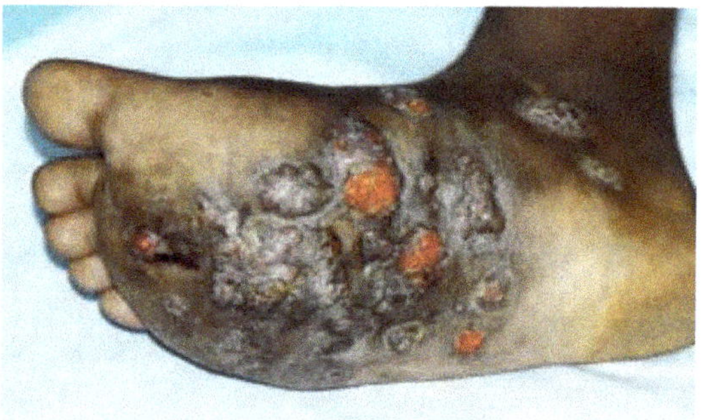

Figure 4. Foot eumycetoma with skin hyperpigmentation, multiple nodules and active sinuses.

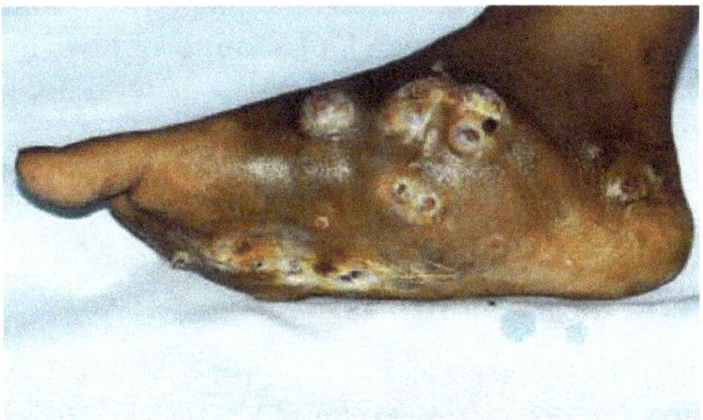

Figure 5. Foot eumycetoma with skin hyperpigmentation, multiple nodules, active sinuses discharging black grains discharge and local hyperhidrosis.

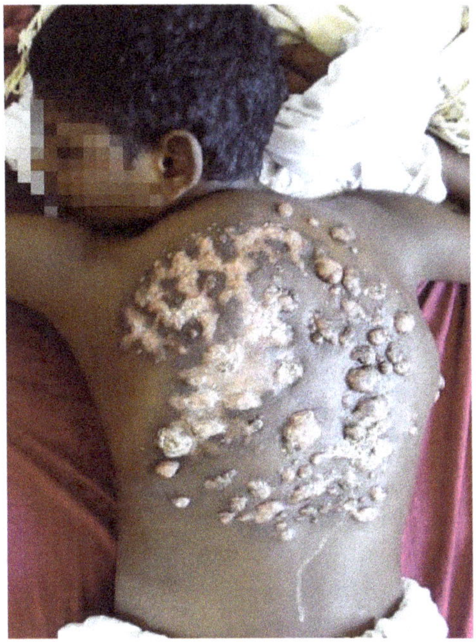

Figure 6. Massive back actinomycetoma with multiple nodules and sinuses.

In long-standing massive mycetoma lesions, dilated tortuous veins at, and proximal to, the mycetoma site are noted. They are frequently confused with varicose veins. They develop as a secondary phenomenon to accommodate the brisk venous return due to the increased arterial blood flow caused by the chronic inflammatory process at the mycetoma site (Figure 7) [33].

Unusually and for unknown reasons, the tendons and the nerves are spared until very late in the disease process; this may explain the rarity of neurological and trophic changes even in patients with long-standing mycetomas. The absence of trophic changes may be explained by the more than adequate blood supply in the mycetoma-infected area [34].

In the majority of patients, the regional lymph nodes are small and shotty. An enlarged regional lymph node is not uncommon and this may be due to secondary bacterial infection, the genuine lymphatic spread of mycetoma or it may be due to immune complex deposition as part of a local immune response to mycetoma infection [35].

In general, the infection remains localised and constitutional disturbances are rare but when they do occur they are generally due to secondary bacterial infection of the open sinus tracts and generalised immunosuppression. Cachexia and anaemia may be seen in late mycetoma. This is often due to malnutrition, sepsis and mental depression [36]. Co-morbidities in mycetoma are rare and the commonest are diabetes mellitus and hypertension, as in the general population. HIV and malignant transformation are not reported in mycetoma [30].

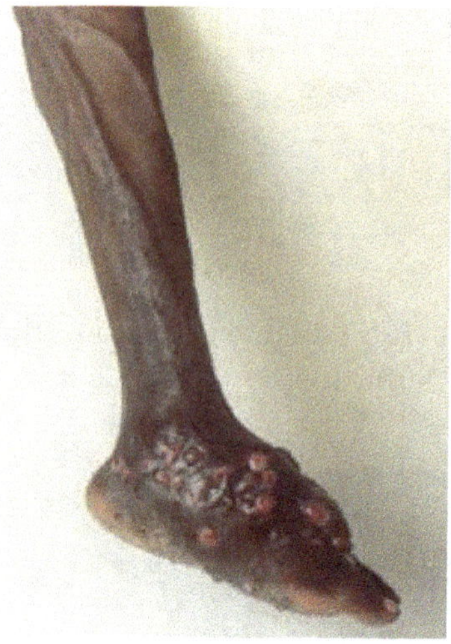

Figure 7. Massive mycetoma foot with dilated tortuous veins at and proximal to the mycetoma site.

Mycetoma is usually painless in nature; it has been suggested that the mycetoma produces substances that have an anaesthetic action. At a late stage of the disease, the pain may also become negligible due to nerve damage by the tense fibrous tissue reaction, endarteritis obliterans or poor vascularisation of the nerves [37]. Pain at the mycetoma site is reported in 20% of patients and it is commonly produced by the secondary bacterial infection or transiently when a new closed sinus is about to open onto the skin surface.

Mycetoma can produce many distortions, deformities and disabilities and that is due to structural impairment that includes bone destruction or periostitis, loss of function and disuse atrophy of the affected limb. The current treatment options are limited and suboptimal; many patients undergo repeated massive surgical excisions leading to more tissue destruction and fibrosis and disability (Figure 8) [38].

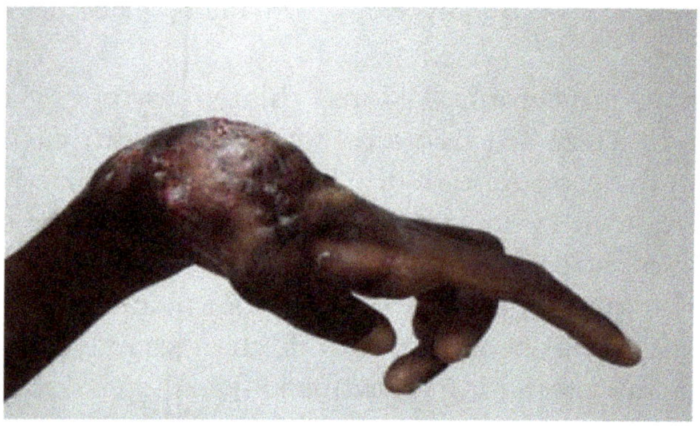

Figure 8. Hand eumycetoma with massive deformity.

4. The Site of Mycetoma

The commonest site for mycetoma is the foot (79.2%); most of the lesions are seen on the dorsal aspect of the forefoot and the left foot is affected slightly more often [39]. The hand ranks as the second commonest site (6.6%), with the right hand is more affected. This may imply a traumatic basis of the infection in this site [40]. In endemic areas, other parts of the body may be involved but less frequently, and these include the knee, arm, leg, head and neck, thigh and the perineum [41–45]. Rarer sites for eumycetomas are the chest and abdominal walls, facial bones, mandible, paranasal sinuses, eyelid, vulva, orbit and scrotum (Figures 9–11) [46–50]. *Nocardia* actinomycetomas are often found on the chest or abdominal wall. Bilateral limb mycetomas, although described, are very rare.

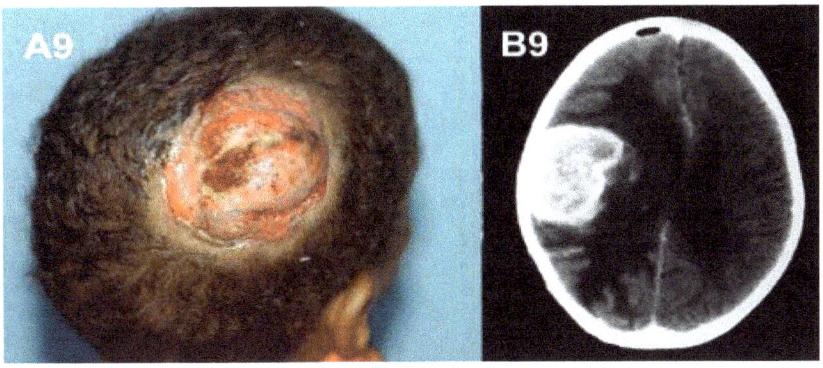

Figure 9. (**A**) massive head eumycetoma. (**B**) CT scan showing intra-cranial extension.

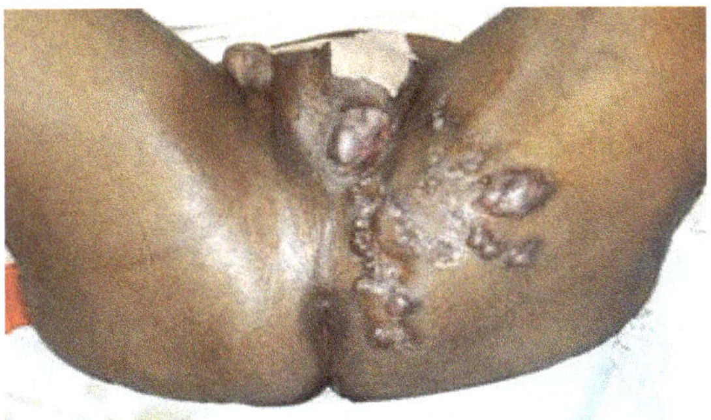

Figure 10. Massive gluteal, perineal and scrotal eumycetoma.

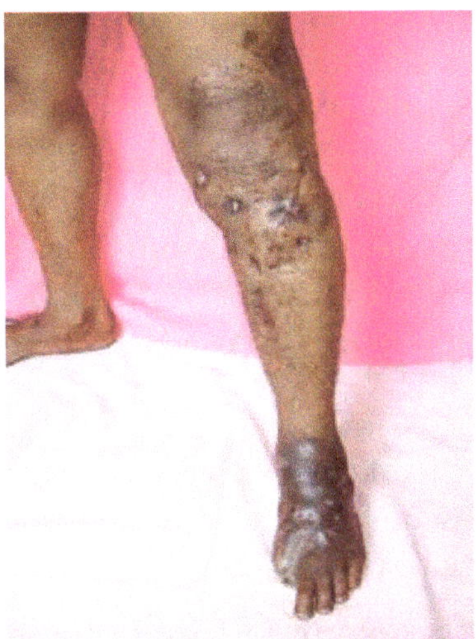

Figure 11. Massive foot actinomycetoma with leg and knee inguinal satellite lesions.

5. Mycetoma Spread

Spread along the lymphatics to the regional lymph nodes is reported and this is more frequent with actinomycetoma [12]. At the regional lymph nodes, the disease progresses; a new disease satellite lesion develops and progresses to form a massive mycetoma, and in some cases, this can cause lymphatic obstruction and lymphedema (Figure 11) [51]. Bloodstream spread in mycetoma is a rare event. It has been reported in some cases, where there was spinal cord compression and paraplegia. In these cases, the skin and subcutaneous tissue were normal and the mycetoma was an unexpected finding at surgery upon opening the spinal dura matter [52]. In these cases, the mycetoma grains were actually seen in the lumen of the intact blood vessel (Figure 12).

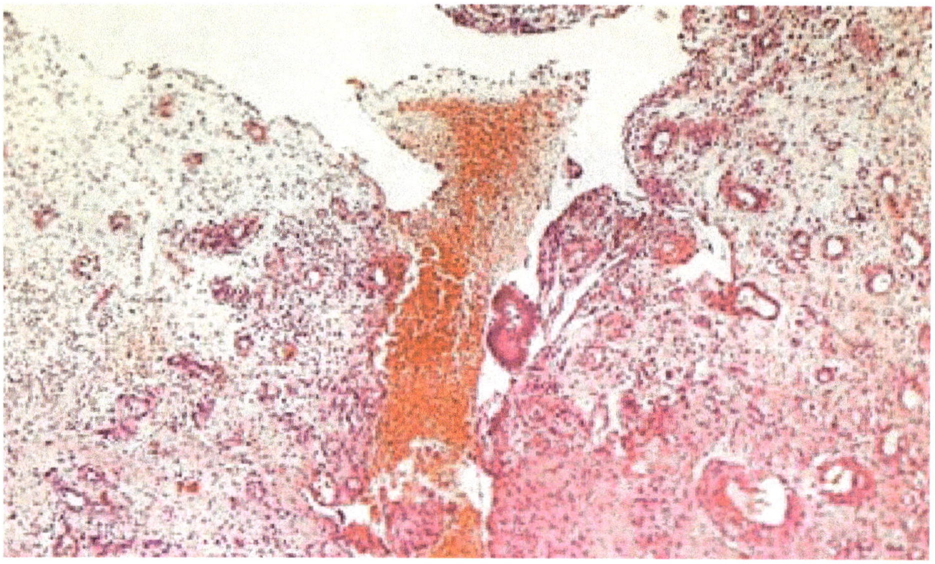

Figure 12. Photomicrograph showing *A. madurae* grains within the lumen of the intact blood vessel (H&E X 200).

6. Aggressive Mycetoma

Although mycetoma is primarily a localised disease of gradual onset and slow progress, some patients present with massive, aggressive, uncontrolled disease and most of these are fatal. In these patients, the disease progressed wildly and aggressively from the subcutaneous tissue to involve the deep organs such as the urinary bladder, pelvic organs, spinal cord, lung and other structures and resulted in fatal outcome [53–56].

Two patients with fatal eumycetoma presented with pulmonary secondaries were reported; one from the knee and the second from gluteal eumycetoma. In these patients, *Madurella mycetomatis* had progressed widely without response to the different medical and surgical treatment modalities. Vascular spread, which is a rare phenomenon in mycetoma, may explain the secondary lung lesions encountered in these patients [52,54–56].

Several cases of mycetoma of the head and neck region have reported. They proved to be serious medical and health problem, with low cure rate and were associated with grave complications and poor outcome due to intra-cranial spread [57].

Pelvic mycetoma spread has also been reported. In these cases, the urinary bladder, rectum, hip bones and other local structures were involved. The disease was complicated by multiple urinary and rectal fistulae, pathological fractures and all patients died from massive sepsis (Figure 13) [52–56].

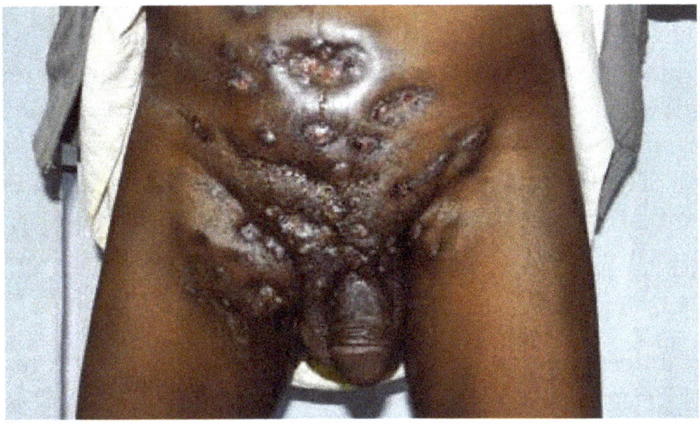

Figure 13. Massive anterior abdominal eumycetoma spreading to both inguinal regions and scrotum.

7. The Differential Diagnosis

In endemic areas, any subcutaneous mass is considered as mycetoma unless proved otherwise. The differential diagnosis of mycetoma includes thorn and foreign body granulomas, particularly in mycetoma endemic areas [57]. Also, it includes many soft tissue tumours such as Kaposi's sarcoma, fibroma, malignant melanoma or fibrolipoma and keloids [1,58]. Many dermatological conditions, such as botryomycosis, sporotrichosis and plantar or acral psoriasis, can mimic mycetoma [59]. In very early mycetomas, before the first appearance of sinuses, the lesion simply resembles a firm subcutaneous nodule, which makes recognition of the earliest signs based on a visual appearance very difficult as the differential encompasses a variety of benign and inflammatory conditions, from dermatofibromas to hypertrophic scars. The radiological features of advanced mycetoma resemble osteogenic sarcoma and bone tuberculosis (Figure 14). Primary osseous mycetoma, without overlying sinuses, is uncommon but must be differentiated from chronic osteomyelitis, osteoclastoma, bone cysts and syphilitic osteitis.

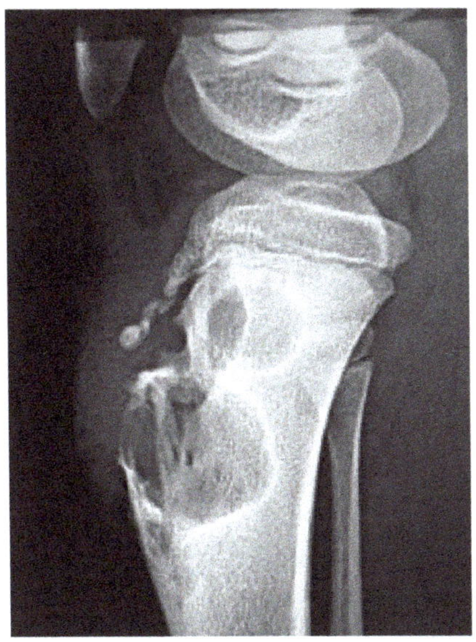

Figure 14. X-ray of thigh and knee eumycetoma showing massive soft tissue shadow, periosteal reaction and multiple bone cavities resembling osteogenic sarcoma.

This paper has concentrated on the variations in the clinical presentation of mycetomas. The currently available treatments for mycetoma are suboptimal and unsatisfactory, characterised by a low cure rate and high patient follow-up dropout and recurrence rates [49]. Furthermore, presently there are neither preventive nor control measures or programs for mycetoma. Moreover, mycetoma affects the most underprivileged population in remote areas and hence most patients present late with advanced disease. To overcome this, early case detection, which depends on detecting the visual warning signs of the disease and treatment is the only available means to prevent the numerous and serious complications of mycetoma. The first step in early case detection is meticulous clinical examination of the suspected patients, as other diagnostics tools, including direct microscopy, culture, histopathology and molecular identification, are commonly not available in mycetoma- endemic regions [60].

Author Contributions: The three authors contributed equally to this review article, and that included conceptualization, literature review, writing of original draft preparation, and review & editing.

References

1. Fahal, A.H. Mycetoma: A thorn in the flesh. *Trans. R. Soc. Trop. Med. Hyg.* **2004**, *98*, 3–11.
2. Fahal, A.H.; Hassan, M.A. Mycetoma. *Br. J. Surg.* **1992**, *79*, 1138–1141. [CrossRef] [PubMed]
3. Bonifaz, A.; Tirado-Sánchez, A.; Calderón, L.; Saúl, A.; Araiza, J.; Hernández, M.; González, G.M.; Ponce, R.M. Mycetoma: Experience of 482 cases in a single center in Mexico. *PLoS Negl. Trop. Dis.* **2014**, *8*, e3102.
4. Ahmed, A.O.; van Leeuwen, W.; Fahal, A.; van de Sande, W.; Verbrugh, H.; van Belkum, A. Mycetoma caused by *Madurella mycetomatis*: A neglected infectious burden. *Lancet Infect. Dis.* **2004**, *4*, 566–574. [CrossRef]
5. Ahmed, A.O.A.; van de Sande, W.W.; Fahal, A.; Bakker-Woudenberg, I.; Verbrugh, H.; van Belkum, A. Management of mycetoma: Major challenge in tropical mycoses with limited international recognition. *Curr. Opin. Infect. Dis.* **2007**, *20*, 146–151. [PubMed]
6. Fahal, A.H.; van de Sandy, W.W. The epidemiology of mycetoma. *Curr. Fungal Infect. Rep.* **2012**, *6*, 320–326. [CrossRef]
7. Fahal, A.H. Mycetoma. In *Tropical Infectious Diseases. Principles, Pathogens and Practice*, 3rd ed.; Guerrant, R.L., Walker, D.H., Weller, P.F., Eds.; Elsevier: Amsterdam, The Netherlands, 2011; pp. 565–568.
8. Williams, N.S.; Bulstrode, C.; O'Connell, P.R. *Bailey and Love's Short Practice of Surgery 26E*, 26th ed.; Taylor & Francis Ltd.: London, UK, 2013; pp. 84–88.
9. Fahal, A.H. *Mycetoma: Clinico-Pathological Monograph*; University of Khartoum Press: Khurtum, Sudan, 2006; pp. 40–49.
10. Hassan, M.A.; Fahal, A.H. *Mycetoma: In Tropical Surgery*; Kamil, R., Lumbly, J., Eds.; Westminster Publication Ltd.: London, UK, 2004; pp. 30–45.
11. Fahal, A.H.; Suliman, S.H.; Gadir, A.F.A.; EL Hag, I.A.; EL Amin, F.I.; Gumaa, S.A.; Mahgoub, E.S. Abdominal wall mycetoma: An unusual presentation. *Trans. R. Soc. Trop. Med. Hyg.* **1994**, *88*, 78–80. [CrossRef]
12. Fahal, A.H.; Suliman, S.H. Clinical presentation of mycetoma. *Sudan Med. J.* **1994**, *32*, 46–66.
13. Fahal, A.H.; El Hassan, A.M.; Abdelalla, A.O.; Sheikh, H.E. Cystic mycetoma: An unusual clinical presentation of *Madurella mycetomatis*. *Trans. R. Soc. Trop. Med. Hyg.* **1998**, *92*, 66–67. [CrossRef]
14. Fahal, A.H.; EL Toum, E.A.; EL Hassan, A.M.; Gumaa, S.A.; Mahgoub, E.S. A preliminary study on the ultrastructure of *Actinomadura pelletieri* and its host tissue reaction. *J. Med. Vet. Mycol.* **1994**, *32*, 343–348. [CrossRef] [PubMed]
15. EL Hassan, A.M.; Fahal, A.H.; EL Hag, I.A.; Khalil, E.A.G. The pathology of mycetoma: Light microscopic and ultrastructural features. *Sudan Med. J.* **1994**, *32*, 23–45.
16. Fahal, A.H.; Hassan, M.A.; Sanhouri, M. Surgical treatment of mycetoma. *Sudan Med. J.* **1994**, *32*, 98–104.
17. Fahal, A.H.; EL Toum, E.A.; EL Hassan, A.M.; Gumaa, S.A.; Mahgoub, E.S. Host tissue reaction to *Madurella mycetomatis*: New classification. *J. Med. Vet. Mycol.* **1995**, *33*, 15–17. [CrossRef] [PubMed]
18. Van de Sande, W.W.; Fahal, A.H.; Goodfellow, M.; Maghoub, E.S.; Welsh, O.; Zijlstra, E.E. The merits and pitfalls of the currently used diagnostic tools in mycetoma. *PLoS Negl. Trop. Dis.* **2014**, *3*, e2918. [CrossRef] [PubMed]

19. Welsh, O.; Al-Abdely, H.M.; Salinas-Carmona, M.C.; Fahal, A.H. Mycetoma medical therapy. *PLoS Negl. Trop. Dis.* **2014**, *8*, e3218. [CrossRef] [PubMed]
20. Welsh, O.; Vera-Cabrera, L.; Welsh, E.; Salinas, M.C. Actinomycetoma and advances in its treatment. *Clin. Dermatol.* **2012**, *30*, 372–381. [CrossRef] [PubMed]
21. Mhmoud, N.A.; Ahmed, S.A.; Fahal, A.H.; de Hoog, G.S.; Gerrits van den Ende, A.H.; van de Sande, W.W. *Pleurostomophora ochracea*, a novel agent of human eumycetoma with yellow grains. *J. Clin. Microbiol.* **2012**, *50*, 2987–2994. [CrossRef] [PubMed]
22. De Hoog, G.S.; Van Diepeningen, A.D.; Mahgoub, E.S.; Van de Sande, W.W. New species of *Madurella*, causative agents of black-grain mycetoma. *Clin. Microbiol.* **2012**, *50*, 988–994. [CrossRef] [PubMed]
23. Mahgoub, E.S.; Gumaa, S.A. Ketoconazole in the treatment of eumycetoma due to *Madurella mycetomi*. *Trans. R. Soc. Trop. Med. Hyg.* **1984**, *78*, 376–379. [CrossRef]
24. Fahal, A.H.; Rahman, I.A.; El-Hassan, A.M.; EL Rahman, M.E.; Zijlstra, E.E. The efficacy of itraconazole in the treatment of patients with eumycetoma due to *Madurella mycetomatis*. *Trans. R. Soc. Trop. Med. Hyg.* **2011**, *105*, 127–132. [CrossRef] [PubMed]
25. Mahgoub, E.S.; Murray, I.G. *Mycetoma*; Medical Books Ltd.: London, UK, 1973; pp. 2–25.
26. Abbott, P.H. Mycetoma in the Sudan. *Trans. R. Soc. Trop. Med. Hyg.* **1956**, *50*, 11–24. [CrossRef]
27. Lynch, J.B. Mycetoma in the Sudan. *Ann. R. Coll. Surg. Engl.* **1964**, *35*, 319–340. [PubMed]
28. EL Moghraby, I.M. Mycetoma in Gezira. *Sudan Med. J.* **1971**, *9*, 77.
29. Mahgoub, E.S. Mycoses in the Sudan. *Trans. R. Soc. Trop. Med. Hyg.* **1977**, *71*, 184–188. [CrossRef]
30. Fahal, A.H.; Mahgoub, E.S.; EL Hassan, A.M.; Abdel-Rahman, M.E.; Alshambaty, Y.; Hashim, A.; Hago, A.; Zijlstra, E.E. A new model for management of mycetoma in the Sudan. *PLoS Negl. Trop. Dis.* **2014**, *8*, e3271. [CrossRef] [PubMed]
31. López-Martínez, R.; Méndez-Tovar, L.J.; Lavalle, P.; Welsh, O.; Saúl, A. Epidemiology of mycetoma in Mexico: Study of 2105 cases. *Gac. Med. Mex.* **1992**, *128*, 477–481. [PubMed]
32. López-Martínez, R.; Méndez-Tovar, L.J.; Bonifaz, A.; Arenas, R.; Mayorga, J.; Welsh, O.; Vera-Cabrera, L.; Padilla-Desgarennes, M.C.; Contreras Pérez, C.; Chávez, G.; et al. Update on the epidemiology of mycetoma in Mexico. A Review of 3933 cases. *Gac. Med. Mex.* **2013**, *149*, 586–592. [PubMed]
33. Ahmed, A.O.A.; Adelmann, D.; Fahal, A.H.; Verbrugh, H.A.; Van Belkum, A.; de Hoog, S.A. Environmental occurrence of *Madurella mycetomatis*, major agent of human eumycetoma in Sudan. *J. Clin. Microbiol.* **2002**, *40*, 1031–1036. [CrossRef] [PubMed]
34. Ahmed, A.O.A.; van Vianen, W.; ten Kate, M.; van de Sande, W.W.J.; Van Belkum, A. A murine model of *Madurella mycetomatis* eumycetoma. *FEMS Immunol. Med. Microbiol.* **2003**, *37*, 29–36. [CrossRef]
35. Fahal, A.H.; Azziz, K.A.A.; Suliman, S.H.; Galib, H.V.; Mahgoub, E.S. Dual infection with mycetoma and tuberculosis. *East Afr. Med. J.* **1995**, *72*, 749–750. [PubMed]
36. Fahal, A.H.; Arbab, M.A.R.; EL Hassan, A.M. Aggressive clinical presentation of mycetoma due to *Actinomadura pelletierii*. *Khartoum Med. J.* **2012**, *5*, 699–702.
37. Ibrahim, A.I.; EL Hassan, A.M.; Fahal, A.H.; van de Sande, W.W. A histopathological exploration of the *Madurella mycetomatis* grain. *PLoS ONE* **2013**, *8*, e57774. [CrossRef] [PubMed]
38. Aounallah, A.; Boussofara, L.; Ben Saïd, Z.; Ghariani, N.; Saidi, W.; Denguezli, M.; Belajouza, C.; Nouira, R. Analysis of 18 Tunisian cases of mycetoma at the Sousse hospital (1974–2010). *Bull. Soc. Pathol. Exot.* **2013**, *106*, 5–8. [CrossRef] [PubMed]
39. Dieng, M.T.; Niang, S.O.; Diop, B.; Ndiaye, B. Actinomycetomas in Senegal: Study of 90 cases. *Bull. Soc. Pathol. Exot.* **2005**, *98*, 18–20. [PubMed]
40. Marc, S.; Meziane, M.; Hamada, S.; Hassam, B.; Benzekri, L. Clinical and epidemiological features of mycetoma in Morocco. *Med. Mal. Infect.* **2011**, *41*, 163–164. [CrossRef] [PubMed]
41. Philippon, M.; Larroque, D.; Ravisse, P. Mycetoma in Mauritania: Species found, epidemiologic characteristics and country distribution. Report of 122 cases. *Bull. Soc. Pathol. Exot.* **1992**, *85*, 107–114. [PubMed]
42. Fahal, A.H.; Sharfy, A.R.A. Vulval mycetoma: A rare cause of bladder outlet obstruction. *Trans. R. Soc. Trop. Med. Hyg.* **1998**, *92*, 652–653. [CrossRef]
43. Mohamed, E.W.; Mohamed, E.N.A.; Yousif, B.M.; Fahal, A.H. Tongue actinomycetoma due to *Actinomadura madurae*: A rare clinical presentation. *J. Oral. Maxillofac. Surg.* **2012**, *70*, e622–e624. [CrossRef] [PubMed]

44. Suleiman, A.M.; Fahal, A.H. Oral eumycetoma: A rare and unusual presentation. *Oral. Surg. Oral. Med. Oral. Pathol. Oral. Radiol.* **2013**, *115*, e23–e25. [CrossRef] [PubMed]
45. Fahal, A.H.; Yagi, H.I.; EL Hassan, A.M. Mycetoma induced palatal deficiency and pharyngeal plexus dysfunction. *Trans. R. Soc. Trop. Med. Hyg.* **1996**, *90*, 676–677. [CrossRef]
46. Fahal, A.H.; Sharfi, A.R.; Sheikh, H.E.; EL Hassan, A.M. Internal fistula formation: An unusual complication of mycetoma. *Trans. R. Soc. Trop. Med. Hyg.* **1996**, *89*, 550–552. [CrossRef]
47. Mohamed, E.W.; Suleiman, H.S.; Fadella, A.I.; Fahal, A.H. Aggressive perineal and pelvic eumycetoma: An unusual and challenging problem to treat. *Khartoum Med. J.* **2012**, *5*, 771–774.
48. Hussein, A.; Ahmed, A.E.M.; Fahal, A.H.; Mahmoud, A.; Sidig, A.; Awad, K. Cervical cord compression secondary to mycetoma infection. *Sud. J. Public Health* **2007**, *2*, 112–115.
49. Zein, H.A.M.; Fahal, A.H.; Mahgoub, E.S.; EL Hassan, T.; Abdel Rahman, M.E. The predictors of cure, amputation & follow-up dropout among mycetoma patients as seen at the Mycetoma Research Centre, University of Khartoum. *Trans R. Soc. Trop. Med. Hyg.* **2012**, *106*, 639–644. [PubMed]
50. Wendy, W.J.; van de Sande, W.W.; Mahgoub, E.S.; Fahal, A.H.; Goodfellow, M.; Welsh, O. The mycetoma knowledge gap: Identification of research priorities. *PLoS Negl. Trop. Dis.* **2014**, *8*, e2667.
51. EL Hassan, A.M.; Mahgoub, E.S. Lymph node involvement in mycetoma. *Trans. R. Soc. Trop. Med. Hyg.* **1972**, *66*, 165–169. [CrossRef]
52. Arbab, M.A.; El Hag, I.A.; Abdul Gadir, A.F.; Siddik, H.E.-R. Intraspinal mycetoma: Report of two cases. *Am. J. Trop. Med. Hyg.* **1997**, *56*, 27–29. [CrossRef] [PubMed]
53. Saad, E.S.A.; Fahal, A.H. Broncho-pleuro-cutaneous fistula and pneumothorax: Rare challenging complications of chest wall eumycetoma. *PLoS Negl. Trop. Dis.* **2017**, *11*, e0005737. [CrossRef] [PubMed]
54. Mohamed, N.A.; Fahal, A.H. Mycetoma pulmonary secondaries from a gluteal eumycetoma: An unusual presentation. *PLoS Negl. Trop. Dis.* **2016**, *10*, e0004945. [CrossRef] [PubMed]
55. Mohamed, E.S.W.; Seif El Din, N.; Fahal, A.H. Multiple mycetoma lung secondaries from knee eumycetoma: An unusual complication. *PLoS Negl. Trop. Dis.* **2016**, *10*, e0004735. [CrossRef] [PubMed]
56. Scolding, P.S.; Abbas, M.A.; Omer, R.F.; Fahal, A.H. *Madurella mycetomatis*-induced massive shoulder joint destruction: A management challenge. *PLoS Negl. Trop. Dis.* **2016**, *10*, e0004849. [CrossRef] [PubMed]
57. Fahal, A.; Mahgoub, E.S.; El Hassan, A.M.; Jacoub, A.O.; Hassan, D. Head and neck mycetoma: The Mycetoma Research Centre experience. *PLoS Negl. Trop. Dis.* **2015**, *9*, e0003587. [CrossRef] [PubMed]
58. Fahal, A.; Mahgoub, E.S.; El Hassan, A.M.; Abdel-Rahman, M.E. Mycetoma in the Sudan: An update from the Mycetoma Research Centre, University of Khartoum, Sudan. *PLoS Negl. Trop. Dis.* **2015**, *9*, e0003679. [CrossRef] [PubMed]
59. Mitjà, O.; Marks, M.; Bertran, L.; Kollie, K.; Argaw, D.; Fahal, A.H. Integrated control and management of neglected tropical skin diseases. *PLoS Negl. Trop. Dis.* **2017**, *11*, e0005136. [CrossRef] [PubMed]
60. Bakhiet, S.M.; Fahal, A.H.; Musa, A.M.; Mohamed, E.S.W.; Omer, R.F.; Ahmed, E.S. A holistic approach to the mycetoma management. *PLoS Negl. Trop. Dis.* **2018**, *12*, e0006391. [CrossRef] [PubMed]

Permissions

All chapters in this book were first published by MDPI; hereby published with permission under the Creative Commons Attribution License or equivalent. Every chapter published in this book has been scrutinized by our experts. Their significance has been extensively debated. The topics covered herein carry significant findings which will fuel the growth of the discipline. They may even be implemented as practical applications or may be referred to as a beginning point for another development.

The contributors of this book come from diverse backgrounds, making this book a truly international effort. This book will bring forth new frontiers with its revolutionizing research information and detailed analysis of the nascent developments around the world.

We would like to thank all the contributing authors for lending their expertise to make the book truly unique. They have played a crucial role in the development of this book. Without their invaluable contributions this book wouldn't have been possible. They have made vital efforts to compile up to date information on the varied aspects of this subject to make this book a valuable addition to the collection of many professionals and students.

This book was conceptualized with the vision of imparting up-to-date information and advanced data in this field. To ensure the same, a matchless editorial board was set up. Every individual on the board went through rigorous rounds of assessment to prove their worth. After which they invested a large part of their time researching and compiling the most relevant data for our readers.

The editorial board has been involved in producing this book since its inception. They have spent rigorous hours researching and exploring the diverse topics which have resulted in the successful publishing of this book. They have passed on their knowledge of decades through this book. To expedite this challenging task, the publisher supported the team at every step. A small team of assistant editors was also appointed to further simplify the editing procedure and attain best results for the readers.

Apart from the editorial board, the designing team has also invested a significant amount of their time in understanding the subject and creating the most relevant covers. They scrutinized every image to scout for the most suitable representation of the subject and create an appropriate cover for the book.

The publishing team has been an ardent support to the editorial, designing and production team. Their endless efforts to recruit the best for this project, has resulted in the accomplishment of this book. They are a veteran in the field of academics and their pool of knowledge is as vast as their experience in printing. Their expertise and guidance has proved useful at every step. Their uncompromising quality standards have made this book an exceptional effort. Their encouragement from time to time has been an inspiration for everyone.

The publisher and the editorial board hope that this book will prove to be a valuable piece of knowledge for researchers, students, practitioners and scholars across the globe.

List of Contributors

Janet Douglass and Daniel Lindsay
Division of Tropical Health and Medicine, James Cook University, Townsville 4811, Australia

Luke Becker
Division of Tropical Health and Medicine, James Cook University, Cairns 4870, Australia

Patricia Graves, Maureen Roineau and Jesse Masson
Division of Tropical Health and Medicine, James Cook University, Cairns 4870, Australia
College of Public Health, Medical and Veterinary Sciences, James Cook University, Cairns, QLD 4870, Australia

Ni Ni Aye, Tint Wai and Yi Yi Win
Department of Health, Myanmar Ministry of Health and Sports, Nay Pyi Taw 15011, Myanmar

San San Win
World Health Organization, Country Office, Yangon 11201, Myanmar

Susan Gordon
Division of Tropical Health and Medicine, James Cook University, Townsville 4811, Australia
College of Nursing & Health Sciences, Flinders University, Bedford Park 5042, Australia

Kenneth B. Yeh, Teresa Martinez Torres, Julie Lucas and Richard Winegar
Global Health Surveillance and Diagnostics, MRIGlobal, Gaithersburg, MD 20878, USA

Jeanne M. Fair
Biosecurity and Public Health, Los Alamos National Laboratory, Los Alamos, NM 87545, USA

Woutrina Smith and Corina Monagin
One Health Institute, University of California, Davis, CA 95616, USA

Jacqueline Fletcher
National Institute for Microbial Forensics & Food and Agricultural Biosecurity, Oklahoma State University, Stillwater, OK 74078, USA

Andrew C. Steer
Tropical Diseases, Murdoch Children's Research Institute, Parkville VIC 3052, Australia
Department of Paediatrics, University of Melbourne, Parkville VIC 3052, Australia
Department of General Medicine, Royal Children's Hospital, Parkville VIC 3052, Australia
International Alliance for the Control of Scabies, Parkville VIC 3052, Australia

Sergio A. Hernández and José A. Gabrie
Department of Health Sciences, Brock University, St. Catharines, ON L3S 2A1, Canada

Carol Anahelka Rodríguez, María Mercedes Rueda and Maritza Canales
Department of Parasitology, School of Microbiology and Institute of Microbiology Research, National Autonomous University of Honduras, Tegucigalpa, Honduras

Gabriela Matamoros and Ana Sanchez
Department of Health Sciences, Brock University, St. Catharines, ON L3S 2A1, Canada
Department of Parasitology, School of Microbiology and Institute of Microbiology Research, National Autonomous University of Honduras, Tegucigalpa, Honduras

Ronald Mergl
Niagara Falls Animal Medical Centre, Niagara Falls, ON L2E 6Z8, Canada

David John Chandler and Lucinda Claire Fuller
Dermatology Department, Brighton General Hospital, East Sussex BN2 3EW, UK

Allen G. Ross and Shu-Kay Ng
Menzies Health Institute Queensland, Griffith University, Gold Coast, QLD 4222, Australia

Keren Papier
National Centre for Epidemiology & Population Health, Australian National University, Canberra, ACT 2601, Australia

Ruby Luceres-Catubig
Department of Health, Research Institute for Tropical Medicine, Muntinlupa 1781, Metro Manila, Philippines

Thao N. Chau
Discipline of Public Health, School of Health Sciences, Flinders University, Adelaide, SA 5001, Australia

Marianette T. Inobaya
Menzies Health Institute Queensland, Griffith University, Gold Coast, QLD 4222, Australia
Department of Health, Research Institute for Tropical Medicine, Muntinlupa 1781, Metro Manila, Philippines

Gaetano Scanni
MD Dermatologist, Dipartimento di Medicina dei Servizi ASL Bari, Via Vico Traversa 11, 70127 Bari, Italy

Michael Marks
Clinical Research Department, London School of Hygiene & Tropical Medicine, Keppel Street, London WC1E 7HT, UK

Gloria M. Mulenga
Department of Veterinary Services, Kakumbi Tsetse and Trypanosomiasis Research Station, Mfuwe 10101, Zambia
Ministry of Fisheries and Livestock, Department of Veterinary Services, Lusaka 10101, Zambia
College of Public Health Medical and Veterinary Services, James Cook University, Townsville, Queensland 4814, Australia

Lars Henning
College of Public Health Medical and Veterinary Services, James Cook University, Townsville, Queensland 4814, Australia

Kalinga Chilongo and Chrisborn Mubamba
Ministry of Fisheries and Livestock, Department of Veterinary Services, Lusaka 10101, Zambia

Boniface Namangala
Institute of distance learning, The University of Zambia, Lusaka 10101, Zambia

Bruce Gummow
College of Public Health Medical and Veterinary Services, James Cook University, Townsville, Queensland 4814, Australia
Faculty of Veterinary Science, University of Pretoria, 0028 Pretoria, South Africa

Hollman Miller
Public Health Service, Vaupes Department, Mitú 97001, Colombia

Julian Trujillo-Trujillo
Department of Neglected Tropical Diseases, Ministry of Health and Social Protection, Bogotá 110311, Colombia

Abebayehu Tora
Department of Sociology, Wolaita Sodo University, Sodo, Ethiopia

Hermann Feldmeier
Institute of Microbiology and Infection Immunology, Campus Benjamin Franklin, Charité—University Medicine Berlin, corporate member of Freie Universität Berlin, Humboldt-Universität zu Berlin and Berlin Institute of Health, 12203 Berlin, Germany

Asrat Mengiste
National Podoconiosis Action Network, Addis Ababa, Ethiopia

Gail Davey and Maya Semrau
Department of Global Health and Infection, Brighton and Sussex Medical School, Falmer Campus, University of Sussex, Brighton BN1 9PX, UK

John Archer
Wolfson Wellcome Biomedical Laboratories, Department of Zoology, Natural History Museum, Cromwell Road, London SW7 5BD, UK
Department of Tropical Disease Biology, Liverpool School of Tropical Medicine, Pembroke Place, Liverpool L3 5QA, UK

Lisa O'Halloran, Martyn Stewart and E. James LaCourse
Department of Tropical Disease Biology, Liverpool School of Tropical Medicine, Pembroke Place, Liverpool L3 5QA, UK

Hajri Al-Shehri
Department of Tropical Disease Biology, Liverpool School of Tropical Medicine, Pembroke Place, Liverpool L3 5QA, UK
Department of Tropical Infectious Diseases, Ministry of Health, Asir District, Abha 61411, Saudi Arabia

Shannan Summers, Tapan Bhattacharyya and Amaya L. Bustinduy
Department of Clinical Research, London School of Hygiene and Tropical Medicine, Keppel Street, London WC1E 7HT, UK

Narcis B. Kabaterine, Aaron Atuhaire, Moses Adriko and Moses Arianaitwe
Vector Control Division, Ministry of Health, Kampala 759125, Uganda

Bonnie L. Webster
Wolfson Wellcome Biomedical Laboratories, Department of Zoology, Natural History Museum, Cromwell Road, London SW7 5BD, UK

J. Russell Stothard
Department of Tropical Disease Biology, Liverpool School of Tropical Medicine, Pembroke Place, Liverpool L3 5QA, UK

Sushma Tatipally and Aparna Srikantam
LEPRA Society, Blue Peter Public Health and Research Centre, Cherlapally, Hyderabad 501301, Telangana, India

Sanjay Kasetty
Formerly at LEPRA Society, Blue Peter Public Health and Research Centre, Cherlapally, Hyderabad 501301, Telangana, India

Kittipong Chaisiri
Department of Helminthology, Faculty of Tropical Medicine, Mahidol University, Bangkok 10400, Thailand

Jean-François Cosson
NRA, Biologie Moléculaire et Immunologie Parasitaires et Fongiques, BIPAR, Ecole Nationale Vétérinaire d'Alfort, 94704 Maisons-Alfort Cedex, France

Serge Morand
CNRS ISEM-CIRAD ASTRE, Faculty of Veterinary Technology, Kasetsart University, Bangkok 10220, Thailand

Guadalupe Estrada-Chávez
Department of Dermatology and Dermato-Oncology, Instituto Estatal de Cancerología "Dr. Arturo Beltrán Ortega", Health Secretary Guerrero, Faculty of Medicine, Universidad Autónoma de Guerrero Mexico, Community Dermatology Mexico C.A., 39850 Acapulco, Guerrero, Mexico

Roberto Estrada
Community Dermatology Mexico C.A.; Health Secretary Guerrero, 39355 Acapulco, Guerrero, Mexico

Daniel Engelman
Centre for International Child Health, University of Melbourne, Melbourne, Australia/Group A Streptococcal Research, Murdoch Children's Research Institute, 3010 Melbourne, Australia
Tropical Diseases, Murdoch Children's Research Institute, Parkville VIC 3052, Australia
Department of Paediatrics, University of Melbourne, Parkville VIC 3052, Australia
Department of General Medicine, Royal Children's Hospital, Parkville VIC 3052, Australia
International Alliance for the Control of Scabies, Parkville VIC 3052, Australia

Jesus Molina
Department of Pediatrics, Acapulco General Hospital, Health Secretary Guerrero, 39901 Acapulco, Guerrero, Mexico

Guadalupe Chávez-López
Department of Dermatology and Mycology Acapulco General Hospital, Health Secretary Guerrero, Community Dermatology Mexico C.A., 39355 Acapulco, Guerrero, Mexico

Jan Douglass and Jeffrey Warner
College of Public Health, Medical and Veterinary Sciences, James Cook University, Cairns, QLD 4870, Australia

Khin Saw Aye and Kyi May Htwe
Department of Medical Research, Myanmar Ministry of Health and Sports, Nay Pyi Taw, Myanmar

Sreejith Radhakrishnan
MRC Centre for Global Infectious Disease Analysis, Department of Infectious Disease Epidemiology, Imperial College London, London W2 1PG, UK
Department of Animal Husbandry, Government of Kerala, Thiruvananthapuram 695 033, India

Abi Tamim Vanak
Ashoka Trust for Research in Ecology and the Environment, Bengaluru 560 064, India
DBT/Wellcome Trust India Alliance Fellow, Hyderabad 500 034, India
School of Life Sciences, University of KwaZulu-Natal, Durban 4001, South Africa

Pierre Nouvellet
MRC Centre for Global Infectious Disease Analysis, Department of Infectious Disease Epidemiology, Imperial College London, London W2 1PG, UK
School of Life Sciences, University of Sussex, Brighton BN1 9QG, UK

Christl A. Donnelly
MRC Centre for Global Infectious Disease Analysis, Department of Infectious Disease Epidemiology, Imperial College London, London W2 1PG, UK
Department of Statistics, University of Oxford, Oxford OX1 3LB, UK

Johanna K. Mayer-Coverdale
Department of Microbiology, Pathology Queensland, Royal Brisbane andWomen's Hospital, Queensland 4001, Australia

Amy Crowe
Infectious Diseases Physician, St Vincent's Hospital, 41 Victoria Pde, Fitzroy 3065, Australia

Pamela Smith and Robert W. Baird
Microbiology, Territory Pathology, Royal Darwin Hospital, Tiwi 0810, Australia

Ahmed Hassan Fahal
The Mycetoma Research Centre, University of Khartoum, Khartoum 11111, Sudan

Suliman Hussein Suliman
Department of Surgery, Faculty of Medicine, University of Khartoum, Khartoum 11111, Sudan

Roderick Hay
The International Foundation for Dermatology, London W1P 5HQ, UK

Index

www.ingramcontent.com/pod-product-compliance
Lightning Source LLC
LaVergne TN
LVHW082142200926
848484LV00008B/2096